A Practical Guide to Laboratory Andrology

Second edition

A Practical Guide to Basic Laboratory Andrology

Second edition

David Mortimer
Oozoa Biomedical Inc., Vancouver

Lars Björndahl
Karolinska Institutet, Stockholm

Christopher L. R. Barratt
University of Dundee

José Antonio Castilla
HU Virgen de las Nieves, Granada

Roelof Menkveld
Stellenbosch University

Ulrik Kvist
Karolinska Institutet, Stockholm

Juan G. Alvarez
Centro Androgen, La Coruña

Trine B. Haugen
Oslo Metropolitan University

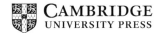

CAMBRIDGE
UNIVERSITY PRESS

University Printing House, Cambridge CB2 8BS, United Kingdom

One Liberty Plaza, 20th Floor, New York, NY 10006, USA

477 Williamstown Road, Port Melbourne, VIC 3207, Australia

314–321, 3rd Floor, Plot 3, Splendor Forum, Jasola District Centre, New Delhi – 110025, India

103 Penang Road, #05–06/07, Visioncrest Commercial, Singapore 238467

Cambridge University Press is part of the University of Cambridge.

It furthers the University's mission by disseminating knowledge in the pursuit of education, learning, and research at the highest international levels of excellence.

www.cambridge.org
Information on this title: www.cambridge.org/9781009181631
DOI: 10.1017/9781009181648

First published 2022

Printed in the United Kingdom by TJ Books Limited, Padstow Cornwall

A catalogue record for this publication is available from the British Library.

Library of Congress Cataloging-in-Publication Data
Names: Mortimer, David, 1953– author. | Björndahl, L. (Lars), author. | Barratt, C. L. R., author. | Castilla, José Antonio, author. | Menkveld, Roelof, author.
Title: A practical guide to basic laboratory andrology / David Mortimer, Lars Björndahl, Christopher L.R. Barratt, José Antonio Castilla, Roelof Menkveld, Ulrik Kvist, Juan G. Alvarez, Trine B. Haugen.
Description: Second edition. | Cambridge, United Kingdom ; New York, NY : Cambridge University Press, 2022. | Preceded by A practical guide to basic laboratory andrology / Lars Björndahl ... [et al.]. 2010. | Includes bibliographical references and index.
Identifiers: LCCN 2021044757 (print) | LCCN 2021044758 (ebook) | ISBN 9781009181631 (paperback) | ISBN 9781009181648 (ebook)
Subjects: MESH: Semen Analysis | Infertility, Male | Spermatozoa | Laboratory Manual
Classification: LCC RC889 (print) | LCC RC889 (ebook) | NLM WJ 709 | DDC 616.6/921–dc23
LC record available at https://lccn.loc.gov/2021044757
LC ebook record available at https://lccn.loc.gov/2021044758

ISBN 978-1-009-18163-1 Paperback

Contents

Abbreviations

A list of abbreviations and acronyms commonly used in andrology and ART laboratories that may be used in this book without further definition is provided below. Standard SI units and chemical formulae are not defined here, nor are standard symbols and many abbreviations that are in general English usage.

A23187	a calcium ionophore
AATB	American Association of Tissue Banks (USA)
AI	artificial insemination (unspecified source of spermatozoa)
AID	artificial insemination by donor (no longer used since the advent of AIDS, see DI and TDI)
AIDS	acquired immunodeficiency syndrome, caused by HIV infection
AIH	artificial insemination homologous, or artificial insemination by husband
ALH	amplitude of lateral head displacement, a sperm kinematic measure (μm)
APAAP	alkaline phosphatase: anti-alkaline phosphatase complex
AR	acrosome reaction
ARIC	acrosome reaction following ionophore challenge
ART	assisted reproductive technology
ASAB(s)	antisperm antibody(ies)
ASRM	American Society for Reproductive Medicine (USA)
ATP	adenosine triphosphate
AZF	azoospermia factor, a region on the Y-chromosome
BBT	basal body temperature
BCF	beat/cross frequency, a sperm kinematic measure (Hz)
BSA	bovine serum albumin (Cohn fraction V)
CAP	College of American Pathologists (USA)
CASA	computer-aided sperm analysis (*not* computer-automated semen analysis)
CBS	Cryo Bio System (Paris, France; part of IMV), the manufacturer of *High Security Straws* for cryobanking spermatozoa
CD (-ROM)	compact disk (read-only memory)
CD45	the 'pan-leucocyte' antigen
C.I.	Colour Index number (for stains)
CJD	Creutzfeldt-Jakob disease
CLIA	Clinical Laboratory Improvement Amendments (USA)
CMV	cytomegalovirus
COLA	Commission on Laboratory Accreditation (USA)
COSHH	control of substances hazardous to health
COVID-19	coronavirus disease 2019, caused by the SARS-CoV-2 virus
CPA	cryoprotective agent *or* Clinical Pathology Accreditation (UK)
CPM	cryoprotectant/cryopreservation medium
cryo	cryopreservation or cryopreserved
CSF	cryosurvival factor, the proportion of motile spermatozoa post-thaw expressed as a percentage of the motile spermatozoa pre-freeze

CV	coefficient of variation
CZBT	competitive (sperm-)zona binding test
–D	sometimes added to acronyms such as IVF to denote the use of donor spermatozoa
D	the fractal dimension, used as a kinematic measure of sperm movement (no units)
DFI	(sperm) DNA fragmentation index, a result provided by the SCSA
DGC	density gradient centrifugation (sperm preparation method)
DHA	docosahexaenoic acid
DI	donor insemination
DMSO	dimethyl sulphoxide (a cryoprotectant and also a carrier molecule for A23187)
DNA	deoxyribonucleic acid
DPX	a microscopy mountant
DSUS	direct swim-up from semen (sperm preparation method)
DTT	dithiothreitol
DVD	digital versatile disc
EBV	Epstein-Barr virus
ECA	European Cooperation for Accreditation
EDTA	ethylenediaminetetraacetic acid, a chelator of divalent cations
EFQM	European Foundation for Quality Management
EGTA	ethyleneglycol tetraacetic acid, a chelating agent with a high affinity for calcium ions
EQA	external quality assurance/assessment
EQAP	external quality assessment programme
EQAS	external quality assessment scheme
EQC	external quality control
ESHRE	European Society of Human Reproduction and Embryology
EtOH	ethyl alcohol or ethanol
EU	European Union (*not* enzyme unit)
FDM	Hamilton Thorne CASA-II software proprietary abbreviation for the fractal dimension 'D'
FITC	fluorescein isothiocyanate, a fluorochrome
FMEA	failure modes and effects analysis
FMLP	formyl-methionyl-leucyl-phenylalanine, a purportedly leucocyte-specific probe to induce the generation of ROS
FNA	fine needle aspirate (a technique for performing TESA)
FSH	follicle stimulating hormone
FW	formula weight of a chemical or compound, see also MW (molecular weight)
GAT	Kibrick gelatin agglutination test for sperm agglutinating antisperm antibodies
GEYC	glycerol-egg yolk-citrate, a modified Ackerman's CPM for human spermatozoa
GLP	Good Laboratory Practice
GMP	Good Manufacturing Practice
H33258	Hoechst dye 33258, a DNA fluorochrome that can be used as a vital stain
HA	hyaluronic acid *or* hyperactivation/hyperactivated (sperm motility)
HBV	hepatitis B virus
hCG	human chorionic gonadotrophin
HCV	hepatitis C virus
H-H	head-to-head sperm agglutination
H-MP	head-to-midpiece sperm agglutination
H-T	head-to-tail sperm agglutination
HEPES	N-(2-hydroxyethyl)piperazine-N'-(2-ethanesulphonic) acid, a zwitterionic pH buffer, pKa at 25°C = 7.5, useful pH range = 6.8–8.2
HEPT	(zona-free) hamster egg penetration test
HFEA	Human Fertilisation and Embryology Authority (UK)
hFF	human follicular fluid

HIV	human immunodeficiency virus, types -1 and -2 (causes AIDS)
HMT	hyaluronate migration test
HOS test	hypo-osmotic swelling test
HPF	high power field (40× objective)
HPM	high power magnification (40× objective)
HPV	human papilloma virus
HSA	human serum albumin (Cohn fraction V)
HSPM	human sperm preservation medium, a particular CPM formulation for human spermatozoa
HSV	herpes simplex virus
HTF	human tubal fluid culture medium
HTLV	human T-cell lymphotropic virus, types -I and -II (HTLV-III was renamed HIV-1)
HZA	hemizona assay
IACC	Inter-American Accreditation Co-operation (USA)
IBT	Immunobead test
ICI	intra-cervical insemination
ICSI	intracytoplasmic sperm injection
ID	identification
Ig	immunoglobulin, also as IgA, IgG and IgM isotypes
ILAC	International Laboratory Accreditation Cooperation
IM	the immotile sperm fraction in WHO5
IMV	Instruments de Medicine Vétérinaire (L'Aigle, France), the original manufacturer of semen straws
IPA	isopropyl alcohol
IQA	internal quality assurance (scheme)
IQC	internal quality control (scheme)
ISO	International Organization for Standardization (Geneva, Switzerland)
IU	International Unit (IU for enzymes refers to the conversion of 1 µmole of substrate/ min at 37°C
IUI	intra-uterine insemination
IVF (-ET)	*in-vitro* fertilization (and embryo transfer)
JCAHO	Joint Commission on Accreditation of Healthcare Organizations (USA)
KPI	Key Performance Indicator (plural = KPIs)
LCR	ligase chain reaction
LH	luteinizing hormone
LIN	linearity, a sperm kinematic measure calculated as VSL/VCL × 100 (%)
LN2	or as LN_2, liquid nitrogen
LPF	low power field (10× objective)
LPM	low power magnification (10× objective)
MAR	mixed antiglobulin reaction
MeOH	methyl alcohol or methanol
MESA	micro(surgical) epididymal sperm aspiration
MI	(sperm) motility index
MOPS	3-(N-morpholino)propanesulphonic acid, a zwitterionic pH buffer, pKa at 25°C = 7.2, useful pH range = 6.5–7.9
MSDS	material safety data sheet
mtDNA	mitochondrial DNA
MW	molecular weight of a compound based on its chemical formula
NA	numerical aperture (of a microscope objective)
NADH	ß-nicotinamide adenine dinucleotide, reduced form
NAFA	Nordic Association for Andrology
NATA	National Association of Testing Authorities (Australia)

NCD	nuclear chromatin decondensation
NH	negative high phase contrast microscope optics
NP	the npn-progressive sperm fraction in WHO5
NPM	non-progressively motile (spermatozoa)
OI	oil immersion
PBS	phosphate buffered saline
PCR	polymerase chain reaction
PCT	post-coital test
PDCA	the Plan-Do-Check-Act quality cycle or Deming wheel
PESA	percutaneous epididymal sperm aspiration
PETG	polyethylene terephthalate glycol
PL	positive low phase contrast microscope optics
PMA	phorbol 12-myristate 13-acetate, an agent that provokes the generation of ROS by leucocytes and spermatozoa
PNA	peanut agglutinin, a lectin from *Arachis hypogea* that binds to the outer acrosomal membrane
PNP	p-nitrophenol
PNPG	4-nitrophenyl α-D-glucopyranoside
PR	(sperm motility) progression rating, also the progressive sperm fraction in WHO5
PSA	prostate specific antigen **or** *Pisum sativum* (pea) agglutinin, a lectin that binds to the acrosomal contents
PT	proficiency testing
PVA	polyvinyl alcohol
PVC	polyvinyl chloride
PVP	polyvinyl pyrolidone
QA	quality assurance
QC	quality control
QI	quality improvement
QMS	quality management system
RBC	red blood cell (erythrocyte)
RCA	root cause analysis
RFID	radio frequency identification (device)
ROS	reactive oxygen species (a type of free radical)
RPLND	retro-peritoneal lymph node dissection
SARS-CoV-2	severe acute respiratory syndrome coronavirus 2, causes COVID-19
SCD test	sperm chromatin dispersion test
SCMC test	sperm-cervical mucus contact test
SCSA	sperm chromatin structure assay
SD	standard deviation
SDF	sperm DNA fragmentation
SDS	sodium dodecyl (lauryl) sulphate
SEM	standard error of the mean **or** scanning electron microscopy
SIG	Special Interest Group (of a professional society)
SIT	Isojima sperm immobilization test for complement-dependent cytotoxic antisperm antibodies
SMIT	sperm-mucus interaction test
SOP	standard operating procedure
SPA	sperm penetration assay (American term for the HEPT)
STD	sexually transmissible disease
STR	straightness, a sperm kinematic measure calculated as VSL/VAP × 100 (%)
TAT	Friberg tray agglutination test for sperm agglutinating antisperm antibodies
TBS	Tris buffered saline

TDI	therapeutic donor insemination (an alternative to DI)
TEM	transmission electron microscopy
TES	N-[Tris(hydroxymethyl)methyl]-2-aminoethanesulphonic acid, a zwitterionic pH buffer, pKa at 25°C = 7.5, useful pH range = 6.8–8.2
TESA	testicular sperm aspiration
TESE	testicular sperm extraction, usually by surgical testicular biopsy
TEST	or TES-Tris, a buffer combination of TES and TRIS
TQM	total quality management
TRIS	N-Tris(hydroxymethyl)aminomethane, pKa at 25°C = 8.1, useful pH range = 7–9
TRITC	tetramethyl rhodamine isothiocyanate, also known simply as rhodamine, a fluorochrome
tt	tail-tip (of the spermatozoon)
T-T	tail-to-tail sperm agglutination
TUNEL	terminal deoxynucleototidyl transferase
TUR	trans-urethral resection, of the prostate
TYG	TEST-yolk-glycerol, a particular CPM formulation for human spermatozoa
TZI	Teratozoospermia Index
U	(International) Unit; see IU
UPS	uninterruptible power supply
u.v.	ultraviolet
VAP	average path velocity, a sperm kinematic measure (μm/s)
vCJD	variant Creutzfeldt-Jakob disease
VCL	curvilinear velocity, a sperm kinematic measure (μm/s)
VCR	videocassette recorder
VHS	the most common standard for domestic and commercial videocassettes
VOC	volatile organic compound
VSL	straight line velocity, a sperm kinematic measure (μm/s)
WBC	white blood cell (leucocyte)
WHMIS	Workplace Hazardous Material Information Scheme (now generally superseded)
WOB	wobble, a sperm kinematic measure calculated as VAP/VCL × 100 (%)
WHO	World Health Organization (Geneva, Switzerland)
XHT	crossed hostility test
ZBT	(sperm-)zona binding test
ZIKV	Zika virus
ZP	zona pellucida
ZP3	zona pellucida glycoprotein 3

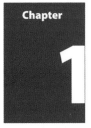

Introduction

Male subfertility is a very significant global problem. Epidemiological data show that approximately one in seven couples are classified as subfertile [1]. Sperm dysfunction is the single most common cause of male subfertility. An older study employing a sperm concentration cut-off of $<20 \times 10^6$/ml found that 20% of 18-year-old men were classed as subfertile [2]. Although it is too simplistic to base a classification of subfertility solely on sperm concentration, the reported frequency of male subfertility points to a high proportion of the population being affected, compared with other prevalent diseases such as diabetes. What is more worrying is the likelihood that sperm counts are falling and the prevalence of male subfertility is increasing [3,4]. Moreover, male fertility has been shown to be a barometer of overall health and longevity [5–7], and significant evidence suggests that the health of future generations may be influenced epigenetically by the quality of their father's spermatozoa, which may have been altered by his diet and/or lifestyle [8–10]; perhaps such effects underlie the fall in sperm counts [4]. In addition, there are many substances and products that are toxic to spermatozoa in our everyday environment [11]. Unfortunately, little progress has been made towards answering fundamental questions in andrology or in developing new diagnostic tools or alternative management strategies for infertile men other than ICSI [12,13]. A recent expert meeting highlighted evidence gaps and important research areas, and proposed a strategic approach whereby andrology might make the rapid progress necessary to address key scientific, clinical, and societal challenges that face our discipline [14]. Andrology is therefore a pivotal discipline in modern medicine, and it is against this background that we have updated this handbook.

Semen analysis provides a comprehensive view of the reproductive functioning of the male partner of the subfertile couple. It includes assessments of sperm count (which reflects sperm production, transport through the male genital tract and ejaculatory function), sperm motility (a basic functional marker of likely sperm competence), sperm vitality (to distinguish between dead spermatozoa and live, immotile spermatozoa), sperm form (aspects of sperm production and maturation), and the physical appearance of the ejaculate (semen production). In addition to this basic semen assessment there are further tests that can be performed – what we have termed extended semen analysis – permitting further analyses that assess more functional aspects of the semen sample. Such tests include biochemical examinations to evaluate the secretions from the auxiliary sex glands, the detection of anti-sperm antibodies, and the use of computer-aided sperm analysis (CASA) to examine sperm motility patterns ('kinematics', see Chapter 6).

A high quality, comprehensive semen assessment is not just the cornerstone of the diagnosis of male subfertility, it is also the starting point for providing prognostic information. While the basic semen assessment has been performed for over 70 years, there have been a number of studies questioning the value of the traditional semen characteristics (sperm concentration, motility and morphology) in the diagnosis and prognosis of male subfertility [15]. Partly, this is the result of an incomplete understanding of what clinical information a semen assessment can provide (see below), but primarily it is because the basic assessments are usually performed using inadequate methods with limited understanding of the technical requirements and poor quality assurance [16]. An enduring example of this is the UK survey of laboratories performing 'andrology tests', which showed dramatic variation from WHO recommended procedures leading to uncritical reporting of results [17,18].

In this handbook we provide a detailed, step-by-step guide using robust methods for examining human semen. We have also included a comprehensive explanation of staff training, and sections on Quality Control, Quality Assurance and Quality Improvement. Adoption of such methods and procedures will lead to a significant improvement in the quality of the data produced by an andrology laboratory, and therefore more robust clinical information. At the time of completing this book (August 2021), during the second year of the COVID-19 pandemic, we have at last seen the convergence of basic semen analysis methodology between the ESHRE Andrology Special Interest Group (SIG) Basic Semen Analysis Course methods (this book), the recommendations of the sixth edition of the World Health Organization manual ('WHO6') [19], and the reference methods for basic human semen examination published in ISO Standard 23162:2021 [20] which should be adopted by ISO 15189-accredited medical laboratories worldwide.

One matter that has been discussed in relation to semen analysis is the number of specimens that must be analysed from each individual. Quite often at least two specimens are said to be required to get a representative result for the individual [21,22]. However, when based on laboratory data, a considerable portion of the variability in results can be ascribed to technical variability due to poor quality laboratory methods. Thus, with poor technical quality (including low numbers of spermatozoa assessed) investigations of multiple specimens from the same subject can, at least in part, compensate – but is not cost-efficient either for the patient and their partner or for the laboratory. The reason why epidemiological studies investigating men for possible reproductive toxicological effects only need to produce one specimen is most likely because the variability in individual specimens 'disappears' when average values are used and differences in averages between groups can be analysed [23]. Although there is a considerable biological variability in semen analysis results (see Chapter 2), especially concerning sperm concentration, the clinical evaluation of the man does not always require analyses of several ejaculates. For the primary investigation of the man in a subfertile relationship, information from the very first 'quality' semen analysis can be enough to direct the continued investigation – either a very poor result indicating the need for direct clinical andrological investigations, or a very good result indicating that further basic semen analyses will not reveal any more pertinent information [24–26]. In those subjects with intermediate results, valuable information can be gained from repeated semen analysis. The methods as described in this handbook are designed to minimize variability due to technical factors, and thereby optimize both the evaluation of the man and the laboratory work [27].

For the proper use of semen analysis results, appropriate interpretation is fundamental. With a few clear exceptions (e.g. azoospermia), the data cannot provide unambiguous information about the chances of future conception, either *in vivo* or *in vitro*. Currently, there is a clear tendency to over-emphasize the value of a single parameter, e.g. strict cut-offs for 'normal' sperm morphology as used in ART clinics to decide that ICSI is 'necessary'. However, as has been known for seven decades, there is a considerable overlap between the semen characteristics of fertile and subfertile men, so no single parameter can be used to provide prognostic information about the fertility potential of the couple [28,29]. A combination of several variables (motility, morphology and concentration) does give more accurate diagnostic and prognostic information, although there will always be overlaps between what is considered fertile and subfertile [26,30,31]. Irrespective of the low predictive value for the reproductive success of the couple, a comprehensive semen analysis provides information about the status of the male reproductive organs, and this is important in the wellbeing of the man. The results of a semen analysis are often used as a sentinel marker for the potential treatment pathway for patients. For example, a primary question in ART clinics remains: is the semen of this man suitable for IUI, or is IVF, or even ICSI, needed? [28] Primarily, what the clinic is trying to do is determine whether there are indications that the man will have a high likelihood of *failure* using a particular treatment modality, i.e. the man's spermatozoa are unsuitable for insemination by IUI, and IVF is indicated. However, despite the plethora of literature surrounding this area, there are still no simple answers. For example, a meta-analysis of the literature trying to ascertain the number of spermatozoa that have been (can be) used as a cut-off for IUI success concluded that there was no such cut-off, and that the data available were of insufficient quality to provide a robust answer [32]. Of course, the quality of the sperm preparation methodology (and also the products used, see Chapter 9) will also impact on treatment outcome, confounding any simple relationship between pre-treatment semen characteristics and treatment outcome.

For the comprehensive investigation of a man's fertility potential, it is essential not only to perform a semen analysis, but also that a physical examination be performed and a complete medical history taken [33]. Accurate interpretation of a semen analysis cannot be made without knowing the patient's history, and having information from a physical examination and other laboratory investigations, e.g. hormone analyses [33]. Reduced fertility potential can be secondary to other diseases that should be properly investigated and treated; it is thus irresponsible and unethical to embark upon an infertility work-up without a complete physical examination and history [14,33].

A common source for misunderstandings and misinterpretations is the use of qualitative terms such as oligozoospermia and asthenozoospermia. Originally, these terms were used to characterize laboratory findings before the quantitative measures had become usable and reliable. But subsequently, these terms have been given precise limits on quantitative scales, creating the false impression of dichotomy (two clearly separated outcomes, like subfertile and fertile), and even a 'diagnosis', based on semen characteristics – as opposed to the true situation of a sliding scale between severely infertile (but not sterile) and fertile. In an effort to reduce such confusion in the future, we have abandoned the use of all such qualitative terms and urge everyone working in the field to do likewise. Just describe what you see, as objectively and quantitatively as possible, and interpret the test results within the holistic medical context for the subject, especially the particular circumstances that exist within the reproductive unit of which he is part, i.e. with the female partner, since (sub)fertility is always a feature of a couple.

References

1. Hull MG, Glazener CM, Kelly NJ, et al. Population study of causes, treatment, and outcome of infertility. *Br Med J (Clin Res Ed)* 1985; **291**: 1693–7.

2. Andersen AG, Jensen TK, Carlsen E, et al. High frequency of sub-optimal semen quality in an unselected population of young men. *Hum Reprod* 2000; **15**: 366–72.

3. Sharpe RM, Irvine DS. How strong is the evidence of a link between environmental chemicals and adverse effects on human reproductive health? *BMJ* 2004; **328**: 447–51.

4. Levine H, Jørgensen N, Martino-Andrade A, et al. Temporal trends in sperm count: a systematic review and meta-regression analysis. *Hum Reprod Update* 2017; **23**: 646–9.

5. Glazer CH, Bonde JP, Eisenberg ML, et al. Male infertility and risk of nonmalignant chronic diseases: a systematic review of the epidemiological evidence. *Semin Reprod Med* 2017; **35**: 282–90.

6. Hanson MB, Eisenberg ML, Hotaling JM. Male infertility: a biomarker of individual and familiar cancer risk. *Fertil Steril* 2018; **109**: 6–19.

7. Kasman AM, Del Giudice F, Eisenberg ML. New insights to guide patient care: the bidirectional relationship between male infertility and male health. *Fertil Steril* 2020; **113**: 469–77.

8. Lane M, Robker RL, Robertson SA. Parenting from before conception. *Science* 2014; **345**: 756–60.

9. Siklenka K, Erkek S, Godmann M, et al. Disruption of histone methylation in developing sperm impairs offspring health transgenerationally. *Science* 2015; **350**: aab2006.

10. Wright C. Lifestyle factors and sperm quality. In: Aitken RJ, Mortimer D, Kovacs G, eds. *Male and Female Factors That Maximize IVF Success*. Cambridge: Cambridge University Press, 2020.

11. Mortimer D, Barratt CL, Björndahl L, et al. What should it take to describe a substance or product as 'sperm-safe'. *Hum Reprod Update* 2013; **19 Suppl 1**: i1–i45.

12. Barratt CLR, De Jonge CJ, Sharpe RM. 'Man Up': the importance and strategy for placing male reproductive health centre stage in the political and research agenda. *Hum Reprod* 2018; **33**: 541–5.

13. Aitken RJ. Not every sperm is sacred; a perspective on male infertility. *Mol Hum Reprod* 2018; **24**: 287–98.

14. Cairo Consensus Workshop Group. The current status and future of andrology: a consensus report from the Cairo workshop group. *Andrology* 2020; **8**: 27–52.

15. Björndahl L, Barratt CL. Semen analysis: setting standards for the measurement of sperm numbers. *J Androl* 2005; **26**: 11.

16. Björndahl L, Barratt CL, Mortimer D, Jouannet P. 'How to count sperm properly': checklist for acceptability of studies based on human semen analysis. *Hum Reprod* 2016; **31**: 227–32.

17. Riddell D, Pacey A, Whittington K. Lack of compliance by UK andrology laboratories with World Health Organization recommendations for sperm morphology assessment. *Hum Reprod* 2005; **20**: 3441–5.

18. Zuvela E, Matson P. Performance of four chambers to measure sperm concentration: results from an external quality assurance programme. *Reprod Biomed Online* 2020; **41**: 671–8.

19. World Health Organization. *WHO Laboratory Manual for the Examination and Processing of*

Human Semen, 6th edn. Geneva: World Health Organization, 2021.

20. International Organization for Standardization. *ISO 23162:2021 Basic Semen Examination – Specification and Test Methods.* Geneva: International Organization for Standardization, 2021.

21. Keel BA. Within- and between-subject variation in semen parameters in infertile men and normal semen donors. *Fertil Steril* 2006; **85**: 128–34.

22. Castilla JA, Alvarez C, Aguilar J, et al. Influence of analytical and biological variation on the clinical interpretation of seminal parameters. *Hum Reprod* 2006; **21**: 847–51.

23. Stokes-Riner A, Thurston SW, Brazil C, et al. One semen sample or 2? Insights from a study of fertile men. *J Androl* 2007; **28**: 638–43.

24. Hirsh A. Male subfertility. *BMJ* 2003; **327**: 669–72.

25. Mishail A, Marshall S, Schulsinger D, Sheynkin Y. Impact of a second semen analysis on a treatment decision making in the infertile man with varicocele. *Fertil Steril* 2009; **91**: 1809–11.

26. Barratt CLR, Björndahl L, De Jonge CJ, et al. The diagnosis of male infertility: an analysis of the evidence to support the development of global WHO guidance – challenges and future research opportunities. *Hum Reprod Update* 2017; **23**: 660–80.

27. Björndahl L. What is normal semen quality? On the use and abuse of reference limits for the interpretation of semen analysis results. *Hum Fertil* 2011; **14**: 179–86.

28. Mortimer D, Mortimer ST. The case against intracytoplasmic sperm injection for all. In: Aitken RJ, Mortimer D, Kovacs G, eds. *Male and Female Factors That Maximize IVF Success.* Cambridge: Cambridge University Press, 2020.

29. MacLeod J, Wang Y. Male fertility potential in terms of semen quality: a review of the past, a study of the present. *Fertil Steril* 1979; **31**: 103–16.

30. Guzick DS, Overstreet JW, Factor-Litvak P, et al. National Cooperative Reproductive Medicine Network. Sperm morphology, motility, and concentration in fertile and infertile men. *N Engl J Med* 2001; **345**: 1388–93.

31. Jedrzejczak P, Taszarek-Hauke G, Hauke J, et al. Prediction of spontaneous conception based on semen parameters. *Int J Androl* 2008; **31**: 499–507.

32. van Weert JM, Repping S, Van Voorhis BJ, et al. Performance of the postwash total motile sperm count as a predictor of pregnancy at the time of intrauterine insemination: a meta-analysis. *Fertil Steril* 2004; **82**: 612–20.

33. Jequier AM. The importance of diagnosis in the clinical management of infertility in the male. *Reprod Biomed Online* 2006; **13**: 331–5.

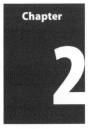

Basic Physiology

What Are Gametes Good For? Protection against Micro-Organisms

One prerequisite for multi-cellular organisms to survive is to be able to repulse attacks by micro-organisms, their DNA, RNA and proteins and prions. Every individual multi-cellular organism has developed an immunological defence system that is directed towards everything but itself. However, to discriminate foreign cells and micro-organisms from cells belonging to itself it is essential to be unique. The problem to become unique was solved some 600 million years ago with the evolution of a new type of cell division, meiosis, which enabled the formation of genetically unique gametes. The fusion (fertilization) of two genetically unique gametes (the spermatozoon and the oocyte) results in a new individual with a unique genetic constitution. Due to meiotic recombination, every gamete is supplied with one out of four unique DNA molecules for every chromosome pair. In human beings there are 23 pairs of chromosomes, so the number of possible DNA combinations in any gamete is 4^{23}, i.e. any gamete achieves 1 out of at least 70×10^{12} combinations (1 out of 70 million millions) of genetic material. At fertilization, gametes from two different individuals fuse and form one new individual; the genetic composition of the child is thus one combination out of 4900×10^{24} possible combinations. A male human produces some 100 million genetically unique lots per day. A woman produces normally one mature oocyte a month, and again each oocyte becomes as genetically unique as any spermatozoon upon when the second meiotic division is completed fertilization.

Thus, the evolution of meiosis and unique gametes was a prerequisite for an individual immune defence, which in turn was a prerequisite for the evolution and survival of multi-cellular organisms exposed to endless attacks of micro-organisms [1,2].

Outside the Body the Laboratory Staff Must Protect the Gametes

Outside the body there is no immune system or reproductive tract to protect the gametes. The laboratory must therefore fulfil these functions to protect gametes and embryos. Assisted reproduction *in vitro* would be impossible if micro-organisms were not actively combatted. Laminar-air-flow benches, sterile and controlled handling and culture media, rooms with controlled air purity, and special clothing for the involved staff are some of the precautions expected for best practice [3,4]. Sometimes chemical weapons like antibiotics are necessary. Nonetheless, micro-organisms with foreign DNA and RNA can invade our culture media and become incorporated into embryos and thereby future generations [1].

Every Man Is a Unique Experiment by Nature

In most multi-cellular organisms two types of gonads, ovaries and testes, have developed that produce two different types of gametes: immotile oocytes and motile spermatozoa, both evolved to fuse with each other. Usually (but not always) only one type of gonad exists within an individual. In evolutionary terms the development of two different types of gametes is an important mechanism for achieving the mixture of genes from two different individuals and counteracting the simple fusion of gametes from a single individual. Hence, among animals, the development of the male and female sexes respectively can be seen as nature's way to improve probabilities for individuals to find an individual with compatible gametes. In plants, access to spermatozoa (pollen) is facilitated via wind, water or other vectors, while in mammals direct contact between the two gamete-bearing individuals is required.

In mammals, some 300 million years ago, the genes controlling sperm production were transferred from one of the two ancient X-chromosomes onto a "shortened X", today called the Y-chromosome. As a consequence, mammals are heterogametic rather than homogametic, i.e. they have two different types of gametes, one carrying the X chromosome the other the Y.

The Y-bearing organism developed into a mobile, sperm-producing individual. In order for the 'species' to survive, the sperm producer must succeed in finding signs of ovulation and be able to deliver spermatozoa for fertilization of the oocytes. In some species of Asian mole, the Y chromosome has disappeared and critical male-determining genes have moved onto a somatic chromosome.

In mammals, the default development (phenotype) is the female development. The development of a fertile man able to react to signs of ovulation requires the selection of a handful of specific male development routes, during embryonic, fetal and childhood development [5,6]. Many of these traits are known to be dependent on testosterone and result in the development of (a) the testes, (b) internal male genital structures, (c) external male genitalia, and (d) male sexual identity.

Production of the Male Gamete, the Spermatozoon

Spermatogenesis is the process by which spermatozoa are produced from spermatogonia in the testis. The light microscopic examination performed during semen analysis aims to give information about the success of spermatogenesis, including the number of spermatozoa, and the success of spermiogenesis by their morphology and motility. A more thorough evaluation of the ejaculate can reveal a variety of disturbances originating in the different steps of spermatogenesis and might shed light on disturbed testicular function or even reveal CIS-cells indicating the presence of early testis cancer [6,7].

Spermatogenesis Is Prepared in the Embryo

Already during the embryonic and fetal stage, preparations for spermatogenesis are being made. Immature germ cells from the epiblast migrate from the yolk sac and invade the seminiferous cords (which will become tubules at puberty) in both testes, and start to proliferate up to week 18 in the fetus. The other cells inside the seminiferous cords, the Sertoli cells, also multiply. The somatic Sertoli cell and its spermatogonia could be regarded as a unit for future sperm production. If the migration of germ cells is disturbed, or if the germ cells degenerate, few or no spermatogonia will be left for sperm production and the only cells left would be the Sertoli cells (known clinically as the 'Sertoli cell only' syndrome).

Spermatogenesis Is Comprised of Five Different Processes

1) *Renewal of stem cells.* There are two types of spermatogonia type A: dark and pale (Figure 2.1). Both belong to the stem cell population and are continuously renewed by mitotic divisions. It is estimated that spermatogonia undergo some 20 mitotic cell divisions a year, so at 35 years of age the spermatogonia have undergone some 400 mitotic cell divisions, whereas the female oocyte rests from embryonic week 10 until ovulation. Thus, hazards linked to cell division events (mutations in the DNA, aneuploidy, mutations and deletions in mitochondrial DNA) are more likely to affect spermatogenesis than oogenesis.

2) *Spermatocytogenesis.* An important process is an exponential increase in number of spermatozoa; in the human testis two consecutive mitotic divisions prepare for the meiotic cell division. One spermatogonium A pale is recruited for sperm production and undergoes two mitotic cell divisions, resulting in a clone of four spermatogonia B. Each of these then differentiates into four primary spermatocytes. The latter two mitotic cell divisions increase the possible number of spermatozoa by a factor of four. If one mitotic division does not occur, then only half the number of spermatozoa can be produced. It means that missing mitotic divisions could be one cause of low sperm numbers. In rodents, there may be 11 mitotic divisions before the meiotic divisions begin, and in the rhesus monkey there may be five mitotic divisions. Thus, in those species, one A-spermatogonium will theoretically result in 8192 and 128 spermatozoa, respectively, whereas the number of resulting spermatozoa in man is 16 [8].

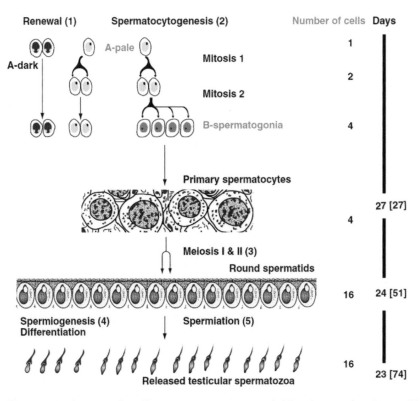

Figure 2.1 A schematic outline of human spermatogenesis compiled from data given by references [7] and [8]. (1) shows that A-pale spermatogonia renew by mitosis and that A-dark spermatogonia mainly rest; (2) outlines that another A-pale spermatogonia are chosen to undergo two mitotic cleavages into four B-spermatogonia and that B-spermatogonia differentiate into primary spermatocytes (spermatocytogenesis); (3) shows the two meiotic divisions of each primary spermatocytes into four round spermatids; and (4) the differentiation of round spermatids into elongated spermatids (spermiogenesis) that through spermiation (5) are released as testicular spermatozoa into the lumen of the seminiferous tubule. Number of cells refers to the number of daughter cells (finally spermatozoa) resulting from one spermatogonium. Days mark the duration of each step and in square brackets the accumulated duration. Illustration by U. Kvist based on illustrations of cells by A. F. Holstein [7]; ©2003 Holstein et al.; licensee BioMed Central Ltd; www.rbej.com/content/1/1/107

3) **Meiosis.** The purpose of this process is to ensure that every spermatozoon achieves (a) a unique combination of DNA and (b) a haploid genome in which the original 23 pairs of chromosomes are reduced to 23 single copies of the DNA. Each of the four primary spermatocytes in a clone undergoes the two meiotic divisions. From eight secondary spermatocytes finally 16 round spermatids are formed.

4) **Spermiogenesis.** This is the process where the round spermatid transforms (differentiates) into a functional messenger cell called the testicular spermatid that is still attached to the Sertoli cell (Figure 2.2).

5) **Spermiation.** Initiated by the Sertoli cell, testicular spermatozoa are released from the Sertoli cells, which take up the surplus cytoplasm and membrane from the sperm midpiece (the residual body).

Spermatogenesis Takes Place in the Seminiferous Tubules

A normal tubule has a diameter of about 180 μm, and the diameter is decreased when spermatogenesis is impaired (Figure 2.3). The tubule walls are composed of five layers of myofibroblasts in connective tissue, which cause peristaltic waves of contraction to transport the immotile testicular spermatozoa to the rete testis for further transportation, via the efferent ducts, to the caput of the epididymis. The thickness of the

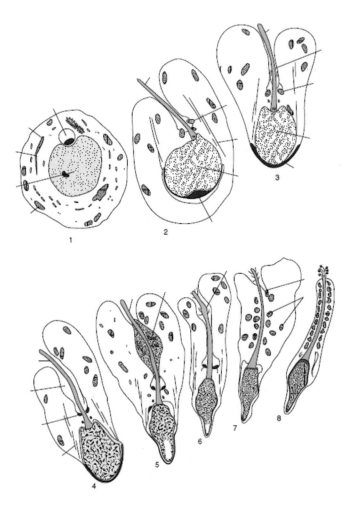

Figure 2.2 The steps of spermiogenesis. (1) Immature spermatid with round-shaped nucleus. The acrosome vesicle is attached to the nucleus, the tail anlage fails to contact the nucleus. (2) The acrosome vesicle is increased and flattened over the nucleus. The tail establishes contact with the nucleus. (3–8) Acrosome formation, nuclear condensation and development of tail structures take place. (8) The mature spermatid is released from the germinal epithelium. Semi-schematic drawing on the basis of electronmicrographs by A. F. Holstein [7]; ©2003 Holstein et al.; licensee BioMed Central Ltd; www.rbej.com /content/1/1/107

peritubular tissue is 8 μm, corresponding to the size of the neighbouring spermatogonia. A thickened wall is associated with impaired spermatogenesis [7].

The Sertoli Cell

The Sertoli cell is the dominating cell in the seminiferous cords and tubules. It is a supporting cell that provides nutrition and mediates paracrine signals for spermatogenesis as well as protection of the developing germs cells from the immune system. The Sertoli cell communicates, via factors and testosterone, with the Leydig cells in the interstitium between the seminiferous tubules. It produces inhibin B, which exerts a negative feedback on the FSH secretion from the pituitary gland. In about half of men with azoospermia, the Sertoli cells produce low levels of inhibin B, resulting in elevated FSH levels in the blood. However, low levels of inhibin B and high levels of FSH do not exclude that focal spermatogenesis can be found at testicular biopsy, making sperm retrieval and ICSI a possible treatment [9,10].

Protection from the immune system is mediated by neighbouring Sertoli cells forming tight junctions between them, thereby dividing the seminiferous tubules into two compartments: (1) the basal compartment

(A)

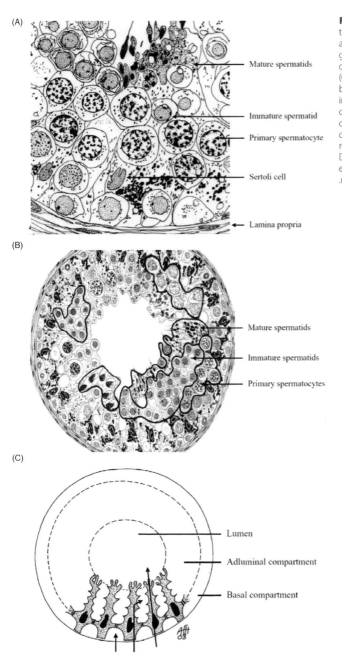

Mature spermatids

Immature spermatid

Primary spermatocyte

Sertoli cell

Lamina propria

(B)

Mature spermatids

Immature spermatids

Primary spermatocytes

(C)

Lumen

Adluminal compartment

Basal compartment

Figure 2.3 (A) Cross-section of a seminiferous tubule of a fertile man 32 years of age. Drawing of a semithin section, ×300. (B) A section of the germinal epithelium in the seminiferous tubule drawn on the basis of a semithin section, ×900. (C) Sertoli cells divide the germinal epithelium in basal and adluminal compartments. Arrows indicate that the passage of substances from the outside stops at the tight junctions in the basal compartment and that the adluminal compartment and the lumen can only be reached by transport through the Sertoli cells. Drawings by A. F. Holstein [7]; ©2003 Holstein et al.; licensee BioMed Central Ltd; www.rbej.com/content/1/1/107

facing the 'inside' where the immune system can act against 'foreign' objects, and (2) the one facing the 'outside world' – the luminal compartment, i.e. the lumen into which the spermatozoa are released and transported out of the man. At meiosis, the primary spermatocytes, which soon are going to give rise to spermatids with unique DNA (and therefore will appear as 'foreign' to the immune system), are transferred from the basal to the luminal (outside) compartment, thus escaping the risk of being attacked by the immune system. The so-called *blood-testis barrier* consists of a combination of these inter-Sertoli cell connections, the peritubular tissue in the walls of the tubules, and the endothelium of the testicular capillaries in the interstitium between the tubules [7].

The Testicular Interstitium and the Leydig Cells

Besides spermatogenesis, the testis has another vital physiological role: testosterone production by the Leydig cells which surround the capillaries in the interstitium.

The Embryonic Male

In response to hCG from the pregnant ovary or the placenta, Leydig cells produce testosterone necessary for the differentiation and development of male genitalia. Disturbed function of the ovary or placenta during critical time intervals during embryonic development can jeopardize the specific male development and hence future male fertility.

The Adult Man

At puberty, GnRH is secreted from the hypothalamus in isolated peaks (one every 90 min), which stimulates the pituitary to secrete FSH and LH (named luteinizing hormone from its effect in females). LH stimulates the Leydig cells to produce testosterone. No less than 90% of the testosterone is taken up by the Sertoli cells in the tubules and is used to support spermatogenesis and by luminal flow for the androgen-specific functions of the excurrent duct system up to the corpus of the epididymis. Some 10% is delivered to the capillary blood and exerts systemic androgen effects on the man, including male secondary sex characteristics like body and facial hair, deep voice, increased muscle mass, decreased body fat, increased male haemoglobin, and enforced skeleton as well as brain function resulting in a 'male temperament' [6].

The Human Spermatozoon

The Messenger Cell

The morphology of the human spermatozoon is depicted in Figure 2.4, drawn by the German scientist Adolph Holstein, based on electron microscopic studies [7]. An extensive review of human sperm structure and function has recently been published by Mortimer [11]. The spermatozoon is a messenger cell – a conveyer of information – carrying the unique paternal messages needed to create a healthy child and grandchildren. As a messenger it needs special properties, such as being motile in order to reach the immotile oocyte and deliver its information after fusion with the oocyte membrane. The motility of the spermatozoon depends on the axoneme structures (e.g. microtubule doublets, dynein arms, spokes), the presence of functional mitochondria, functional centrioles (tail insertion), and fibrous tail sheath (rigid tail movements).

The Sperm Chromatin, DNA, Protamines and Zinc

The DNA of the spermatozoon is temporarily well-protected in a semi-crystalline structure stabilized by zinc (Figure 2.5). This unique, dense packaging of sperm chromatin offers protection and could compensate for the lack of DNA repair systems. The sperm chromatin is primarily arranged like a 'rope' with three intermingled strands: the two DNA strands constitute two strands while the third strand is constituted of protamines. There is one zinc ion for every protamine molecule and turn of the DNA helix, i.e. for every 10 base-pairs of DNA. Zinc withdrawal enables a quick unwrapping of the chromatin into separate DNA

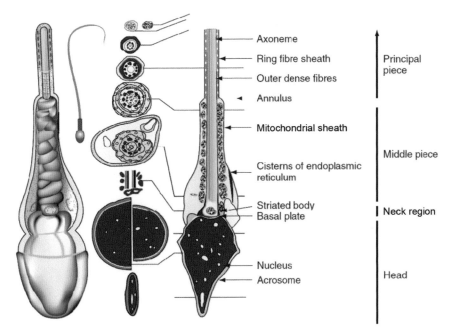

Figure 2.4 The human spermatozoon. Left = cut-away representation of the spermatozoon showing the acrosome, the nucleus and nuclear envelope, the mitochondrial sheath of the main piece of the flagellum. Middle = cross-sections at different levels indicated in the longitudinal section of the human spermatozoon shown on the right. Semi-schematic drawing by A. F. Holstein on the basis of electronmicrographs [7]; ©2003 Holstein et al.; licensee BioMed Central Ltd; www.rbej.com/content/1/1/107

threads (double-stranded helices), when studied almost immediately after ejaculation. This ability promptly declines among spermatozoa left in the liquefying ejaculate *in vitro* [1,12–14].

This unique, dense packaging of the sperm genome is due to exchange of DNA-binding histones in the nucleus. During the late phases of spermiogenesis, somatic histones are replaced first by temporary proteins and then by protamines. At the same time, zinc is incorporated into the sperm nucleus. The positive amino groups ($-NH_3^+$) of arginine in the protamines neutralize the negative phosphate groups ($-PO_4^{3-}$) of the DNA-backbone, which is the basis for the tight packing of the DNA-protamine complex [15,16].

This allows chromatin fibres to be closely aligned side by side and coiled into toroids with a diameter of 50–100 nm with 50 000 base pairs of DNA [16–19]. It appears that starting from the centromere, the p- and q-arms of the chromosomes separately form rows of piled toroids (see, for example, Figure 6 in [20]).

In human sperm chromatin there are mainly two types of protamines, protamine 1 and protamine 2. Besides arginine, these protamines contain the amino acids cysteine and histidine that can form stable temporary salt-bridges with zinc. The NH group of the imidazole ring of histidine and the reduced SH group of the cysteine have high affinity for zinc (*c.f.* zinc-fingers). Moreover, the presence of zinc facilitates the binding of DNA to protamine [15,21,22]. Sperm nuclear zinc deficiency induced *in vitro* provokes liberated sulfhydryl groups to form disulfide-bridges and thereby changing the type of chromatin stability from zinc-dependent to non-zinc-dependent chromatin stability caused by disulphide-bridges leading to an abnormal (covalently bonded) and less easily reversible stabilization of the chromatin (Figure 2.6). This is likely to hinder or at least delay sperm chromatin decondensation in the ooplasm and could therefore be an important cause for male factor infertility.

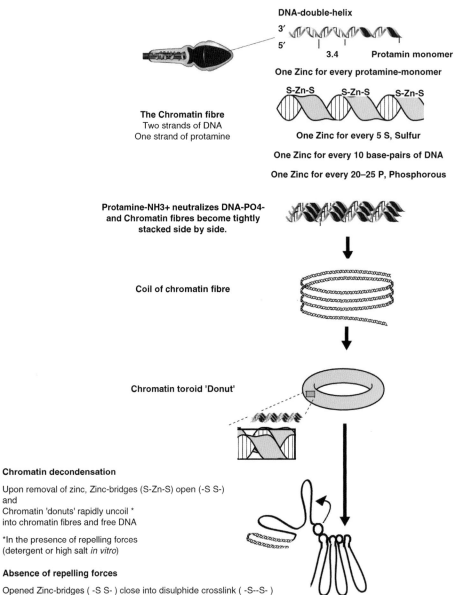

DNA-double-helix

3′
5′
3.4   **Protamin monomer**

One Zinc for every protamine-monomer

S-Zn-S   S-Zn-S   S-Zn-S

The Chromatin fibre
Two strands of DNA
One strand of protamine

One Zinc for every 5 S, Sulfur

One Zinc for every 10 base-pairs of DNA

One Zinc for every 20–25 P, Phosphorous

**Protamine-NH3+ neutralizes DNA-PO4-
and Chromatin fibres become tightly
stacked side by side.**

Coil of chromatin fibre

Chromatin toroid 'Donut'

Chromatin decondensation

Upon removal of zinc, Zinc-bridges (S-Zn-S) open (-S S-)
and
Chromatin 'donuts' rapidly uncoil *
into chromatin fibres and free DNA

*In the presence of repelling forces
(detergent or high salt *in vitro*)

Absence of repelling forces

Opened Zinc-bridges (-S S-) close into disulphide crosslink (-S--S-)
resulting in a superstabilized partly closed chromatin.

Figure 2.5 Outline of a model for human sperm chromatin stabilization. The chromatin fibre is arranged by three strands; two are the two DNA strands of the DNA-double helix and the third is a strand of protamine composed of zinc-linked protamine-monomers. One zinc is present for every protamine-monomer for every turn of the DNA helix, i.e. for every 10 base pairs. There is one zinc for every 5 thiols (S) of protamine cysteine residues and for every 20–25 phosphorus (in phosphate groups of mainly the DNA backbone). Chromatin fibres are arranged condensed, side by side, and coiled into donut-like toroids, when the negative charges of DNA phosphate groups have been neutralized by the positive charges of the NH^{3+} of arginine residues of protamines [from 15,17]. Chromatin decondensation involves uncoiling of toroids. This can be effectuated by repelling forces once the stabilizing bridges connecting protamine monomers have been interrupted by, e.g., withdrawal of zinc from the zinc-bridges (-S-Zn-S-) leaving them open (-S S-). In the absence of repelling forces, open bridges (-S S-) rapidly close into disulphide crosslinks (-S–S-) resulting in a superstabilized, partly closed chromatin. This can be re-opened by reductive cleavage by disulphide-bridge cleaving agents. Illustration compiled by U. Kvist, based on [15,17].

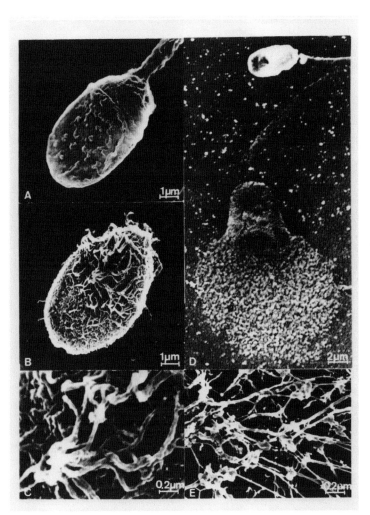

Figure 2.6 Scanning electron microscope (SEM) images of human spermatozoa. Sperm preparation by U. Kvist, 1980; SEM images by L Nilsson. (A) Human sperm head in buffered salt solution containing 0.15 mM zinc; the sperm head plasma membrane is intact. (B) Human sperm exposed to sodium dodecyl sulphate (SDS) with 0.15 mM zinc; the plasma and nuclear membranes are lost and nuclear chromatin is visible, but still intact not decondensing (some dispersing chromatin fibres are seen in the caudal region of the head). (C) Higher magnification detail of image B; note nodular chromatin with diameter 100 nm, corresponding to unravelling chromatin toroids. (D) Human spermatozoa exposed to SDS with 6 mM EDTA; the upper sperm head as an intact superstabilized nucleus that does not decondense in SDS-EDTA, while the lower sperm head is grossly swollen and decondensed. (E) Human spermatozoon decondensed in SDS-EDTA showing highly decondensed chromatin with nodular structures corresponding to chromatin toroids (donuts) in various degrees of unravelling.

Sperm Mitochondrial DNA and Impaired Spermatogenesis

Each mitochondrion in the body contains several copies of circular mitochondrial DNA (mtDNA). Although most of the genome is packaged into the chromosomes within the nucleus, mitochondria also have a small amount of their own DNA. In humans, mitochondrial DNA comprises 16,559 base pairs which constitute 37 genes, all of which are essential for normal mitochondrial function: 13 are for enzymes involved in oxidative phosphorylation (OXPHOS), while the remaining 24 code for transfer and ribosomal RNAs (i.e. tRNA and rRNA molecules). The OXPHOS enzymes are not coded for within the nuclear genome of mammalian cells.

At fertilization, the spermatozoon brings some 100 copies of mitochondrial DNA, whereas the oocyte has some 100,000 copies. Sperm mtDNA has passed up to 400 cell divisions and is more likely to be mutated than the mtDNA in the oocyte that have been selected, multiplied and then kept resting since the tenth fetal week. Sperm mitochondrial DNA is ubiquitin-targeted already in the testis to be destroyed upon entrance into the oocyte [23,24]. Thus, mitochondria are inherited through the female germ cell line. There are reports suggesting that mutated sperm mitochondrial

DNA may escape destruction and cause mitochondrial disease in the offspring. If so, it seems to be an extremely rare event.

Mutagenic damage to mitochondrial DNA (mtDNA) is a condition that limits the lifespan of each individual. By regeneration of mitochondria with undamaged native mtDNA in the oocyte, a new individual is provided with fully functional mitochondria from the one cell stage or zygote. This appears to be the evolutionary mechanism for family eternity, by which every new generation can start off with fresh mitochondria.

Mutagenic deletions of mitochondrial DNA are likely to propagate relatively rapidly in cells with frequent cell divisions. For a 35-year-old man, his spermatogonia have undergone some 400 mitotic divisions. This means that a deletion of the mtDNA in a spermatogonium would lead to a metabolic exhaustion of the processes involved in spermatogenesis and could therefore be manifested by, for example, severely reduced sperm concentration, motility and morphology. Thus, genetic characterization of germ cell mtDNA or sperm mtDNA could be a future tool to estimate whether disorders in spermatogenesis are due to inadequate mitochondrial functions.

Efficiency of Spermatogenesis

Spermatogenesis in man appears to be a process of redundancy. Developing germ cells and spermatozoa are lost during and after spermatogenesis, and only some 25% of spermatozoa formed reach the ejaculate [7]. Among them, the proportion of malformed spermatozoa is extremely high. One can argue that if the man has at least some morphologically 'ideal' (previously referred to as 'morphologically normal') spermatozoa (i.e. the structure and form of the spermatozoa makes them able to pass through cervical mucus and bind to the zona pellucida), then the genetic 'blueprints' for a typical spermatozoon are present. But, control of the process is apparently of very low priority for fertility, and is therefore not given high efficiency in terms of biological quality management. This type of pleiomorphism (large range of sperm forms in the ejaculate) is almost never seen in laboratory animals or inbred farming animals, where spermatozoa have excellent morphology. This may be due to natural selection when males compete for the oocytes at the sperm level, or human selection of animals with good sperm morphology. Besides humans, gorillas and some monogamous mouse strains have pleiomorphic spermatozoa. A plausible explanation for this could be that the performance (and thereby the structure and function) of spermatozoa is not critical when the competition for reproduction is between males (the female only receives spermatozoa from one male), rather than between their spermatozoa (the female receive spermatozoa from several males during an ovulatory cycle) [24]. It should be emphasized that if a man has only 1% of spermatozoa with morphology typical for those spermatozoa that reach the site for fertilization, an ejaculate of 100 million spermatozoa still contains 1 million spermatozoa with 'ideal' morphology.

Note that pleiomorphism means that many different types of morphological variants exist in an ejaculate. This must be distinguished from conditions where most spermatozoa have the same type of atypical morphology. In such cases a genetic reason might be suspected and a chromosomal analysis (karyotype) can rule out chromosomal translocations and inversions. In fact, sperm morphology screening in mice is used as a method to monitor toxicological exposures that induce chromosomal translocations.

Sperm Transport: From Testis to Urethra

Testicular spermatozoa are transported from the seminiferous tubules in the testis by the flow of fluid to the rete testis and then by the 15–20 efferent ducts to the convoluted, approximately 6 m long, epididymal duct on each side (Figure 2.7). The epididymis is anatomically divided into the caput, corpus and cauda regions (Figure 2.8). There is also a more functional subdivision of the epididymal duct into the initial, middle and terminal segments. The epididymal duct, and its continuation into the vas deferens and the seminal vesicles, is developed from the embryonic Wolffian duct. In the vas deferens, the spermatozoa are transported from the distal cauda to the urethra. Before passing through the prostate, the vas deferens widens to form the ampulla of the vas deferens, from which the seminal

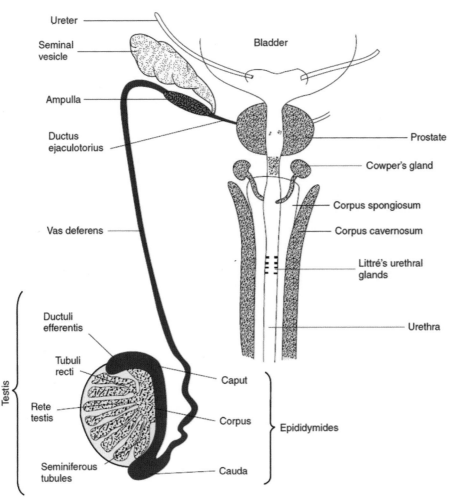

Figure 2.7 Diagram of the human male reproductive tract. Illustration created by U. Kvist ©2021.

vesicles develop. The ampulla and the seminal vesicle on each side have a common excurrent duct named the ejaculatory duct, which opens into the urethra [5,6].

The differentiation, development and secretory function of these organs are dependent on androgens. From the testes to corpus of the epididymis, most androgens are provided by the local fluid transportation from the testis (luminal fluid, lymphatic fluid, and local venous plexa), while the systemic circulation provides androgens to the cauda, vas deferens, seminal vesicles and prostate. The prostate has developed from the embryonic genitourinary sinus.

The Epididymis and Sperm Transport

In most mammals the epididymal transit time has been reported to be 7–10 days. However, the transit time is dependent on the amount of spermatozoa to be transported (i.e. daily sperm production). Men with high sperm output (>200 × 10^6 spermatozoa per day) had an average transit time of two days, whereas men with lower output (mean approximately 70 × 10^6 per day) reached six days of transit time [25]. The luminal transport from corpus to cauda seems independent of nervous regulation but involves local spontaneous waves of contraction, 7–9 per min. In the distal cauda and vas deferens, the spontaneous contractility is only 1–2 waves per min, resulting in an accumulation of spermatozoa in the distal cauda (i.e. it is a region of sperm storage).

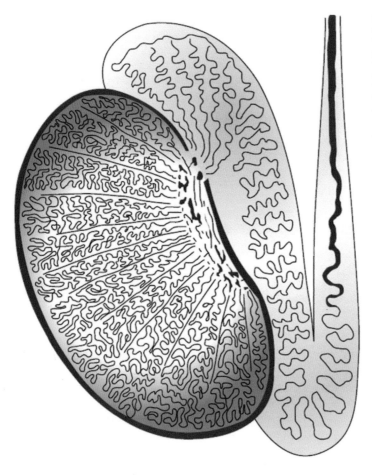

Figure 2.8 A semi-schematic drawing by A. F. Holstein [7] showing the arrangement of the seminiferoustubules in the human testis, the efferent ductules (6 tubules shown of the 10–15 tubules that the testis contains) connecting the rete testis to the epididymal duct, and the continuation of the epididymal duct into the vas deferens. Illustration by A. F. Holstein [7].

Transit time through the caput, corpus and proximal cauda is independent of ejaculatory frequency. The transport of spermatozoa from the distal cauda to the urethra is dependent on neurogenic activity, and frequent ejaculation results in a decline in sperm numbers there, while sexual abstinence results in increased numbers stored. One ejaculation a day for two days seems enough to normalize and equalize an increased or depleted sperm storage to the level of the daily sperm output [26].

The Epididymis, Sperm Maturation and Sperm Fertilization Capacity

During epididymal transit, the spermatozoon undergoes a maturation process by which it acquires capabilities as a messenger cell to traverse and survive the female genital tract and eventually deliver its genetic information to the embryo-to-be. Among these properties are progressive motility, the ability to fuse with and fertilize the oocyte, and the ability to sustain embryonic development into a viable offspring. The maturation process appears not to be restricted to particular parts of the epididymis but occurs as a function of time. Thus, spermatozoa withheld in the caput by occlusion of the duct in the corpus develop fertilizing capacity. Normal development and function of the caput and corpus epididymides is dependent of luminal flow of testosterone, which is locally transformed to the active dihydrotestosterone by the converting enzyme 5-α-reductase type 1.

Epididymis and Sperm Storage

The cauda epididymidis has evolved as the sperm storage organ in animals forced to wait for female ovulation. Is seems that when reaching the proximal cauda, the spermatozoa have achieved 'conservation factors' enabling prolonged storage. Two major factors contributing to this sperm storage are: (1) a low temperature (34°C) and (2) an androgen-dependent environment, including secretory products, created in the cauda epididymidis. The androgen acting in the cauda epididymidis is testosterone, transported by the systemic circulation and taken up by the epididymal epithelial cells and locally converted to dihydrotestosterone by 5-α-reductase type 2, (5-αR2). Factors jeopardizing the scrotal temperature and the testosterone effects (e.g. compounds interacting with 5-αR2) would decrease the functional storage time.

Conservation and Capacitation

The conservation processes involve inactivation of motility and metabolism, and the stabilization of various sperm structures and membranes. At ejaculation, the mixing of spermatozoa with the prostatic fluid restores motility, and it is plausible that the capacitation process needed to activate mammalian spermatozoa for fertilization involves restoration of conserved mechanisms [27].

The Size of the Sperm Storage

As a species, humans exhibit relatively low sperm production, a mere $100–500 \times 10^6$ per day. Sperm production is continuous and, like the ram, a man can have several ejaculations a day with fertile spermatozoa. Ejaculation every fourth hour after three days of abstinence can give results like 1000×10^6 in the first ejaculation, 125×10^6 just 4 h later, and 20×10^6 another 4 h later. It is worth noting that a decline from 1000×10^6 to 20×10^6 fresh spermatozoa due to sexual activity has no negative impact on the man's fertility. In this respect the evaluation of sperm number is totally different from the evaluation of red and white cells in blood. Therefore, when evaluating sperm counts, the ejaculatory frequency (i.e. sexual behaviour) is of critical importance: not only the time interval between the preceding ejaculation to that collected for investigation, but also the frequency of ejaculations preceding collection for investigation. Of all the spermatozoa in the epididymis, 50–80% are localized in the cauda epididymidis, and half of them are available for ejaculation.

DNA Damage upon Sperm Storage

Experiments show that spermatozoa aged within the epididymis (or in the laboratory or within the female genital tract) first lose their potential to contribute to a normal embryonic development (probably due to the fact that prolonged sperm storage results in sperm DNA strand breaks and chromosomal aberrations of the embryos [15]). Thereafter, they lose the ability to fully decondense their nuclear chromatin within the oocyte; followed by the ability to fertilize the oocyte and, long thereafter, they have a reduction in motility.

Animal studies have shown that if the transport of fresh spermatozoa from the testis to the cauda epididymidis is hindered, those spermatozoa remaining in the cauda more frequently cause aneuploidies in resulting embryos after only six days in the epididymis. The question arises, therefore, how those spermatozoa that upon aging in the epididymis have damaged DNA, are eliminated and hindered in reaching the site of fertilization. Possible explanations include:

1) That old spermatozoa are mixed with fresh ones in the cauda epididymidis, and these fresh gametes with undamaged DNA are more likely to reach the oocyte. There is so far no evidence that the female genital tract can select spermatozoa based upon their genomes, and about 0.5–1% of newborns have chromosomal aberrations. Moreover, DNA damage occurs before the ability to fertilize is decreased.

2) Male sexual drive could result in nocturnal emissions, masturbation and non-ovulation-related intercourse, which in turn would eliminate old spermatozoa, making way for fresh ones.

3) Local muscle contractions of the cauda epididymidis/vas deferens can emit spermatozoa to the urethra where they are voided with the urine. Spermatozoa in morning urine is diagnostic for spermarche in boys [25,28].

4) An as yet unexplored possibility might be the existence of an intrinsic system for eliminating aged spermatozoa.

Vas Deferens

The vas deferens can be palpated as a 3–5 mm thick 'string' in both sides of the scrotum. The vas has three robust layers of smooth muscle, one outer longitudinal, one circular and one inner longitudinal, and facing the lumen is a convoluted mucosal layer. The epithelium has one layer with secretory cells. Stimulation of sympathetic neurons releases noradrenalin which stimulates adrenergic α_1-receptors on the smooth muscles leading to a mass-contraction that, within a second, transports spermatozoa from the distal cauda epididymidis to the urethra.

Seminal Vesicles, Ampullae and Ejaculatory Ducts

The seminal vesicles and the ampullae have one layer of secretory epithelium of common origin that is highly convoluted. The secretory cells are stimulated by sympathetic neurons using acetylcholine as the transmitter; acetylcholine stimulates the formation of androgen-specific secretory products like fructose. The smooth muscles of the walls are stimulated to contract by the sympathetic adrenergic neurons; noradrenalin stimulates adrenergic α_1-receptors which initiates contraction whereby the contents are emitted to the urethra. The ejaculatory ducts open in the prostatic part of the urethra. In cases of agenesis of the Wolffian duct system (epididymides, vasa deferentia, seminal vesicles and ejaculatory ducts), either parts of the system or the whole system is missing. The ejaculate then lacks secretory markers for the missing parts (neutral α-glucosidase for the epididymis, fructose for the seminal vesicles and ampullae).

The Physiological Role of the Seminal Vesicles in Humans Is Unknown

Human spermatozoa ejaculated in, or incubated in, seminal vesicular fluid show decreased motility, vitality, decreased chromatin zinc content, and profound changes in chromatin stability.

Importance of Fructose and Prostaglandins Are Unknown

In many textbooks, fructose is mentioned as a substrate for sperm metabolism. However, considering the negative effects that seminal vesicular fluid has on spermatozoa (decrease in vitality, motility and affected chromatin packaging), and that *in vivo* spermatozoa normally do not come into contact with seminal vesicular fluid, the paradigm of seminal fructose being a substrate for human spermatozoa should be challenged [29]. Another role for fructose, and other 'unusual' sugar-types in semen of other animals could be to normalize the osmotic pressure to 290 mOsm/l. The seminal vesicles contain 40 million times higher concentrations of prostaglandins than the blood, and their physiological role also remains to be clearly determined.

The Prostate

The prostate is composed of 20 to 30 different glandular acini that open into the urethra. These glands evolved as branching buds from the sinus urogenitalis (i.e. an origin similar to the lower parts of the vagina). Testosterone from the systemic circulation is locally transformed to 5-α dihydro-testosterone by 5-αR2. Sympathetic cholinergic nerves stimulate the formation of androgen-specific secretory products as zinc, magnesium, calcium, citrate, acid phosphatase, and prostate specific antigen (PSA) [29]. Anti-cholinergic compounds thus counteract the formation of prostatic secretion, as do inhibitors of testosterone-dehydrogenase type 2. At emission, smooth muscle cells surrounding the glands are contracted and the fluid from the 20 to 30 glands is expelled and mixed with spermatozoa in the urethra. Emission is mediated by the adrenergic α_1-receptors on the smooth muscle cells stimulated by noradrenalin released from sympathetic adrenergic neurons.

Prostatic fluid also contains many substances that are normally present in blood plasma and are transudated from the blood plasma to the prostatic fluid. An acute inflammatory reaction in the prostate increases the transudated part, resulting in higher semen volume with lower concentration of androgen-specific compounds.

The Bladder Neck and Emission

Emission involves emptying of spermatozoa and the various fluids into the urethra. The sympathetic neurons also release noradrenalin on the smooth muscles surrounding the urinary bladder neck, which results in a closure of the urethra, preventing the emitted spermatozoa and fluid from passing up into the urinary bladder.

Diseases or surgery affecting the sympathetic neurons, e.g. diabetes, transurethral resection of the prostate (TUR) or retro-peritoneal-lymph-node-dissection (RPLND), can result in disturbed emission. Either there is no, or decreased, emptying of spermatozoa and fluid into the urethra, or fluid is expelled up into the urinary bladder. This condition results in lower or no volume expelled at ejaculation, with little or no antegrade ejaculation. Presence of large numbers of spermatozoa in urine collected after orgasm means that there has been a retrograde ejaculation.

Often, low or no antegrade ejaculation is associated with impaired emission from the epididymis and the glands, and no or few spermatozoa are found in the urine. In some cases, α_1-agonists can stimulate emission, bladder neck closure and result in antegrade ejaculation.

Innervations of the Smooth Muscles of the Emission Organs

The ductuli efferentes, the Wolffian duct system, the prostate and the bladder neck constitute a functional transport system of smooth muscles. In the efferent ducts, caput, corpus and proximal cauda epididymides, the smooth muscles are rich in intercellular tight junctions. The consequence is that spontaneous electrical depolarizations can be spread and induce waves of spontaneous contractions transporting spermatozoa and fluids without regulation by nerves. In contrast, the smooth muscles of the distal cauda, the vas deferens, the seminal vesicles, the ejaculatory ducts, the prostate and the bladder neck, have fewer junctions and are therefore dependent on neurogenic stimulation to induce waves of contraction [31].

The post-synaptic nerves stimulating the smooth muscles are specific to the genital tract and are called short adrenergic neurons. The pre-synaptic sympathetic neurons emanate from the lateral horns of the thoracic and lumbar regions of the spinal cord. They reach the genitalia through the hypogastric plexus and the hypogastric nerves running lateral to the rectum. Inside the genital organs they are connected to the post-synaptic short neurons. Ejaculation induced by vibrators uses, as do masturbation or coitus, the whole emission reflex. Electric stimulation of the hypogastric plexus or hypogastric nerves result in contractions in the distal cauda, vas deferens, the seminal vesicles, the ejaculatory ducts, the prostate and the bladder neck. By rectal electro-stimulation, various parts of the system can be activated to cause emission without the normal ejaculatory sequence.

The smooth muscles in the whole system respond to noradrenergic α_1-stimulation. Emission can be partially or completely blocked by α_1-receptor blockers (e.g. phentolamine and some anti-depressive agents) and is augmented by α_1-agonists (e.g. phenylpropanolamine, as used against oedema in the nasal mucosa). The adrenergic neurons are inhibited by the cholinergic neurons that stimulate secretion. Thus, during formation of fluid during sexual arousal, emission can be partly inhibited.

Innervations of Secretory Cells

The secretory cells in the epididymis, the vas deferens, the ampulla, the seminal vesicles and the prostate are innervated by short sympathetic cholinergic neurons releasing acetylcholine. The secretory neurons are inhibited by the adrenergic neurons. Thus, secretory stimulation decreases upon emission.

Ejaculation

At orgasm, spermatozoa in the cauda of the epididymis are emitted into the urethra and suspended in prostatic fluid. Striated muscles in the pelvis contract and increase the pressure in the urethra so that its contents are expelled. Later expelled fractions are mainly composed of a fluid from the seminal vesicles, which form a gel. Spermatozoa in the zinc-rich prostatic fluid preserve motility, vitality and a zinc-dependent stabilization of their nuclear chromatin. Spermatozoa that meet seminal vesicular fluid lose motility, vitality and zinc and the normal stabilization of the nuclear chromatin [1,14].

Ejaculatory Muscles

The urethral walls are extended by prostatic fluid with spermatozoa. This extension evokes somatic reflexes of rhythmic contractions in the bulbo- and ischio-cavernosus muscles and also in the muscles of the pelvic floor. The bulbocavernosus muscle surrounds the corpus spongiosum of the penis and inserts into the corpus cavernosum of both sides. The ischio-cavernosus muscles insert into the crus of the penis on both sides. These striated muscles of the perineum are innervated by the pudendal nerve. Note that whereas emission is controlled by autonomic nerves, ejaculation is governed by striated muscles under 'voluntary' control. However, men seldom practice to train these muscles, as done with the striated muscles controlling the bladder and the rectum, so ejaculation is experienced as an involuntary process once orgasm is reached.

Intra-Urethral Pressure and Ejaculatory Flow Speed

The contractions create an increase in intra-urethral pressure which forces the urethral contents outwards through the penis (when the bladder neck is closed). The flow speed of the ejaculate portions is dependent on how effectively the contraction force is transduced into increased pressure in the urethra lumen. The more powerful the erection the more of the force is transferred to pressure, giving a high flow velocity and a good separation of the ejaculate fractions. In contrast, a poor erection means more penile plasticity and less separation of ejaculatory fractions.

The high ejaculatory flow-speed is physiological, but also one reason why the sperm-containing first fraction of an ejaculate is often lost at semen collection by masturbation. Such ejaculates, where many (most?) of the spermatozoa have escaped collection, should not, of course, be used to evaluate sperm production.

The Sequence of Ejaculation

Our knowledge of the normal ejaculatory sequence comes from studies using split-ejaculates [14,29,32]. At ejaculation, each fraction was collected and characterized by counting the spermatozoa and measuring secretory markers for the prostate (zinc) and the seminal vesicles (fructose). Such studies revealed that spermatozoa from the distal cauda epididymidis are suspended in the simultaneously emitted fluid from the prostatic glands and expelled in a first ejaculatory portion: thus, the physiological ejaculate that is deposited onto the cervical mucus comprises spermatozoa in prostatic fluid. Shortly thereafter, fluid from the seminal vesicles is expelled. A specific sequence of ejaculation is also true for several animals; for example, in the boar, where the sperm-rich fraction is collected for assisted reproduction.

Abnormal Ejaculatory Sequence

A common, but often neglected, disorder is delayed emptying of the prostatic fluid, seen especially in men with inflammatory reaction of the prostate [32–34]. The spermatozoa are then primarily expelled mixed with the seminal vesicular fluid, which has the potential to affect sperm motility, vitality and chromatin packaging. Amelar and Hotchkiss noted that some 6% of infertile men had a delayed expulsion of spermatozoa and that the sperm-rich fraction of the ejaculate was more successful for insemination [32].

Redistribution of Zinc at Ejaculation

Zinc is secreted as both free ions and ions bound to citrate in the prostatic fluid. Seminal vesicular fluid contains powerful zinc-binding, high-molecular weight proteins which can extract zinc from spermatozoa and redistribute the citrate-bound and free zinc to the proteins of vesicular origin during and after liquefaction [33–36]. The proportion of zinc bound to high molecular weight proteins shows huge variations between men and ejaculates (2–67%) [37]. Although a semen sample might have high zinc concentration, compounds in the liquefied ejaculate can act as zinc chelators, thereby adversely affecting the sperm chromatin.

The Ejaculatory Sequence, Ejaculate Composition and Sperm Chromatin Stability

Forces that normally stabilize the sperm chromatin seem essential for a safe transfer of the genetic material to the oocyte. Fertile sperm donors have been shown to have higher sperm chromatin zinc content than infertile men, and some 25% of infertile men can have altered chromatin stability. The chance for pregnancy at IVF is severely reduced among men with low seminal zinc concentration. Zinc withdrawal enables a quick unwrapping of the whole nucleus into separate threads, when studied within minutes after ejaculation. This ability promptly declines when spermatozoa are stored *in vitro* [12,15]. Compounds from the seminal vesicles can deprive the sperm chromatin of zinc, affecting the normal protective packaging of the sperm DNA. It should be recalled that *in vivo* the spermatozoa are expelled in the zinc-rich prostatic fluid and enter the cervical mucus immediately at ejaculation without exposure to zinc-depriving seminal vesicular fluid.

Recently, it was reported that ejaculates with a high proportion of spermatozoa that had acquired chromatin zinc deficiency during or after liquefaction were the ejaculates that contained high proportions of spermatozoa with fragmentated sperm DNA [38,39]. Hence it appears that the unphysiological way in which we collect semen and expose spermatozoa to seminal vesicular fluid during liquefaction can cause semen samples for use in ART to undergo oxidative sperm DNA damage.

The 'Standardized' Methods for Semen Analysis and Sperm Handling

In reality, the 'standardized' semen sample only exists in the laboratory, when the entire ejaculate is collected and mixed in a single container. From a physiological perspective, the 'standard semen sample' is therefore an artefact that forces spermatozoa in the prostatic fluid to be trapped by the expanding vesicular gel for up to 20 min. Prostate Specific Antigen (PSA) from the prostate degrades the gel-forming seminogelins of vesicular origin. Due to this process, and to the general conditions during the *in vitro* handling procedures, the spermatozoa are exposed to increasing osmolarity, increased oxygen tension and elevated levels of free radicals [1,14].

A Change in Semen Osmolarity *In Vitro* Affects Sperm Selection *In Vitro*

In vivo, spermatozoa are expelled in the isotonic prostatic fluid onto the isotonic cervical mucus extruding from the cervical opening into the vagina. *In vitro*, enzymatic digestion of macromolecules starts at ejaculation, resulting in a rapid increase of the semen osmolarity from 290 up to 450 mOsmol/l by 3 h later [14,39–42].

There are two implications of this: (1) the possible direct effect of the increasing osmolarity on spermatozoa; and (2) the risk and effects of hypo-osmotic stress, when spermatozoa in hypertonic seminal plasma later are exposed to isotonic culture media used for sperm selection.

Increasing osmolarity in the liquefied ejaculate: The actual osmolarity reached and its rate of increase vary between samples [41]. Increased semen osmolarity is strongly associated with decreased sperm motility [41]. When semen osmolarity increases the spermatozoon loses water, which activates volume-regulating mechanisms to restore the cellular volume, a process that requires energy. Continuously increasing osmolarity evokes continuous volume regulation that could exhaust the spermatozoa by consuming their intracellular ATP, which is also needed for other cellular functions such as motility. Ejaculates incubated at higher osmolality therefore show reduced sperm motility and velocity [43], and semen samples with impaired motility had higher osmolality than controls [44–46].

Abruptly decreased osmolarity – the unintended hypo-osmotic shock at sperm selection: This hypo-osmotic challenge occurs when the spermatozoon that had adjusted to increasing osmolality abruptly are exposed to isotonic (~290 mOsm/l) selection media. After semen liquefaction and before sperm selection osmolarity levels increase from 290mOsm/l at ejaculation to 330–350–380 mOsm/l. Thus, the hypo-osmotic shock varies conspicuously between various samples ranging from 40–90 mOsm/l [41].

Living spermatozoa with intact membranes take up water and swell, an almost instantaneous effect described by Kölliker in 1856 [41]. The size of the osmotic shock is the main factor that determines the amount of water to be taken up. The amount of water taken up determines the degree of swelling response seen in the tail, causing a variable degree of distal tail coiling and tail folding within its plasma membrane: tail tip coiling being the mildest effect. Up to now this iatrogenic osmotic shock has unintendedly been imposed on the spermatozoon in most samples used for ART.

The Hypo-osmotic Swelling Test

In contrast to the inadvertent osmotic shock, the osmotic difference that spermatozoa are exposed to in the hypo-osmotic swelling (HOS) test is fully intended. The HOS test was developed to reveal which spermatozoa are alive and able to take up water, swell and coil their tails in response to exposure to an osmolarity of 175 mOsm/l [47], i.e. an osmotic shock of 155–205 mOsm/l (which is far greater than the 40–90 mOsm/l shock that occurs during sperm selection for ART.

The HOS test will cause excessive water uptake and results in more advanced sperm swelling and many spermatozoa react with full coiling of the tail that can be seen either as a circular structure at the base of the head or as total coiling of the tail around the sperm head.

Since the osmotic shock induced at sperm selection seldom results in totally coiled tails, the consequences of exposing spermatozoa in the ejaculate to 'isotonic' selection media has unfortunately remained unrecognized until recently [43]. It was observed that ejaculated spermatozoa exposed to isotonic selection media swam in a jerky fashion. Freeze-frame video recordings of jerky swimming spermatozoa revealed spermatozoa with morphological deformed tails that were coiled at the tips or partly folded, irreversible morphological changes that did not change within an hour [43].

One approach to eliminate the effects of increasing osmolarity would be to apply the selection provided by nature, i.e. to select spermatozoa at ejaculation, for instance by using the first, non-coagulated split ejaculate fraction for density gradient centrifugation within minutes after ejaculation, or by early dilution of the ejaculate [14,43].

The Importance of Sperm Number Is Overestimated

Just 10–200 spermatozoa normally reach the ampullar parts of the oviducts; of which only one will fertilize [48,49]. Fatherhood has been proven among vasectomized men without any detectable spermatozoa in the ejaculate. Finding no spermatozoa in one 10 μm deep chamber only tells us that the probability is 95% that the sample has less than 720,000 spermatozoa. No spermatozoa observed in a centrifuged sample after examination of microscope 400 fields tells us, with the same probability, that there are less than 200 spermatozoa in the sample. Thus, if no spermatozoa are found under the microscope it does not exclude the possibility that there were spermatozoa present in the ejaculate.

In a study from Norway, men contributing to pregnancy within one month had higher total sperm number (mean 410×10^6 per ejaculate) compared to men needing up to 12 months to contribute to a pregnancy (mean 254×10^6 per ejaculate). Of all men contributing to a pregnancy within one year, 95% had $\geq 22 \times 10^6$ sperm per ejaculate [50]. Among infertile couples in France, studied after a period of at least six months of infertility, those with $<5 \times 10^6$ spermatozoa per ml, i.e. approximately corresponding to a total number of 22×10^6 per ejaculate in the study above, had a low (11%) chance of achieving a pregnancy within the next year whereas men with $>5 \times 10^6$/ml had a 62% probability of contributing to a pregnancy during the same time [51]. A cut-off of 5×10^6/ml was also found in a Danish study [52], while another Danish study advocated a cut-off concentration of 40×10^6 per ml (corresponding to ~170 $\times 10^6$ spermatozoa per ejaculate). However, the confidence interval for this chosen level was zero to infinity, and the data given allowed the reader to recalculate a cut-off level close to 10×10^6/ml. Moreover, some 20% of the men included in this study failed to collect the first, sperm-rich fraction, biasing the results and conclusions [53]. Thus, a clinical cut-off for the chance to achieve pregnancy within one year seems close to 20×10^6 spermatozoa per ejaculate.

The Risk for Damaged Sperm DNA Is Increased among Men with Low Sperm Number

Studies of the integrity of sperm DNA show that men with few spermatozoa have spermatozoa with more chromosomal aberrations and more DNA strand breaks.

The spermatozoon is the only cell in the body that lacks DNA repair systems. This means that damage to the DNA during sperm formation, maturation, storage, ejaculation, *in vitro* handling, and transfer to the oocyte cannot be repaired by the spermatozoon itself. DNA damage does occur and can be repaired by the oocyte, although this repair could be complete, wrong or incomplete. Faulty repair might result in *de novo* translocations (chromosome strand sections containing genes that are wrongly transferred onto other chromosomes) or inversions (chromosome strand sections containing genes that are inserted onto the right chromosome but in the opposite direction). If all the genetic material is still present, the translocation or inversion is called balanced, but if not, it is unbalanced. If DNA strand breaks are left unrepaired, genes can be lost and the condition is called a chromosome deletion. Deletions and unbalanced aberrations often result in miscarriage or malformations, and can also affect psychomotor development after birth. A balanced translocation results in a healthy child with normal psychomotor development and normal puberty. However, its own fertility could be reduced and it has higher risk of contributing to miscarriage, fetal death, malformations and affected psychomotor development in the subsequent generation. This is because individuals with balanced translocation produce gametes with variable genomes: some gametes have too much DNA, some too little, some have normal DNA, and some have the same balanced translocation as the individual himself.

A spermatozoon used for fertilization that has an acquired DNA damage might therefore not only affect the child-to-be but also, or only, affect the generation thereafter. Consequently, the full safety of any assisted reproduction method can only be judged using a two-generation perspective [1,54–56].

Female Reproductive Physiology from a Sperm Perspective

Sperm Invasion Threatens the Human Oocyte: A Hundred Million against One

With the evolution from external to internal fertilization, and internal embryonic and fetal development, the numbers of embryos and fetuses must be limited. Females who ovulated multiple oocytes were at an evolutionary disadvantage. Males are, in this evolutionary aspect, still at primitive invertebrate level, i.e. 100 million genetic lots are produced each day and released in vast numbers. Human females are anatomically unsuited for multiple pregnancies. The increased prevalence of obstetrical problems and adverse outcomes in spontaneous twin pregnancies are eloquent expressions of humans being an essentially monotocous species

However, in some 1% of families there is a hereditary propensity for spontaneous twin pregnancies. In these cases, the survival of females and fetuses has been less incompatible with twin pregnancies. This is, however, not the case for the twin pregnancies produced by ART [1].

The evolutionary pressure on the female side that resulted in the ovulation of a single oocyte created another problem for nature. The single oocyte is threatened by an invasion, 100×10^6 spermatozoa against one single oocyte, and evolutionary biologists discuss the need for the female to protect her oocyte from this invasion. The cervical mucus, the isthmus of the Fallopian tubes, and the barriers protecting the oocyte can be viewed as central components of this defence.

Passage through the Cervical Mucus, the Uterus and the Fallopian Tubes

From a physiological point of view the cervical mucus is where the male deposits the first expelled population of spermatozoa suspended in prostatic fluid (Figure 2.9). Thereafter, the gel-forming seminal vesicular fluid is expelled – and there is no evidence that these two secretions are mixed in the vagina as they are mixed in a semen collection vessel. Rather, it seems that *in vivo* the freely swimming spermatozoa in the prostatic fluid, some of which enter the cervical mucus, and the gel-formed vesicular secretion form two separate compartments. In many other mammalian species, the seminal vesicular secretion forms a firm copulatory plug that

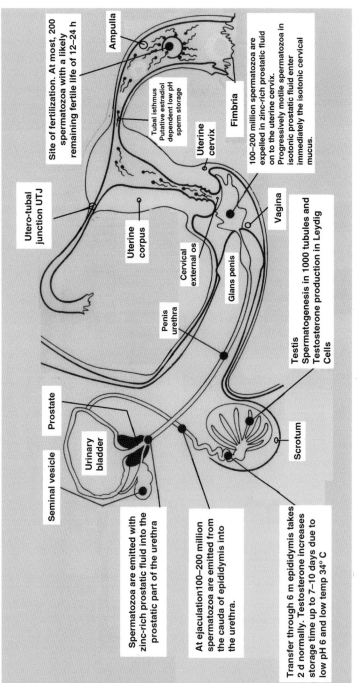
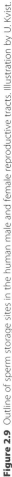

Ampulla

Site of fertilization. At most, 200 spermatozoa with a likely remaining fertile life of 12–24 h

Tubal isthmus
Putative estradiol dependent low pH sperm storage

Uterine cervix

Fimbria

100–200 million spermatozoa are expelled in zinc-rich prostatic fluid on to the uterine cervix.
Progressively motile spermatozoa in isotonic prostatic fluid enter immediately the isotonic cervical mucus.

Utero-tubal junction UTJ

Uterine corpus

Cervical external os

Vagina

Glans penis

Penis urethra

Testis
Spermatogenesis in 1000 tubules and Testosterone production in Leydig Cells

Scrotum

Seminal vesicle **Prostate**

Urinary bladder

Spermatozoa are emitted with zinc-rich prostatic fluid into the prostatic part of the urethra

At ejaculation100–200 million spermatozoa are emitted from the cauda of epididymis into the urethra.

Transfer through 6 m epididymis takes 2 d normally. Testosterone increases storage time up to 7–10 days due to low pH 6 and low temp 34° C

Figure 2.9 Outline of sperm storage sites in the human male and female reproductive tracts. Illustration by U. Kvist.

prevents other males from mating successfully with the female, so in this respect the human seminal vesicular contribution can be seen as being vestigial.

The cervix, its mostly impermeable mucus, and the low pH of the vagina, which is created by the vaginal microbiome [57,58], are barriers in the female between micro-organisms in the outside world and the interior of the female reproductive tract and the peritoneal compartment.

To enable fertilization, these barriers must allow penetration of motile male gametes at ovulation. FSH leading to follicular development also results in increased levels of estradiol (E2) which stimulate the cervical glands to produce mucus that (1) does not kill the spermatozoa and (2) allows them to penetrate using their own power (motility). At ovulation, the cervical mucus has conditions optimal for sperm passage, the highest anti-bacterial activity and, at the same time, the pH of the vagina is the lowest. Soon after ovulation, increased levels of progesterone affect the cervical glands and make the mucus they secrete impenetrable to spermatozoa.

The textbook picture of the vagina as an open tube with cervical mucus restricted to the cervical canal must also be challenged. Close to ovulation the narrow, collapsed lumen of the vagina contains the 'sperm-catching' cervical mucus protruding from the external cervical os into the vagina – unless it has been interfered with by, for instance, hygiene procedures. Using natural family planning procedures, samples of cervical mucus are collected at the vulva. Clinical protocols for vaginal examination prescribe that this expression of physiology – protruding cervical mucus – should be removed to give the examiner a clear view of the cervix. However, the procedure can give the examiner the wrong impression that cervical mucus is restricted to the cervix only.

It has been suggested that the cervix functions as a sperm reservoir. However, while spermatozoa might have been found to survive deep up in the crypts of cervical mucus, this does not prove that spermatozoa temporarily surviving in the crypts actually constitute a reservoir since there is no evidence that these spermatozoa ever re-emerge from the crypts into the cervical canal [49,59,60].

The progressive motility of the spermatozoon is essential for it to penetrate into and pass through cervical mucus, and hence spermatozoa with poor motility are excluded or filtered out during their passage through it. Concomitantly, spermatozoa with abnormal morphology are also removed [30], resulting in only a minority of ejaculated spermatozoa actually entering the cervix [49,59,60]. Some hours after ejaculation, the uterus is invaded by leucocytes that attack the spermatozoa. It is therefore reasonable to assume that the fertilizing spermatozoon has to traverse the uterus and reach the immune-privileged oviductal epithelium in the isthmus of the oviduct ahead of this elimination of spermatozoa in the uterus. Uterine muscular contractions might enhance passage of spermatozoa through the uterine cavity to the utero-tubal junctions since radio-labelled spheres placed in the vagina can be translocated to the oviductal isthmus during the late follicular phase [59].

The Utero-Tubal Junction and the Isthmic Sperm Reservoir

The anatomy of the utero-tubal junction, the folded mucosa and contracted smooth muscle layer, along with a mucus secretion that flows towards the uterus, together constitute a functional barrier for the spermatozoa to pass, as well as a barrier that can prevent a fertilized oocyte reaching the uterine cavity too soon. Short adrenergic neurons release noradrenalin that triggers the smooth muscles of the isthmus to contract when dominated by estradiol during the follicular phase before ovulation. Following ovulation, increased levels of progesterone hyperpolarize the smooth muscles, thus counteracting the adrenergic action and the muscles relax, allowing the zygote to pass at Day 3 to 4 after fertilization. There is some evidence indicating that more than good sperm morphology and progressive motility is needed to pass into the isthmus of the Fallopian tubes. A few thousand spermatozoa may swim through the utero-tubal junctions to reach the isthmus region of the oviducts. Whereas other mammals reveal a distinct sperm reservoir, the human isthmus constitutes at least a functional reservoir that could prolong the availability of spermatozoa maintained in a fertile state, by interacting with the oviductal epithelium. The perceived difference might be due to the fact that the proximal isthmus, which is the likely site of the sperm reservoir within the human female reproductive tract, is embedded within the thick muscular wall of the uterus, and therefore difficult to access for observational studies. Subpopulations of small numbers of spermatozoa become capacitated and hyperactivated, which enables them to proceed towards the tubal ampulla [61]. At any time only some 10–200 spermatozoa could be flushed from normal human oviducts, while some thousands could be recovered in distally obstructed oviducts [49,59,60].

Which Are the Few Spermatozoa that Reach the Oviductal Ampulla?

These spermatozoa constitute a subpopulation of those few thousands that traversed the utero-tubal junction and became attached to the oviductal epithelium in the isthmus. So, which are they?

- Spermatozoa that reach the oviducts before the uterine invasion defence system reacts and impedes later arriving spermatozoa?
- A subpopulation of spermatozoa that reaches the isthmus and has a special additional competence to pass?
- A subpopulation that is invisible to the uterine invasion defence system?

If it is the first two groups, then spermatozoa in the first expelled ejaculate fraction would be more representative for these than the spermatozoa residing in the liquefied whole ejaculate. But if it is the latter two groups, then these spermatozoa would be true subpopulations that we need to be able to identify. In the future we might be able to identify and select spermatozoa that can reach the oviducts from within the first expelled fraction. But we can never truly predict whether a man will become a father or not, regardless of the sophistication of methods we use, as long as we only assess the 'messenger' functions of the spermatozoa. Also, the messages could only be studied in a number of spermatozoa representative of the selected subpopulations, since it is doubtful that we will ever be able to study the messages of a single spermatozoon without affecting its integrity [1].

When Will Competent Spermatozoa Reach the Site of Fertilization?

There is no valid support for a rapid (minutes) sperm transport, although some early observations indicated that human and rabbit spermatozoa could reach the ampulla minutes after insemination – although these spermatozoa were mostly dead and did not contribute to fertilization [59,60]. Experimental studies to clarify the physiological situation, especially in humans, are lacking, and will be extremely difficult to perform.

Allowing speculation, a sperm progression velocity of 25–50 µm/s corresponds to 1.5–3.0 mm/min. Considering that the distance from the external cervical os to the oviductal ampulla is some 150 mm, theoretically a spermatozoon would take 50–100 min to swim the distance unaided. Adding a delay (minutes to days) in transport through the isthmus, it being a functional barrier and reservoir that is also influenced by the female hormonal status and ovulation, competent spermatozoa might arrive in the ampulla from perhaps 1 h up to several days after ejaculation at intercourse.

At insemination, sperm transport is further delayed because selection of spermatozoa from hypertonic liquefied semen into isotonic cervical mucus or isotonic preparation medium induces irreversible sperm tail-tip coiling and tail bending that reduces the proportion of motile spermatozoa as well as sperm velocity (see above) [43].

Considering artificial insemination, at intra-cervical insemination (ICI) the hypotonic shock occurs when spermatozoa in hypertonic liquefied raw semen are placed onto or into the isotonic cervical mucus. This will in turn delay sperm transport to the Fallopian tubes and affect their efforts to approach the oocyte. At intrauterine insemination (IUI) or Fallopian tube sperm perfusion (FSP), sperm distribution to the Fallopian tubes appears to be facilitated by the insemination technique. However, the hypotonic shock and its irreversible effect on sperm morphology and motility, would have occurred when the spermatozoa were selected from hypertonic liquefied semen into the isotonic preparation medium. Although flushed into the Fallopian tubes, their already impaired motility might hamper and delay the spermatozoa's final approach to the oocyte [14,43].

Sperm Storage

The human oocyte has a fertilization window of some 8–12 h after ovulation. It appears essential that a relatively small number of spermatozoa with full fertilizing potential are at hand in the Fallopian tubes to penetrate the cumulus and corona cells, the zona pellucida, and fuse with the oocyte to achieve fertilization within this short time window.

Normally around 70% of couples achieve pregnancy within six months after having randomly timed intercourse, so it can be argued that the conditions for sperm storage in these men and women are satisfactory. On the other hand, couples that do not achieve pregnancy spontaneously within a year of trying appear more likely to have impaired conditions for sperm storage: in theses couples the timing of ejaculation/insemination and ovulation seems to be of greater importance when treated with ART.

As illustrated in Figure 2.9, the proximal cauda of the epididymis and the isthmus of the Fallopian tube have evolved to be sites for sperm storage. In a man with full sperm production, the transit time through the epididymis is 2 days, with two main factors appearing essential to prolong sperm storage from 2 to 7–10 days: (a) low temperature (34°C), and (b) a normal testosterone-dependent environment in the proximal cauda epididymidis that causes low pH. Concordantly, the storage of spermatozoa in the Fallopian tube isthmus appears to be up to about 5 days if a normal estradiol-dependent environment creates a lower pH within the heavily convoluted lining of the isthmus where spermatozoa reside until ovulation [62]. The reduced pH is effectuated by carbonic anhydrase activity in the proximal cauda and in the isthmus.

Thus, the key players for sperm storage are (a) the gonadal production of testosterone and estradiol that, via blood perfusion, induce the low pH; and (b) the lower temperature achieved via a countercurrent blood flow system that achieves and maintains a temperature gradient from the 37°C core temperature of the body to 34°C at the base of the scrotum.

Sperm Responses to Signals from the Female Genital Tract

Capacitation

At ejaculation, the mammalian spermatozoon has not yet acquired full fertilizing capacity. The bio-chemical, molecular and physiological changes that the spermatozoon experiences within the female genital tract are collectively referred to as capacitation, a complex process that results in a spermatozoon fully competent for fertilization. During capacitation, changes occur in membrane properties, enzyme activities, and motility which together make spermatozoa responsive to stimuli that induce hyperacti-vated motility and, later, the acrosome reaction, and thereby prepare the spermatozoon for penetration of the egg investments prior to fertilization [11,61]. These changes are accompanied by the activation of cell signalling cascades *in vivo* or in defined culture media *in vitro* [63–67], although the full nature of these signalling complexes, and their temporal and spatial activations, remain to be elucidated.

Hyperactivated Motility

Hyperactivation is usually considered a part and expression of the capacitation process seen in all Eutherian mammals studied. However, the regulatory pathway that finally gives rise to an increase in flagellar Ca^{2+} and triggers hyperactivation can also operate independently from capacitation [68,69].

Hyperactivation is characterized by high amplitude, asymmetrical flagellar bending, and robust assessment of hyperactivation needs parameters measured by CASA. Besides promoting the passage through the zona pellucida, hyperactivation may also facilitate release of sperm from the oviductal storage reservoir in the isthmus and may propel sperm through mucus in the oviductal lumen and the matrix of the cumulus oophorus [61].

The Acrosome Reaction

The acrosome reaction is a 'metamorphosis event' that must be completed by the spermatozoa of many animal species prior to fusion with eggs [11]. In Eutherian mammals it follows capacitation and is triggered by the spermatozoon binding to zona pellucida. It involves multiple fusions between the sperm plasma membrane and the underlying outer acrosomal membrane, resulting in many small vesicles allowing release of the acrosomal content. In the mouse, this exocytosis is triggered by one of the three the zona pellucida glycoproteins, ZP3 (there is also a fourth ZP glycoprotein in the human ZP). Following binding of the spermatozoon to the zona ZP3 promotes a sustained influx of Ca^{2+} into the spermatozoon that is necessary for the acrosome reaction [70]. Among substances released during the acrosome reaction are hyaluronidase and acrosin. These are enzymes capable of degrading the cumulus mass and the zona pellucida, respectively. However, the hyaluronidase is apparently released at the zona pellucida, i.e. after the cumulus mass has already been traversed, and interestingly spermatozoa lacking acrosin can still fertilize, although they are less efficient [71]. In a sea-snail, acrosin helps the spermatozoon open the oocyte-surrounding gel without acting as an enzyme. Thus, the presence of a molecule that can act as an enzyme does not necessarily mean that it actually has a physiologically important enzymatic effect.

The Barriers of the Oocyte Allow the Passage of Competent Spermatozoa

The mammalian oocyte is surrounded by a thick glycoprotein layer, the zona pellucida, which the spermatozoon takes some 3–4 min to penetrate. Furthermore, around the zona pellucida is the huge cumulus mass, which is composed of about 50 layers of cumulus cells surrounded by the matrix produced by these cells. Hyaluronic acid is the predominant matrix macromolecule. The cumulus mass contains progesterone (secreted by the cumulus cells, which are follicular granulosa cells that underwent luteinization before ovulation) and nitric oxide, both of which induce calcium signalling within the spermatozoon [72]. Most spermatozoa fail to pass through, and become stuck in the cumulus, although exactly why some spermatozoa do not pass remains to be elucidated.

One factor could be lack of hyperactivated motility. Sperm penetration through the cumulus matrix, as well as through the zona pellucida (ZP), are dependent on hyperactivated motility, which is a type of motility characterized by high amplitude flagellar waves that generate powerful propulsive force, capable even of breaking covalent bonds [61]. After passage through the cumulus, the fertilizing spermatozoon must bind to the ZP (a largely species-specific process), undergo the acrosome reaction, and then penetrate through the matrix of the ZP. Thus, the ZP constitutes a barrier which, in most mammals, evolved to admit only spermatozoa of the same species. Following the acrosome reaction, new ligands are exposed on the equatorial segment of the sperm head by which the spermatozoon can bind to the oocyte plasma membrane after passing through the ZP [11].

In conclusion, the spermatozoon that finally fuses with the oocyte is one that underwent capacitation, developed hyperactivated motility, had the competence to pass the cumulus matrix, bore the right code to bind to the ZP, underwent the acrosome reaction, traversed the ZP, and finally showed the right code for binding to the oocyte membrane and was able to fuse with it.

The Spermatozoon Does Not Penetrate the Oocyte – It Fuses with It

Fertilization by fusion of the gametes is a fundamental mechanism and was the first evolutionary step towards sexual reproduction some 600 million years ago. After fusion, the sperm membrane and the oocyte membrane are contiguous [11]. The internal parts of the spermatozoon are then automatically inside and surrounded by the ooplasm. The contaminated outside of the sperm plasma membrane remains on the outside surface of the fertilized oocyte, although after ICSI it is also introduced into the ooplasm [1,11,73].

ICSI Penetrates and Bypasses Fusion

In biological terms ICSI, the injection of a spermatozoon directly into the ooplasm, is a new concept. From an evolutionary perspective, injection of spermatozoa (with their membranes intact) and some suspending medium means that the barriers of the oocyte are breached, raising the possibility of by-passing the natural barriers without physiological control, potentially exposing both the zygote and future generations to the entrance of compounds or organisms that otherwise would not have had access to the inside of the oocyte [73]. This new evolutionary concept requires that we use controlled conditions, especially not using culture media that contain biological material from other species [1,73].

After Fusion – Sperm Messages

As far as is known at present, the spermatozoon brings four messages to the zygote:

1) Factors for oocyte activation;
2) An intact haploid genome;
3) The centrosomes (needed for mitotic divisions in the new individual); and
4) Factors necessary for the initiation of placental development.

Besides DNA, the spermatozoon also brings proteins and mRNA to the oocyte, but the specific functions of these compounds still remain to be elucidated.

1. Activation of the Oocyte

The exact signals are unknown, but electrical events in the oocyte membrane and a rise in calcium in the ooplasm must occur. There is also the release of the cortical granules, which induce changes in the oocyte membrane so that it cannot fuse with other spermatozoa. Only if two spermatozoa are fusing with the oocyte almost simultaneously would polyspermic fertilization occur. Fertilization by two spermatozoa usually results in three pronuclei and a diandric 'dispermic' triploid zygote, which can develop to term (although human triploids always die within hours of birth). Fertilization by a diploid spermatozoon would create a 'diplospermic' diandric triploid zygote; this is very rare *in vivo*, more likely at IVF, and is avoided at ICSI by not injecting spermatozoa with large heads.

The oocyte then completes its second meiotic division, which is followed by the fusion of the male and female pronuclei and, some hours later, the first mitotic cell division. However, the oocyte can also be activated spontaneously, or by chemicals such as ethanol or even physical manipulation with a glass pipette. This capacity for such parthenogenetic development means that even if an oocyte divides into two cells there is no guarantee that it was fertilized by a spermatozoon.

2. An Intact Haploid Genome

Immediately upon sperm-egg fusion, the nuclear envelope surrounding the sperm nucleus dissolves and the tightly condensed nucleus rapidly decondenses to form the male pronucleus.

3. Two Male Centrioles Are Needed for Mitoses of the Zygote

Until recently, it was believed that the spermatozoon in most mammals contributed one centriole to the zygote and that this centriole duplicated into two that organized the first mitosis of the zygote. This was because it was believed that while the mammalian spermatid has two typical centrioles, the proximal and the distal, the distal was lost during late spermiogenesis.

Recently, however, it was demonstrated that the distal centriole seen in the elongating spermatid becomes remodeled in the mature spermatozoon into a functional-but-atypical centriole that is composed of microtubules surrounding earlier undescribed rods of centriole luminal proteins [74]. Consequently, the ejaculated spermatozoon actually carries two functional centrioles, and both are transferred to the zygote. Both the proximal and the atypical distal centriole duplicate within the ooplasm and one of each origin forms a centrosome together with the oocyte pericentriolar material. The centrosomes organize γ-tubulin molecules in the ooplasm into long tubular threads starting at the centrosomes. The threads grow rapidly and can radiate like a 'sperm aster' throughout the ooplasm. The sperm asters anchor to the male and female pronuclei containing the paternal and maternal chromosomes. By contraction of the threads the sperm centrosome drags the pronuclei in close connection. At mitosis, one daughter centriole of the proximal and one of the atypical distal centriole forms the cell spindle of the first mitotic division. If this fails, the blastocyst will die.

The functional importance of the transition from a typical distal centriole to an atypical centriole is not yet understood [74]. However, these new insights clearly provide new possibilities for diagnostics and therapeutic strategies for male infertility, and insights into early embryo development.

A sperm centriole that has been seriously damaged during sperm transfer might fail to sustain embryonic development. Fertilized oocytes that do not divide, or divide only slowly, could have a damaged sperm centriole. Even dividing fertilized oocytes chosen for embryo transfer could be destined to die due to sperm centriolar failure. The anti-cough drug noskapin, and also diazepams, interfere with sperm aster formation, but the extent to which drugs that interfere with centrosome function might have affected human fertility is not known.

Basic Centrosome Physiology

The centrosome is a self-replicating organelle which in most mammals (including humans) is inherited from the male. Interestingly, in mice and other rodents, the zygote does not receive a centriole from the spermatozoon, but the whole centrosome (two perpendicularly oriented cylindrical centrioles and the pericentriolar material, or PCM) comes from the oocyte, a fundamental difference in mammalian evolution [75]. Hence, the centriole is a specialized expression of the centrosome that serves as the main microtubular organizing centre in the zygote and a regulator of cell-cycle progression. It can initiate the aggregation, orientation and function of certain intracytoplasmic threads or tubules for movement and transport, and can also reproduce and is claimed to carry its own RNA-genome, necessary for aster formation for example. A centriole can in turn give rise to a cilium or a flagellum as the sperm tail. In some cells, the centrosome forms many centrioles (basal bodies), each giving rise to a cilium, as in ciliated cells in, e.g., the Fallopian tubes and in the respiratory epithelium. The round spermatid carries one typical centrosome, which has given rise to two centrioles, the proximal and distal centrioles in the connecting piece of the elongating spermatids. The distal centriole gives rise to the sperm flagellum, the basic element of the tail, and can be seen posterior to the connecting piece by transmission electron microscopy in the elongating spermatids. The proximal centriole may have helped in the organization of the chromosomes in the nucleus and shaping of the head by the manchette [76].

4.   Factors Necessary for Initiation of Placental Development

In placental mammals like humans, the nutritional capacity of the oocyte lasts for a few days only. Chorionic villi grow out from the surface of the embryo in all directions, and upon meeting the endometrium these villi actively transform the endometrium into the maternal part of the placenta-to-be. Thus, the embryo plays the active role in placentation. The acceptance of a foreign individual intermingling with the tissue of the host (here the endometrium) was a step taken in evolution and its full consequences are not fully elucidated, e.g. for acceptance of invasive cancer growth.

Two sperm nuclei in a frog oocyte will result in a frog. Two oocyte nuclei in a frog oocyte also will result in a frog. In a placental mammal the situation is different: two sperm nuclei in a mouse oocyte will result in mainly placental tissue. The human equivalent has been known for several years, although its implications were not understood. Two sperm nuclei in a human oocyte result in a hydatidiform mole. In contrast, two oocyte nuclei in an oocyte result in mainly embryonic tissue without initiation of proper placental tissue and the embryo will die. The mechanism by which the spermatozoon initiates placental growth is not understood. Genomic imprinting, i.e. different inactivation of genes by epigenetic control within the male or female gonad, is a favourable candidate for this mechanism.

Evolution of placental animals thus has given the spermatozoon a 'new' important function. Paternal factors thus secure a passage of nutrients and other vital substances to the fetus while the block for placental formation within the oocyte genome protects the female from offspring achieved through parthenogenesis. A consequence of this is that research on factors contributing to subfertility must also consider the possibility that damages to the sperm and its messages might disturb placental formation and function and therefore also be involved in problems related to growth and development a long time after fertilization.

Sperm Mitochondria and their DNA Are Targeted to be Destroyed by the Oocyte

Because sperm mitochondria were already ubiquitin-tagged in the testis, marking them and their DNA for destruction after entry into the oocyte [23], in evolutionary terms mitochondria are inherited through the female germ cell line. While there are reports suggesting that mutated sperm mitochondrial DNA may escape destruction and cause mitochondrial disease in the offspring, it seems to be an extremely rare event.

Concluding Remarks

This chapter has summarized how nature creates, stores and transfers spermatozoa, and how those spermatozoa with intact DNA, mitochondria, centrioles and placental factors give rise to healthy progeny. There are challenges for ART labs to comprehend and always act in concordance with nature, especially the early critical moment of collecting and selecting spermatozoa for use in ART treatments. Nature immediately selects motile spermatozoa from the isotonic, zinc-rich prostatic fluid into the isotonic cervical mucus. But before the human spermatozoon reaches the oocyte in the ART lab it experiences two major non-physiological challenges that can affect its full fertilizing potential: (a) exposure to seminal vesicular fluid (causing chromatin zinc-deficiency and a vulnerable chromatin with increased risk for oxidative DNA damage); and (b) exposure to an osmotic roller-coaster that causes sperm ATP-depletion, tail coiling, impaired sperm motility and low sperm density (as measured in g/ml, not to be confused with sperm concentration), that affect sperm functional properties and sperm selection procedures by swim-up and density gradient centrifugation. These two unphysiological challenges are unintentionally forced upon the spermatozoa when collected as a whole ejaculate and then subjected to diagnostic assessments or sperm selection for ART [38–43].

Obviously, the causes and consequences of these stresses need to be considered and eliminated in order to improve our skills in diagnostics and assisted reproduction. So, for the future, we should consider paying more attention to replicating biophysical and biochemical conditions, as well as practical handling steps, that better support sperm physiology.

References

1. Kvist U. Genetics, ethics and the gametes – on reproductive biology, multiple pregnancies and ICSI. *Acta Obstet Gynecol Scand* 2000; **79**: 913–20.

2. Graves JA. How to evolve new vertebrate sex determining genes. *Dev Dynam* 2013; **242**: 354–9.

3. Mortimer D, Cohen J, Mortimer ST, et al. Cairo consensus on the IVF laboratory environment and air quality: report of an expert meeting. *Reprod Biomed Online* 2018; **36**: 658–74.

4. Cairo 2018 Consensus Group. There is only one thing that is truly important in an IVF lab: everything. *Reprod Biomed Online* 2020; **40**: 33–59.

5. Neill JD, ed. *Knobil and Neill's Physiology of Reproduction*, 3rd edn. Amsterdam: Elsevier Academic Press, 2005.

6. Nieschlag E, Behre HM, Nieschlag S, eds. *Andrology: Male Reproductive Health and Dysfunction*, 2nd edn. Berlin and Heidelberg: Springer-Verlag GmbH, 2001.

7. Holstein AF, Schulze W, Davidoff M. Understanding spermatogenesis is a prerequisite for treatment. *Reprod Biol Endocrinol* 2003; **1**: 107. ©2003 Holstein et al.; licensee BioMed Central Ltd. www.rbej.com/content/1/1/107

8. Ehmcke J, Schlatt S. A revised model for spermatogonial expansion in man: lessons from non-human primates. *Reproduction* 2006; **132**: 673–80.

9. Westlander G, Ekerhovd E, Bergh C. Low levels of serum inhibin B do not exclude successful sperm recovery in men with nonmosaic Klinefelter syndrome. *Fertil Steril* 2003; **79 Suppl 3**: 1680–2.

10. Rosenlund B, Kvist U, Ploen L, et al. Percutaneous cutting needle biopsies for histopathological assessment and sperm retrieval in men with azoospermia. *Hum Reprod* 2001; **16**: 2154–9.

11. Mortimer D. The functional anatomy of the human spermatozoon: relating ultrastructure and function. *Mol Hum Reprod* 2018; **24**: 567–92.

12. Kvist U, Björndahl L, Kjellberg S. Sperm nuclear zinc, chromatin stability, and male fertility. *Scanning Microsc* 1987; **1**: 1241–7.

13. Björndahl L, Kvist U. Loss of an intrinsic capacity for human sperm chromatin decondensation. *Acta Physiol Scand* 1985; **124**: 189–94.

14. Björndahl L, Kvist U. Sequence of ejaculation affects the spermatozoon as a carrier and its message. *Reprod Biomed Online* 2003; 7: 440–8.

15. Björndahl L, Kvist U. A model for the importance of zinc in the dynamics of human sperm chromatin stabilization after ejaculation in relation to sperm DNA vulnerability. *Syst Biol Reprod Med* 2011; **57**: 86–92.

16. Björndahl L, Kvist U. Human sperm chromatin stabilization: a proposed model including zinc bridges. *Mol Hum Reprod* 2010; **16**: 23–9.

17. Ward WS. The structure of the sleeping genome: implications of sperm DNA organization for somatic cells. *J Cell Biochem* 1994; **55**: 77–82.

18. Ward WS. Function of sperm chromatin structural elements in fertilization and development. *Mol Hum Reprod* 2010; **16**: 30–6.

19. Kvist U, Afzelius BA, Nilsson, L. The intrinsic mechanism of chromatin decondensation and its

activation in human spermatozoa. *Devel Growth Differ* 1980; **22**: 543–54.

20. Mudrak O, Tomilin N, Zalensky A. Chromosome architecture in the decondensing human sperm nucleus. *J Cell Sci* 2005; **118**: 4541–50.

21. Bal W, Dyba M, Szewczuk Z, et al. Differential zinc and DNA binding by partial peptides of human protamine HP2. *Mol Cell Biochem* 2001; **222**: 97–106.

22. Brewer L, Corzett M, Balhorn R. Condensation of DNA by spermatid basic nuclear proteins. *J Biol Chem* 2002; **277**: 38895–900.

23. Sutovsky P, Song W-H. Post-fertilisation sperm mitophagy: the tale of Mitochondrial Eve and Steve. *Reprod Fertil Dev* 2017; **31**: 56–63.

24. Birkhead TR, Immler S. Making sperm: design, quality control and sperm competition. *Soc Reprod Fertil* Suppl 2007; **65**: 175–81.

25. Johnson L, Varner DD. Effect of daily spermatozoan production but not age on transit time of spermatozoa through the human epididymis. *Biol Reprod* 1988; **39**: 812–17.

26. Johnson L. A re-evaluation of daily sperm output of men. *Fertil Steril* 1982; **37**: 811–16.

27. Bedford JM. Enigmas of mammalian gamete form and function. *Biol Rev Camb Phil Soc* 2004; **79**: 429–60.

28. Richardson DW, Short RV. Time of onset of sperm production in boys. *J Biosoc Sci Suppl* 1978: **5**: 15–25.

29. Mann T, Lutwak-Mann C. *Male Reproductive Function and Semen.* Berlin and Heidelberg: Springer-Verlag GmbH, 1981.

30. Eggert-Kruse W, Reimann-Andersen J, Rohr G, et al. Clinical relevance of sperm morphology assessment using strict criteria and relationship with sperm-mucus interaction *in vivo* and *in vitro*. *Fertil Steril* 1995; **63**: 612–24.

31. Wagner G, Sjöstrand NO. Autonomic pharmacology and sexual function. In: Sjösten A, ed. *The Pharmacology and Endocrinology of Sexual Function.* Amsterdam: Elsevier Science Publishers, 1988.

32. Amelar RD, Hotchkiss RS. The split ejaculate: its use in the management of male infertility. *Fertil Steril* 1965; **16**: 46–60.

33. Björndahl L, Kjellberg S, Kvist U. Ejaculatory sequence in men with low sperm chromatin-zinc. *Int J Androl* 1991; **14**: 174–8.

34. Kvist U. Sperm nuclear chromatin decondensation ability. An in vitro study on ejaculated human spermatozoa. *Acta Physiol Scand* Suppl 1980; **486**: 1–24.

35. Kvist U. Can disturbances of the ejaculatory sequence contribute to male infertility? *Int J Androl* 1991; **14**: 389–93.

36. Arver S. Studies on zinc and calcium in human seminal plasma. *Acta Physiol Scand Suppl* 1982; **507**: 1–21.

37. Kjellberg S, Björndahl L, Kvist U. Sperm chromatin stability and zinc binding properties in semen from men in barren unions. *Int J Androl* 1992; **15**: 103–13.

38. Houska P, et al. DTT treatment identifies samples with impaired sperm chromatin stability which have increased risk for DNA strand breaks. In: Flanagan J, Björndahl L, Kvist U, eds. *Proceedings of the 13th International Symposium on Spermatology, Stockholm, 2018.* New York: Springer, 2021 (in press).

39. Kvist U. Common challenges for sperm in vitro – causes and consequences. In: Flanagan J, Björndahl L, Kvist U, eds. *Proceedings of the 13th International Symposium on Spermatology, Stockholm, 2018.* New York: Springer, 2021 (in press).

40. Holmes E, Bjorndahl L, Kvist U. Possible factors influencing post-ejaculatory changes of the osmolality of human semen in vitro. *Andrologia* 2019; **51**: e13443.

41. Holmes E, Bjorndahl L, Kvist U. Post-ejaculatory increase in human semen osmolality in vitro. *Andrologia* 2019; **51**: e13311.

42. Holmes E, Björndahl L, Kvist U. Hypotonic challenge reduces human sperm motility through coiling and folding of the tail. *Andrologia* 2020; **52**: e13859.

43. Holmes E, et al. Osmolality changes in human semen in vitro and its implications for sperm density and motility. In: Flanagan J, Björndahl L, Kvist U, eds. *Proceedings of the 13th International Symposium on Spermatology, Stockholm, 2018.* New York: Springer, 2021 (in press).

44. Makler A, David R, Blumenfeld Z, Better OS. Factors affecting sperm motility. VII. Sperm viability as affected by change of pH and osmolarity of semen and urine specimens. *Fertil Steril* 1981; **36**: 507–11.

45. Rossato M, Balercia G, Lucarelli G, et al. Role of seminal osmolarity in the reduction of human sperm motility. *Int J Androl* 2002; **25**: 230–5.

46. Velazquez A, Pedron N, Delgado NM, Rosado A. Osmolality and conductance of normal and abnormal human seminal plasma. *Int J Fertil* 1977; **22**: 92–7.

47. Jeyendran RS, Van der Ven HH, Zaneveld LJ. The hypoosmotic swelling test: an update. *Arch Androl* 1992; **29**: 105–16.

48. Ahlgren M. Sperm transport to and survival in the human Fallopian tube. *Gynecol Invest* 1975; **6**: 206–14.

49. Mortimer D, Templeton AA. Sperm transport in the human female reproductive tract in relation to semen analysis characteristics and time of ovulation. *J Reprod Fertil* 1982; **64**: 401–8.

50. Haugen TB, Egeland T, Magnus O. Semen parameters in Norwegian fertile men. *J Androl* 2006; **27**: 66–71.

51. Jouannet P, Ducot B, Feneux D, Spira A. Male factors and the likelihood of pregnancy in infertile couples. I. Study of sperm characteristics. *Int J Androl* 1988; **11**: 379–94.

52. Bostofte E, Serup J, Rebbe H. Relation between sperm count and semen volume, and pregnancies obtained during a twenty-year follow-up period. *Int J Androl* 1982; **5**: 267–75.

53. Bonde JP, Ernst E, Jensen TK, et al. Relation between semen quality and fertility: a population-based study of 430 first-pregnancy planners. *Lancet* 1998; **352**: 1172–7.

54. Aitken RJ, Bakos HW. Should we be measuring DNA damage in human spermatozoa? New light on an old question. *Hum Reprod* 2021; **36**: 1175–85.

55. Evenson DP, Djira G, Kasperson K, Christianson J. Relationships between the age of 25,445 men attending infertility clinics and sperm chromatin structure assay (SCSAVR) defined sperm DNA and chromatin integrity. *Fertil Steril* 2020; **114**: 311–20.

56. Vaughan DA, Tirado E, Garcia D, et al. DNA fragmentation of sperm: a radical examination of the contribution of oxidative stress and age in 16 945 semen samples. *Hum Reprod* 2020; **35**: 2188–96.

57. Hong X, Ma J, Yin J, et al. The association between vaginal microbiota and female infertility: a systematic review and meta-analysis. *Arch Gynecol Obstet* 2020; **302**: 569–78.

58. Tsonis O, Gkrozou F, Paschopoulos M. Microbiome affecting reproductive outcome in ARTs. *J Gynecol Obstet Hum Reprod* 2021; **50**: 102036.

59. Suarez SS, Pacey AA. Sperm transport in the female reproductive tract. *Hum Reprod Update* 2006; **12**: 23–37.

60. Mortimer D. Sperm transport in the female genital tract. In: Grudzinskas JG, Yovich JL, eds. *Gametes – The Spermatozoon*. Cambridge: Cambridge University Press, 1995.

61. Mortimer ST. A critical review of the physiological importance and analysis of sperm movement in mammals. *Hum Reprod Update* 1997; **3**: 403–39.

62. Kölle S. From mouse to human: new aspects of sperm transport and fertilization using cutting edge technologies. In: Flanagan J, Björndahl L, Kvist U, eds. *Proceedings of the 13th International Symposium on Spermatology, Stockholm, 2018.* New York: Springer, 2021 (in press).

63. Salicioni AM, Platt MD, Wertheimer EV, et al. Signalling pathways involved in sperm capacitation. *Soc Reprod Fertil Suppl* 2007; **65**: 245–59.

64. Gadella BM, Tsai PS, Boerke A, Brewis IA. Sperm head membrane reorganisation during capacitation. *Int J Dev Biol* 2008; **52**: 473–80.

65. De Jonge C. Biological basis for human capacitation—revisited. *Hum Reprod Update* 2017; **23**: 289–99.

66. Puga Molina LC, Luque GM, Balestrini PA, et al. Molecular basis of human sperm capacitation. *Front Cell Dev Biol* 2018. https://doi.org/10.3389/fcell.2018.00072

67. Bosakova T, Tockstein A, Sebkova N, et al. New insight into sperm capacitation: a novel mechanism of 17β-estradiol signalling. *Int J Mol Sci* 2018; **19**: 4011.

68. Suarez SS. Control of hyperactivation in sperm. *Hum Reprod Update* 2008; **14**: 647–57.

69. Publicover S, Harper CV, Barratt C. $[Ca^{2+}]_i$ signalling in sperm–making the most of what you've got. *Nat Cell Biol* 2007; **9**: 235–42.

70. Florman HM, Jungnickel MK, Sutton KA. Regulating the acrosome reaction. *Int J Dev Biol* 2008; **52**: 503–10.

71. Raterman D, Springer MS. The molecular evolution of acrosin in placental mammals. *Mol Reprod Dev* 2008; **75**: 1196–207.

72. Nagyova E. The biological role of hyaluronan-rich oocyte-cumulus extracellular matrix in female reproduction. *Int J Mol Sci* 2018; **19**: 283.

73. Mortimer D, Mortimer ST. The case against intracytoplasmic sperm injection for all. In: Aitken J, Mortimer D, Kovacs G, eds. *Male and Sperm Factors That Maximize IVF Success*. Cambridge: Cambridge University Press, 2020, 130–40.

74. Fishman EL, Jo K, Nguyen QPH, et al. A novel atypical sperm centriole is functional during human fertilization. *Nature Commun* 2018; **9**: 2210. https://doi:10.1038/s41467-018-04678-8

75. Schatten G. The centrosome and its mode of inheritance: the reduction of the centrosome during gametogenesis and its restoration during fertilization. *Dev Biol* 1994; **165**: 299–335.

76. Lehti MS, Sironen A. Formation and function of the manchette and flagellum during spermatogenesis. *Reproduction* 2016; **151**: R43–54.

Basic Semen Examination

This chapter describes the steps involved in performing a basic semen examination. Table 3.1 shows an overview of the entire recommended working process for basic semen examination: following the recommended order for the different component procedures will provide a basis for efficient and high-quality working [1].

Note that semen, like other bodily fluids, must be treated as potentially biohazardous and handled with care, see Chapter 15 on andrology laboratory safety.

Specimen Collection and Delivery

Principles

The circumstances under which a semen specimen is collected and delivered to the laboratory can influence the results of the analysis. Since the time that spermatozoa are held in semen can reduce their survival, motility and fertilizing ability, it is essential that the start of diagnostic investigations is standardized to 30 min after ejaculation (in order to allow most ejaculates to liquefy properly) [1,2]. If the specimen can be collected in a special room adjacent to the laboratory there is a significant reduction of the risk for delays during transportation, and for cooling of the specimen with concomitant loss of motility. This situation calls for proper design and equipping of the semen collection room, and for situations that might cause stress for the subjects, such as long waiting times,

Table 3.1 The component analytical procedures of a complete semen examination is a sequence optimized for efficiency and quality in the laboratory work. Details of the individual procedures are given in this and following chapters. Some steps can be considered optional

Time from ejaculation	Procedure
Immediately	Weigh the sample container with the semen sample, ascertain correct labelling and place it in 37°C incubator Register and label the corresponding laboratory documents
25–30 min	Assess semen liquefaction, visual appearance and smell
30–60 min	Semen viscosity assessment Prepare and examine the wet preparations to assess the other cells, debris, aggregates and sperm agglutination; assess sperm motility; selection of dilution for haemocytometry Perform antisperm antibody test(s) Make smears for sperm vitality testing, if sperm motility is <40% Make dilutions for sperm concentration determination by haemocytometry Make smears for sperm morphology assessment Take a 100 μl aliquot of semen for assessment of inflammatory cells, if necessary Centrifuge and freeze semen/seminal plasma for any requested biochemical analyses
Later	Sperm concentration determination by haemocytometry If there are ≥1 × 10⁶/ml round cells, perform an assessment of inflammatory cells Biochemical analyses of the secretory contributions from the prostate (e.g. zinc), seminal vesicles (e.g. fructose) and epididymis (e.g. α-glucosidase), if required Mount the smears for sperm vitality assessment (if prepared) Perform the sperm vitality assessment (if required) Stain and mount the smears for sperm morphology assessment Perform the sperm morphology assessment

embarrassing encounters, and disturbing noise from outside the room, to be avoided. Duration of stimulation can be important for the outcome, and subjects should be allowed ample time so as not to feel rushed to produce their specimens [3].

Note: In the era of COVID-19 it is recommended that all on-site semen specimen collections should be by appointment. While allowing subjects to bring specimens from home might seem a safer approach, this must be balanced against the risk of specimen degradation as a result of prolonged ejaculation-to-analysis delays. This would be especially important for semen specimens that are to be used for cryopreservation, treatment (IUI, IVF or ICSI) or the assessment of sperm function.

In general, subjects are expected to collect a semen specimen for investigation after between 2 and 7 days of ejaculatory abstinence. However, if the abstinence time can be held to 3–4 days the variability due to abstinence duration can be kept reasonably low [1].

Equipment and Materials
- Waiting area with patient flow minimizing embarrassing contacts between subjects
- Secluded semen collection room
- Semen specimen collection container – non-toxic plastic (Figure 3.1)
- Self-adhesive labels for secure identification of the specimen collection container
- Special condoms (non-toxic, non-spermicidal) if necessary

Notes
1. Specimen identification must involve the use of at least two unique identifiers for its provenance, typically the subject's name and a second numeric or alphanumeric identifier. A specimen accession or reference number is often also employed within the laboratory.

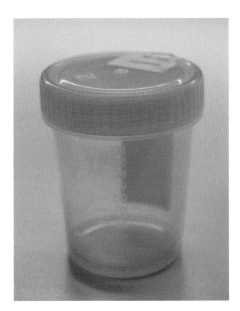

Figure 3.1 Example of a specimen collection container with a tight-fitting lid and ample place for at least two separate unique identifiers as well as space to write the container weight and the time of ejaculation.

2. Electronic specimen identification systems are now available and might be used to integrate patient identify verification and maintenance of specimen chain of custody; refer to Chapter 13 *Risk Management*.

3. In case of difficulties collecting a specimen at the laboratory, a subject might be allowed to produce a first specimen at home and transport it (protected from cooling by keeping the specimen close to the body, and not exposed to excessive heat) to the laboratory for investigation, preferably within 30 min after ejaculation, but at most within 1 hr. In cases where the main problem is to produce a specimen by masturbation, a special, non-spermicidal condom can be used to collect a specimen at intercourse [4].

4. Retrograde ejaculation can be suspected if no ejaculate is expelled at orgasm. In some cases, antegrade ejaculation can be achieved if the subject ejaculates with a full bladder. Other cases might be helped by drugs that counteract parasympathetic activity (e.g. Imipramin 50 mg; in most countries such drugs require prescription by a physician). In other cases, it will probably be necessary to alkalinize the urine in order to be able to retrieve live spermatozoa in urine after ejaculation [5].

5. If a lubricant must be used then it must not show any toxicity to spermatozoa. Currently, the only suitable commercial product for this particular purpose is the vaginal lubricant Pre-Seed™ (see www.firstresponse.com/en/product-listings/fertility-friendly-lubricant).

Patient Instructions

Principles

Written information for the layperson about the purpose of the investigation and circumstances that could interfere with the analysis and with the interpretation of the results should be supplied either directly from the referring physician or by letter to the patient when an appointment for the semen analysis is made with the laboratory. This information should also include a short explanation of the male reproductive organs and their functions. Special attention should be given to the relevance of correct abstinence time and the importance of collecting the entire ejaculate [1,6]. Further oral information should be given when the subject comes to the laboratory to deliver the specimen. On the day of specimen collection, relevant information about specimen collection and abstinence time should be recorded, and other pertinent questions regarding, for instance, recent periods of high fever or inflammatory diseases should be asked and the subject's responses noted [7].

Equipment and Disposable Materials

- Information sheet on the purpose of semen analysis (written for the layperson)
- Information sheet about the male reproductive organs and their functions (written for the layperson)
- Checklist for laboratory staff regarding the verbal information to be given to patients when the appointment is made
- Checklist for laboratory staff regarding the verbal information to be given to, and obtained from, patients when the specimen is collected
- Questionnaire for the patient at the time of specimen collection and delivery

Semen Volume and Handling of the Specimen Container

Background

The first part of the investigation of a semen specimen is its physical examination, which includes measurement of semen volume as well as assessment of viscosity, general visual appearance and smell (odour).

Assessments that follow measurement of the ejaculate volume are best done after full liquefaction of the specimen, and then followed by the microscopic investigations. For an efficient flow of procedures optimizing the quality of the analytical steps (to reduce variability and any negative influence of post-ejaculatory factors), it is recommended that the component investigations are performed in the order shown in Table 3.1 (above).

Principle

Even before the coagulated specimen has liquefied, the volume can be determined by weighing, provided that the specimen collection container has been weighed before the specimen was collected. If at least 30 different containers from a batch have been weighed, and the variation in weight between containers is less than 0.1 g, then all containers can be assumed to have the same weight and then it is not necessary to weigh each one before use. For every new batch of containers, a set of 30 should be tested to establish the consistency of their weight for that specific batch. The specific gravity of semen can be assumed to be 1.0 g/ml, and weighing is preferred to using measuring pipettes since no semen is lost by the weighing procedure [8].

The specimen container should be uniquely labelled, in accordance with all laboratory documentation. It is recommended that the container be given two independent but unique identifiers (one of which must be a number), for example subject identity and laboratory specimen number. To facilitate the proper work sequence in the laboratory, the time for specimen collection should be clearly marked on the container and also recorded in the specimen record form.

The specimen should be placed in a temperature-controlled (37°C) incubator, if possible, on an orbital mixer. The specimen is left in the incubator until 25–30 min after ejaculation, so that examination can be initiated at 30 min after ejaculation. The mixing of the specimen is checked by swirling the specimen around the bottom of the container for 15–20 s, being careful not to introduce air into the semen. When the specimen has been transported to the laboratory after collection at another location, it must be allowed to warm up to 37°C in the incubator (e.g. for 5–10 min) before examination.

Specimen

- Freshly ejaculated human semen

Equipment and Disposable Materials

See also Appendix 2.
- Top-load balance reading to 0.01 g accuracy
- Air incubator at 37°C
- Marker pen for laboratory use, and labels for secure identification
- Calculator to calculate specimen weight

Calibration and Quality Control

The balance should be serviced by the manufacturer/supplier or other specialist at least annually. Balance accuracy should be verified at least monthly to ensure that it delivers reliable results. If deviating results are found, servicing and recalibration of the balance must be carried out as soon as possible. Procedures for balance service and testing should be described in the laboratory's Quality Manual.

Procedure

1. After the ejaculate has been collected the container is weighed. Calculate the specimen volume by subtracting the tare weight from the result of weighing after specimen collection and record the value on the form.
2. Time of ejaculation is written clearly on the vial.
3. Immediately place the specimen container in the incubator and record the time on the form; leave in the incubator until 25–30 min after ejaculation.

Calculations and Results

The initial specimen container weight is subtracted from the total weight measured after specimen collection. The weight of the specimen in grams (g) is recorded as volume (ml) on the specimen record form to one decimal place (i.e. 0.1 g accuracy).

Interpretation Guidelines

A low volume (<2 ml) could have different explanations:

- Incomplete specimen collection
- Secretory dysfunction of accessory sex glands (infections, agenesis of seminal vesicles)
- Stress during specimen collection

A high ejaculate volume (>6 ml) could be due to different causes, although no general, direct relationship has been shown between high semen volume and male infertility. A high volume can cause a relatively high dilution of the spermatozoa, causing a relatively low sperm concentration. High semen volume has also been associated with a high risk for semen loss from the vagina. Causes for increased semen volume can be:

- Inflammatory exudate from, for instance, an infected prostate during the acute (exudative) phase of inflammation
- Extensive sexual stimulation, possibly combined with long abstinence time

Semen Liquefaction

Principles

The ejaculate coagulates due to macro proteins originating from the seminal vesicles. In the laboratory the entire ejaculate is brought together in one collection container, including the first, sperm-rich fraction, and all fractions are involved in the coagulum. Most ejaculates are fully liquefied within 15–20 min, at least when stored at 37°C, due to enzymes (proteases) originating from the prostate.

The physiological importance of ejaculate liquefaction in humans is not known, and it has been suggested that the formation of a coagulum is a collection artefact, and does not represent the normal physiology for the human spermatozoa [9,10]. Disturbances of the process are most probably markers for pathological processes in the male accessory sex glands, which could also result in a negative effect on sperm functions.

Specimen

- Ejaculated semen, ideally 25 min after ejaculation, stored for at least 15 min in an incubator at 37°C

Equipment and Disposable Materials

See also Appendix 2.

- Air incubator at 37°C

Procedure

1. Take the specimen collection container from the incubator 25–30 min after ejaculation.
2. Swirl the semen around the bottom of the container for 15–20 s to ensure that mixing is complete. Be careful not to cause any frothing of the semen.
3. Inspect the specimen for signs of incomplete liquefaction, e.g. gel clumps or streaks.
4. In case considerable parts of the ejaculate are still not liquefied, the specimen should be returned to the incubator and re-inspected 15 and 30 min later.

5. Specimens still not liquefied 60 min after ejaculation are evaluated to the best extent possible. Lack of liquefaction is noted in the laboratory report, as well as a note that further investigations have been done on any material available outside the coagulum.

Results

Results are reported as normal, delayed (fully liquefied at 60 min, but not at 30 min), incomplete (still not completed at 60 min), or not liquefied (intact coagulum at 60 min). Comments should describe whether solitary gel clumps and/or streaks are visible in the otherwise liquefied semen.

Interpretation Guidelines

Since the end result of coagulation and liquefaction mainly depends on the actions of compounds secreted from two different glands, both general and localized infections and inflammatory reactions in the male reproductive tract are likely to interfere and possibly cause changes in the process.

It is therefore advisable that a subject with disturbed liquefaction is given a full clinical examination by a clinical andrologist or a urologist.

Note

Do not confuse incomplete liquefaction and increased viscosity.

Visual Appearance

Principle

A normal semen specimen is usually greyish-white and opalescent. While certain observations regarding unusual colouration or translucence of an ejaculate can have clinical relevance concerning the provenance of the specimen or the subject's medical status, in the absence of any metrological standards for semen colour it is not possible to standardize this observation or establish measurement uncertainty. Consequently, any such comments included in a semen analysis report are considered as having been 'reported by exception', i.e. as describing an observation that is outside the expected.

Specimen

- As for the assessment of semen liquefaction

Equipment and Disposable Materials

- None required

Procedure

While examining the extent of liquefaction, the colour and opalescence (clear appearance) of the specimen are also assessed.

Results

A normal semen specimen is usually greyish-white and opalescent; lack of opalescence should be recorded. Any difference in colour (red, brownish or yellowish) should be recorded.

Interpretation Guidelines

- It is not uncommon that a very clear or translucent specimen is azoospermic or has a very low sperm concentration (severe oligozoospermia).
- Human semen can have a pale yellow colouration that is not necessarily abnormal. Yellowish colour can be due to an increased concentration of flavoproteins of seminal vesicular origin, often related to

39

long abstinence time. A combination of very low volume and yellow colour can appear in acute infections with high concentration of inflammatory cells in semen. On rare occasions yellow semen can be due to jaundice, which should be properly investigated medically.

- The presence of erythrocytes or haemoglobin (red or brownish appearance of the semen) as a solitary finding is not considered to reflect any pathological condition. Red staining of semen is an indication of blood and can be due to a skin injury while producing the ejaculate, or the blood might originate from one of the accessory glands, and hence might be a sign of infection. If the finding is consistent, the subject should be investigated further to establish the source for the blood.

Semen Odour

Principle

Perception of the smell of normal semen is subjective, and generally quite variable, but semen that smells strongly, especially of urine or putrescence can usually be perceived by most laboratory staff members.

Specimen

- As for the assessment of semen liquefaction

Equipment and Disposable Materials

- None required

Procedure

When the specimen is inspected for liquefaction, the lid of the container is removed and the smell of the semen evaluated. While certain observations can have clinical relevance concerning the provenance of the specimen or the subject's medical status, in the absence of any metrological standards for semen odour it is not possible to standardize this observation or establish measurement uncertainty. Consequently, any such comments included in a semen analysis report are considered as having been 'reported by exception', i.e. as describing an observation that is outside the expected.

Results

If present, a strong, disgusting smell (putrescent), or a urine smell is recorded in the sample form.

Interpretation Guidelines

A strong and repugnant smell can be caused, for instance, by a bacterial infection. The patient should be examined by a clinician to decide whether medical treatment of an infection is indicated.

Semen Viscosity

Principle

A viscous semen specimen forms long threads instead of discrete drops when it is allowed to run out of a pipette. This is not the same phenomenon as coagulation and liquefaction, but abnormalities can have the same cause – disturbed accessory gland function causing both viscosity problems and problems with coagulation and liquefaction. In the absence of established metrological standards for semen viscosity it is not possible to standardize this observation or establish an uncertainty of measurement.

Specimen

- As for the assessment of semen liquefaction

Equipment and Disposable Materials

- Wide bore serological pipette, or glass or plastic rod, validated for lack of sperm toxicity
- Measuring scale (e.g. rule) of 20 mm to facilitate assessment

Procedure

1. Aspirate the semen into (for example) a 5 ml plastic volumetric pipette.
2. Let the semen run out of the pipette back into the sample collection container.
3. Estimate the length of the threads formed between the droplets.

Results

If threads >20 mm long are formed when the semen drops from the pipette the sample is considered to have an abnormal viscosity, and this finding should be recorded on the report form. The longer the thread the more severe the abnormal viscosity.

Interpretation Guidelines

The main problem with a highly viscous semen specimen is the difficulty it creates for performing proper assessments of sperm motility, concentration, and anti-sperm antibodies, as well as for the preparation of good smears for sperm morphology assessment.

Notes

1. Do not confuse increased viscosity and incomplete liquefaction.
2. Addition of a known volume of saline or suitable culture medium followed by careful mixing can often give a sufficiently homogenous dilution to allow proper investigations. The original volume should be used to give the true original sperm concentration in the undiluted semen. Since the motility characteristics will change due to the dilution (an effect of reduced viscosity), it is essential that it is clearly stated on the specimen record form that the motility assessment was performed on a diluted sample. For specimens intended for treatment (assisted reproductive techniques) the risk for contamination should be minimized by using the same culture medium as will be used for clinical sperm preparation.

Semen pH

Principle

Semen pH is the result of hydrogen ion content in prostatic secretion (acidic), seminal vesicular secretion (alkaline), carbon dioxide evaporation after ejaculation, and effects of chemical reactions occurring from ejaculation until the time of pH assessment. In contrast to the situation in, for instance, blood, there are no homeostatic control systems in the ejaculate, making it extremely difficult to standardize measurements – and hence there are no reliable, useful reference ranges. Therefore, measurement of pH does not provide much information for the basic semen analysis.

There is, however, one situation when measurement of pH can contribute significantly to the investigation: in cases with no spermatozoa in the ejaculate and a relatively low volume, a low pH (≤ 7.0) points to a lack of the alkaline secretions from the seminal vesicles, indicating agenesis of the Wolffian duct system (including the seminal vesicles) as a cause for the azoospermia. Biochemical analysis (zinc and fructose as markers for prostatic and seminal vesicular fluid, respectively) will strengthen this diagnosis (see Chapter 4).

Specimen

- As for the assessment of semen viscosity

Equipment and Disposable Materials

- Merck/EM Science ColorpHast pH test strips, range 6.5 to 10.0. These have been found to be the most accurate pH test strips; they comprise a plastic strip with a single piece of indicator paper attached to one side at one end.

Procedure

1. Using an air-displacement pipetter, transfer a small droplet of semen onto the test strip.
2. Allow the colour to develop.
3. Compare the colour of the test strip with the appropriate color scale to read the pH.

Interpretation Guidelines

1. Azoospermia, low volume (usually <1.0 ml), and pH <7.0 is often indicative of obstructive azoospermia due to agenesis of the Wolffian duct system, provided the semen specimen was completely collected.
2. A pH above 7.5 indicates a significant contribution of seminal vesicular fluid which indicates that the seminal vesicles, at least in part, can contribute to the ejaculate, but does not rule out agenesis of other parts of the Wolffian duct system.

Making a Wet Preparation

Background

A wet preparation is used for direct observation of spermatozoa, along with the other cells and particles in the native semen specimen. The primary methods of investigation are observation, classification and counting.

Principle

For proper evaluation of sperm motility, it is essential that the depth of the preparation is about 20 μm. The depth of a preparation can be calculated by dividing the aliquot volume by the coverslip size (area). Using a 22×22 mm coverslip requires an aliquot volume of 10 μl, while an 18×18 mm coverslip requires a semen aliquot of 6 μl.

It is essential that the coverslip is applied immediately after the semen droplet is placed on the slide – if delayed there is a considerable risk for errors due to desiccation, resulting in a ring of dead spermatozoa and debris around the periphery of the preparation.

Specimen

- As for the assessment of semen liquefaction.

Equipment

See also Appendix 2.
- Air displacement pipetter, 0–20 μl

Disposable Materials

- Glass microscope slides
- Coverslips, 22×22 or 18×18 mm #1½ or #2 thickness (i.e. heavy enough to spread the semen)
- Disposable tips for the automatic pipetter (sterile if the sample is for treatment purposes)
- Gloves

Procedure

1. Use a clean microscope slide that has been pre-warmed to 37°C; store the slide warm during the making of the preparation and ideally keep it at 37°C during the entire investigation of the preparation.
2. Make sure the specimen is well mixed by swirling the semen before taking the aliquot for the wet preparation.
3. Aspirate the appropriate volume with an air-displacement pipetter and deposit it as a droplet in the middle of the microscope slide.
4. Apply the coverslip to the droplet immediately.

Results

No results are recorded at this stage.

Notes

If air bubbles appear centrally under the coverslip it must be discarded and a new preparation made.

Hint: If the pipetter plunger is depressed past the first stop before releasing it to take the sample aliquot, the volume in the pipette tip will be slightly larger than the desired volume. Then, when the aliquot is dispensed onto the slide by depressing the pipetter plunger only to the first stop, the extra material will stay in the pipette tip, greatly reducing the risk of air bubble formation on the top of the dispended droplet.

Initial Evaluation of a Wet Preparation

Principle

Observation under the microscope of spermatozoa, cells and other particulate material.

Specimen

- A freshly prepared, wet preparation from the semen specimen being analysed

Equipment

See also Appendix 2.

- Microscope with 10×, 20× and 40× phase contrast objectives, ideally equipped with a heated stage set at 37°C

Procedure and Results

1. The examination of the wet preparation should begin as soon as the flow has ceased, which should happen within 1 min after placing the coverslip on the semen droplet; if not, then the preparation should be discarded and a new one prepared (Figure 3.2).
2. Count the number of spermatozoa visible in randomly chosen microscope fields. If less than one spermatozoon is observed per 'high power' field of vision (40× objective with wide field eyepieces) the sample should be treated as an azoospermic or severely oligozoospermic sample (see Notes).
3. If spermatozoa are observed then assess their motility (for details, see below).
4. Assess the presence of sperm aggregation and agglutination: The degree of sperm aggregation or agglutination is determined in 10 randomly chosen microscope fields not adjacent to the coverslip edges. The proportion of spermatozoa trapped in clumps is estimated to the nearest 5%.

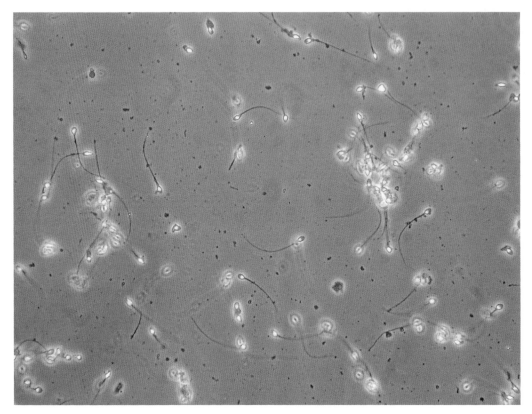

Figure 3.2 Typical appearance of normal semen under phase contrast optics (positive low phase contrast). Note the presence of small and larger particulate debris as well as a few aggregates of debris and dead (immotile) spermatozoa.

- Agglutination is defined as at least some motile spermatozoa adhering without other cells and debris, most likely due to the presence of multivalent anti-sperm antibodies. If the agglutinates are very large, it may be difficult to assess whether the spermatozoa are specifically (e.g. head-to-head or tail-to-tail) or more randomly bound to each other.
- Clumps comprising immotile (dead) spermatozoa and debris are described as aggregation. Small aggregates are common in normal samples, while large aggregates, which can contain hundreds of spermatozoa each, are considered as abnormal.
- In samples where the proportion of spermatozoa involved in clumping is estimated to be 25% or more, motility is assessed on the free spermatozoa only. The proportion of spermatozoa involved in clumping, and a note that motility was assessed on the free spermatozoa only, must be recorded on the specimen form.

5. Assess the presence of other cells and debris: It is common to find other cells and debris in semen samples. Therefore, only the increased presence of such material should be reported if seen in multiple fields. Such abnormalities should be commented upon in the report form using a few different, standardized expressions:

'*Round cells*' are common in semen specimens. '*Leucocytes*' must be differentiated from immature germinal epithelium cells or precursors, or large cell bodies (often without nuclei) consisting of cytoplasm that has become exfoliated from the seminiferous epithelium of the testis. Other round cells can be of prostatic origin. There are two equally valid methods to assess the number of round cells present in semen. Round cells can be counted in the same fields used for motility assessments or, alternatively, in the Neubauer haemocytometer chamber at the same time as the assessment of sperm concentration (see

Calculations). If more than 1×10^6/ml round cells are found, a method for the specific determination of leucocytes should be used to assess the concentration of inflammatory cells in semen (see later in this chapter). However, some authorities recommend performing this investigation when only ≥1 round cell is seen per HPF as a precautionary measure.

'Debris' (differentiate between particulate debris and motile bacteria):

- *No* debris at all is quite rare
- *Some* debris is very common
- *Moderate* contamination with debris is not considered abnormal
- *A large amount* of debris should be regarded as abnormal

'Erythrocytes' (red blood cells) should not be found in semen, although the presence of a few does not indicate pathology.

'Epithelial cells' (squamous, cubic and transitional) can often be found in low numbers in semen specimens; their increased presence has not been linked to any specific pathology. They can be present in large numbers in ejaculates collected by withdrawal (coitus interruptus).

'Bacteria' and *'protozoa'* should not be found in normal semen when examined under a phase contrast light microscope. However, if small motile particles are seen in fresh semen (not to be confused with debris showing Brownian motion), high contamination with bacteria should be suspected and reported. Any observation of easily recognizable *Trichomonas* protozoa should also be reported (Figure 3.3).

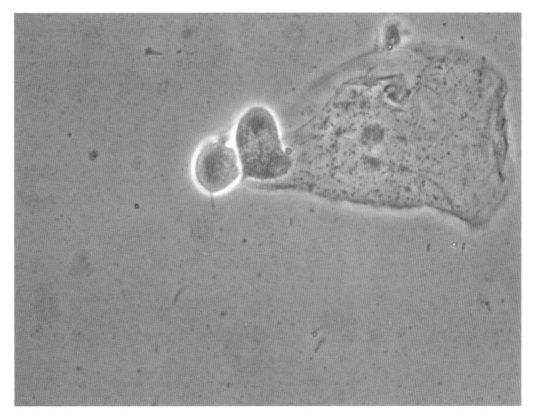

Figure 3.3 Protozoon (left) adjacent to a squamous epithelium cell (right); note the shadow of the beating flagellum at the top of the *Trichomonas* organism.

Calculations

The concentration of round cells/ml semen can be estimated by comparing the relative prevalence of these cells and spermatozoa in the microscope fields observed to the known sperm concentration:

Round cell concentration = sperm concentration × (# round cells per field/# spermatozoa per field)

Notes

Handling of azoospermic and severely oligozoospermic specimens: When no or only very few spermatozoa have been observed in multiple microscope fields of the wet preparation, the sperm concentration cannot be determined using the standard quality-controlled quantitative technique (see below) and it is recommended that this be recorded on the report form and that the observed numbers of motile and immotile spermatozoa are given as free text comments.

A semen specimen containing very few spermatozoa could be centrifuged (at least 1000 *g* for 15 min) and the pellet examined under the microscope (phase contrast optics, 40× objective). The presence of motile or immotile spermatozoa is assessed by scanning the whole area of the coverslip (corresponding to about 400 fields under a 22 × 22 mm coverslip) and the numbers of motile and immotile spermatozoa are recorded on the specimen report form.

Sperm Motility Assessment

Background

Manual/visual sperm motility assessment is performed on duplicate wet preparations as soon as possible after the presence of spermatozoa has been confirmed. Preparations should always be made and assessed in sequence, so that the second preparation is fresh when its motility assessment is started.

Sperm Motility Assessment – Motility Categories

Principle

If possible, it is recommended that motility assessments are made using a video monitor in order to minimize the difference between daily routine and quality control assessment. If video equipment is not available then assessments are done under phase contrast microscopy, ideally using a 10× objective with intermediate magnification (to give a larger image while preserving the depth of focus) or if not available then using a 20× (or 40×) objective.

It is essential that the motility assessment be commenced as soon as possible after the wet preparation has been made (see above) in order to minimize any negative influence of temperature decrease or dehydration.

Sperm motility is assessed by classifying each spermatozoon into one of three classes of motile spermatozoa, or as immotile, in at least five randomly chosen fields away from the edges of each wet preparation; at least 200 spermatozoa should be classified in each preparation. Rapidly progressive spermatozoa (WHO4 (1999) and WHO6 (2021) class *a*) move forward with a speed of at least 25 µm/s (equivalent to half a tail length or five head lengths), slowly progressive (WHO4/6 class *b*) move forward more than 5 µm/s (equivalent to one head length) but less than 25 µm/s, non-progressive spermatozoa (WHO4/6 class *c*) move less than 5 µm/s, and immotile spermatozoa (WHO4/6 class *d*) show no active tail movements [1,11–14].

If at least 25% of the spermatozoa are estimated to be involved in clumps then the motility assessment is made only on the free spermatozoa, and a comment is recorded on the sample report form. Only complete spermatozoa (head with tail) are included in the counts. Do not count 'pinheads', although spermatozoa with no or extremely small sperm heads should be commented upon if estimated to correspond to at least 20% of the intact spermatozoa.

In order to minimize the influence of random errors, motility assessments should always be done in duplicate. If comparison of the duplicate results does not show sufficient similarity, the assessments are discarded and new preparations made and assessed.

Specimen
- Freshly made wet preparations on warm microscope slides (see above)

Equipment
See also Appendix 2.
- Microscope with 10×, 20× and 40× phase contrast objectives, ideally equipped with a heated stage set at 37°C
- Tally counter with at least four channels

Quality Control
- Comparison of duplicate assessments for each specimen
- For novices: repeated training with experienced staff, and using archived reference material with known results
- For all staff members: Internal Quality Control (IQC) monitoring of the variation between staff members and over time (assessment of precision)
- For the laboratory as a unit: External Quality Assurance (EQA) monitoring of the laboratory's performance in relation to other laboratories (assessment of accuracy)

Procedure
1. A wet preparation is prepared as described earlier.
2. Assessment is started as soon as any flow in the preparation has ceased.
3. First, count the rapid and slow progressive spermatozoa, and then count the non-progressive and immotile spermatozoa in the same microscope field. If the concentration of spermatozoa is very high, it is advisable to only count spermatozoa in a smaller field, e.g. in the area of four central squares in an eyepiece grid (eyepiece graticule or reticle).
4. Assess at least five different fields, and count at least 200 spermatozoa in each preparation.
5. Repeat the assessment of the motility of at least 200 spermatozoa in a second wet preparation from the same semen specimen.

Calculations and Results
First calculate the proportions for the four categories (WHO4/6 a,b,c,d) for each of the two preparations: the total number of spermatozoa in each motility group is divided by the total number of spermatozoa assessed in that preparation. Then take the results for the dominant (largest) group and calculate the average proportion for the two duplicates and the difference between the duplicates. Refer to Table App5.1 to establish whether the difference is small enough to accept the replicate assessments: if the difference between the duplicates is less than the limit value in the table the assessments can be accepted, otherwise the data are discarded and two new preparations are made and assessed.

When duplicate counts are accepted, all the category proportions (i.e. proportions of WHO a, b, c, and d, respectively) are calculated from the duplicate results, as well as the proportions of motile ($a+b+c$) and progressively motile ($a+b$) spermatozoa.

All motility results are presented as integer percentage values. The sum of the four motility categories (a,b,c,d) in a sample should be 100. If, due to rounding errors, the sum is 99 or 101, adjust the dominant group to get a sum of 100.

Interpretation Guidelines
- Decreased motility (poor progression, reduced overall motility) can be due to disorders such as infections with inflammatory processes in the excretory glands (prostate and seminal vesicles).
- The presence of some types of anti-sperm antibodies (especially spermotoxic antibodies) can reduce sperm motility.

- Complete absence of sperm motility can be seen in men with cytotoxic anti-sperm antibodies, but also among men with ciliary dyskinesia (immotile cilia syndrome or Kartagener syndrome).

Notes

The proportion of rapid progressive spermatozoa (WHO4/6 category *a*) at 37°C is an important functional sperm property related to fertility and fertilization success [13–17]. It is possible to do repeatable manual assessments of the proportion of rapid progressive spermatozoa, provided staff members are trained using a visual scale for the 25 µm. Although there is no need to record all specimens, there is a major advantage using a video screen for motility assessments. Furthermore, the use of video recordings for training and Quality Control / Quality Assessment is of additional value.

Sperm Motility Assessment Using a Video Display

Principle

The use of a video display for assessing sperm motility has many advantages. Training in small groups assessing the same screen simultaneously is more efficient than individual training. The use of video displays for routine analysis also eliminates the difference between assessments of 'live' samples and QC assessments of recorded samples, which increases the validity of all recorded samples used for training and QC (Figure 3.4).

To obtain the same help in estimating sperm velocity that a grid in a microscope ocular gives, a black acetate with a central circular transparent field showing with a grid with squares corresponding to 25 × 25 µm is attached in front of the video display [13].

To avoid the problem of spermatozoa swimming in and out of focus in the 20 µm-deep preparation, it is best to use a 10×-phase contrast objective combined with additional 'intermediate' magnification in the camera tube to obtain a suitable final magnification on the video display.

Specimen

- The same preparation as for the basic sperm motility assessment

Equipment

See also Appendix 2.
- Videomicrography system
- Stage micrometer

Disposable Materials

- As for the basic sperm motility assessment

Calibration

Ideally, the total magnification on the video display screen should be adjusted so that 100 µm in the sample equals 70–90 mm on the screen (total magnification is adjusted by choosing appropriate intermediate magnification in the photo tube). Check the overall on-screen magnification using a ruler to measure the microscope image of a micrometer scale on the video display.

Quality Control

- Duplicate assessments with comparisons are used to reduce the risk for random sampling errors

Procedure

1. Adjust the microscope for optimal function (correct settings for phase contrast optics or adjusted Köhler bright field illumination).

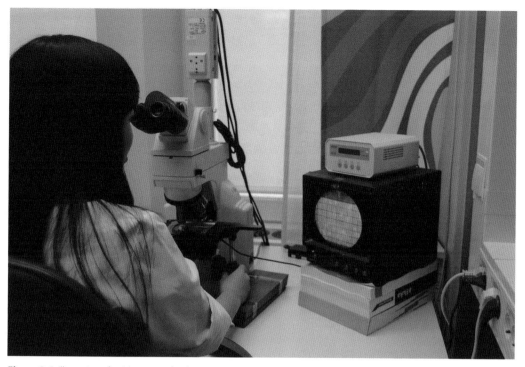

Figure 3.4 Illustration of a video set-up for the routine assessment of sperm motility.

2. Adjust the focus through the oculars of the microscope and then adjust the focus while looking at the image on the video monitor.
3. Chose a microscope field at random.
4. First, count the rapid and slow progressive spermatozoa, and then count the non-progressive and immotile spermatozoa in the same field. If the concentration of spermatozoa is very high, it is advisable to only count spermatozoa in a part of the field, e.g. in the area of four squares at the centre of the overlay grid.
5. Assess at least five different fields and count at least 200 spermatozoa in each preparation.
6. Repeat the assessment of the motility of at least 200 spermatozoa in a second wet preparation from the same semen specimen.

Calculations and Results

Calculations are done in the same way as for a sperm motility assessment performed by looking down the microscope, and the same results are reported.

Interpretation Guidelines

The same interpretation guidelines as for standard motility assessment.

Notes

The video display should not be too large since it is being viewed close-up and the individual pixels can be distracting to the observer. A display as small as 7" (17.5 cm) can be sufficient, although such small displays are increasingly difficult to source.

Video Recording of Sperm Motility

Principle

Recording samples for motility assessments gives extra value for the laboratory by generating training material for novices and other staff members requiring qualitative training, as well as providing an archive of material that can be used for IQC and exchange with other laboratories (EQC/EQA).

Specimen

- As for a basic sperm motility assessment

Equipment

See also Appendix 2.

In addition to the equipment needed for motility assessment on a video display the following capabilities are needed:

- Recording facilities (e.g. DVD recorder, computer with video clip facilities) with the ability to replay the recordings frame-by-frame.
- The ability to superimpose identifying text into the video image, e.g. using a text generator connected between the video camera and the video recorder, or computer software to integrate text into the recordings.

Disposable Materials

- As for a basic sperm motility assessment
- Recording medium for video clips (e.g. recordable DVDs) if not stored directly onto a computer hard drive

Calibration

- As for motility assessment using a video display

Quality Control

- Recorded samples should be examined by all trained members of staff and the average results from experienced members used as target (or 'true') values.
- In recorded semen samples, the velocity of individual spermatozoa can be measured frame-by-frame to classify spermatozoa objectively into the four groups (WHO4/6 *a–d*).
- Recorded samples can also be used for training and QC exchange with other laboratories.
- When using older analogue video recordings, especially when copies are made of the master recording (and even more critically if converted to other formats), it is important to check that the copy gives the same results. This should be done by comparing results from blinded assessments of original and transferred versions of the recording. This problem is minimal with digital recordings.

Procedure

1. Turn on the video system (e.g. camera, display, text generator if used, perhaps a video analog to digital converter or 'grabber', and video recording device or computer with appropriate software).
2. First record, for about 10 s, an image of a micrometer scale as a calibration image.
3. Then record a 5–10 s long segment without the microscope image, preferably showing a specimen identifying text (e.g. 'Andrology Laboratory, X Hospital, Quality Control').
4. Make a fresh wet preparation using a pre-warmed (37°C) microscope slide and coverslip and make sure that there is no flow in the preparation.

5. Using the text superimposition function, create a unique ID for the sample being recorded but which does not reveal the identity of the patient. Either record the ID for 5 s before the first sample clip or align the text so that it does not interfere with the central field of the view where the motility assessments will be made.

6. Make recordings:
   - Check the focus
   - Record for 15–20 s and then add a 5 s blank segment
   - Estimate the number of spermatozoa that could be counted in that field; at least 200 'valid' spermatozoa must be recorded over at least five different fields
   - Change the microscope field and repeat this step; remember to check the focus and that there is no flow before recording each field

7. Record a final blank segment after the last field of the sample for 10–15 s, preferably with a text saying 'End of sample ###' where ### is the sample ID.

8. If appropriate, also record a message 'End of recording' directly after the last specimen on the recording medium.

Sperm Concentration

Principle

Diluted and immobilized spermatozoa are easy to count under the microscope. The difficult part is to ascertain that the aliquot examined is adequate and representative for the entire semen specimen. Spermatozoa should not be lost by sedimentation, aggregation or by adhesion to the walls of the specimen container, pipette tips, or secondary containers, and there must be no dilution errors. Therefore, thorough mixing is essential both before semen dilution and before loading the counting chamber.

It is also important that the dilution is exact. Positive displacement pipetters are necessary to measure exact aliquot volumes of semen due to its higher viscosity.

The next critical step is ensuring an accurate sub-sample volume. In practice, this is achieved by the depth of the counting chamber, so to ensure the correct depth the coverslip must be mounted tightly, and in order to examine the expected volume of the diluted sample the chamber must be filled correctly.

With a 'wet' preparation depth of about 20 µm and a field of vision diameter of about 500 µm under the microscope, the observed numbers of spermatozoa per microscope field gives the appropriate dilution in Table 3.2. The correct area of the microscopic field can be determined using a stage micrometer to measure the diameter of the field of view and calculating its area using the formula: area = πr^2

Standard dilutions for semen are $1 + 19$ and $1 + 9$. For swim-up preparations with $<10 \times 10^6$ spermatozoa/ml, a dilution of $1 + 1$ can be used, and for extremely high concentration semen samples, $1 + 49$ can be used. Although some texts continue to describe making duplicate dilutions, if an accurate minimum 50 µl aliquot of semen is taken carefully from a well-mixed, liquefied ejaculate using a positive displacement pipettor, as described below, this practice does not improve accuracy [18,19].

Table 3.2 Diluting the ejaculate for determining sperm concentration by haemocytometry. The most common dilutions are shown in bold

Spermatozoa per 40× objective field	Dilution to use		Semen (µl)	Diluent (µl)
Swim up	1:2	1 + 1	100	100
<15	1:5	1 + 4	100	400
15–40	**1:10**	**1 + 9**	**50**	**450**
40–200	**1:20**	**1 + 19**	**50**	**950**
>200	1:50	1 + 49	50	2450

Dilutions can be stored for a maximum of four weeks in tested vials (see Note, below) at +4°C, but should preferably be assessed the same day. The problems that can occur upon prolonged storage are sperm clumping and sperm adhesion to the container walls.

Specimen
- Well-mixed liquefied semen

Equipment and Materials

See also Appendix 2.
- Vortex mixer
- Microscope with 10×, 20× and 40× phase contrast objectives
- Humid chamber for haemocytometers
- Counting chamber: haemocytometer with improved Neubauer ruling with proper coverslips
- Positive displacement pipetter: 0–50 µl; with tips (ideally sterile)
- Calibrated, adjustable air-displacement pipetter: 200–1000 µl with tips (ideally sterile)
- Centrifuge
- Tally counter
- Calculator

Disposable Materials
- Working/calculation sheet
- Test tubes or vials with air-tight caps, e.g. Technicon 2 ml autoanalyser vials
  Note: Test these secondary containers to see that spermatozoa do not stick to their inner surfaces, e.g. by performing repeat assessments over a period of, say, four weeks.

Reagents

Diluent for Sperm Concentration

50.0 g $NaHCO_3$
10.0 ml   36–40% formaldehyde solution (a saturated formaldehyde solution)

- Dissolve the constituents in distilled or deionized water (>10 MΩ/cm) and dilute to 1000 ml
- Filter the solution into a clean bottle to eliminate crystals (use a filter paper suitable for retention of coarse and gelatinous precipitates); the diluent should not contain any solid particles
- Store the diluent at +4°C (maximum 12 months)

Quality Control
- Calibration of pipetters should be done regularly. Pipetters showing erroneous results should be recalibrated according to the manufacturer's instructions or sent for repair and recalibration. Results of calibration controls as well as records of repairs and adjustments should be kept in a separate log for each pipetter.
- Counting chambers should be checked for accuracy when new and regularly after use (risk for wear causing reduced chamber depth).
- Comparison of duplicate assessments for each specimen analysed.
- For novices: repeated training with experienced staff and using archive material with known results.
- For all staff members: Internal Quality Control (IQC) monitoring of the variation between staff members and over time (assessment of precision).

- For the laboratory as one unit: External Quality Assurance (EQA) monitoring of the laboratory's performance in relation to other laboratories using reference materials (assessment of accuracy).

Procedure

1. The dilution is prepared according to Table 3.2 (if there are quality issues with the dilution step, it is advisable to make duplicate dilutions from each specimen). Using a positive displacement pipetter, take the exact volume of well-mixed semen and add it to the diluent. To avoid transfer of additional semen on the outside of the pipette tip it is essential to carefully wipe off all fluid from the outside of the tip without extracting any volume from the inside of the tip before (wipe backwards from the open end of the tip) the aliquot is dispensed into the diluent.

2. A special haemocytometer coverslip is mounted on the haemocytometer with Improved Neubauer ruling so that interference patterns are seen between the surfaces where the coverslip is attached. Several Newton's rings/fringes or iridescent lines should be visible in the contact areas when the coverslip is properly attached.

3. Immediately before withdrawing the aliquot of diluted spermatozoa, the diluted sample must be mixed for at least 10 s on a vortex mixer. After mixing, take one aliquot of about 10 µl (the volume should be sufficient to fill one side of a haemocytometer) and load it into one side of a haemocytometer with improved Neubauer ruling, then take a second aliquot of the diluted sample and load it into the other side of the haemocytometer. Each chamber must be completely filled, but not over-filled.

4. Place the haemocytometer horizontally in a humid chamber for 10–15 min to allow sedimentation of the spermatozoa onto the grid of the counting chamber.

5. Spermatozoa are usually counted under a 20× phase contrast objective (most 40× objectives have working distances that are too short). One 'large square' in the Improved Neubauer ruling haemocytometer chamber is limited on all four sides by triple lines (Figure 3.5A, see below). The middle of the three lines defines the border of the large square. When spermatozoa are lying on, or in contact with, the borders of the square, only count those spermatozoa on the upper or left borders, do not count those on the lower or right borders.

   a) Decide the number of squares that should be counted. First count the number of spermatozoa in the large square in the upper left corner of the central grid area (marked as '1' in Figure 3.5A). Based on this number, determine how many squares will be counted in each side of the chamber:

<10 spermatozoa	count all the grid (25 squares in each chamber)
10–40 spermatozoa	count 10 squares in each chamber (2 rows or columns)
>40 spermatozoa	count 5 squares in each chamber (e.g. 4 corners and centre).

   The goal is that typically more than 200 spermatozoa should be counted in each chamber (this number is sufficient for a comparison between the two counts); if the total number of cells counted is less than 200 when all 25 large squares have been assessed, another of the 8 peripheral areas surrounding the central grid can also be counted.

   b) Only if a free sperm head can be recognized with certainty should it be included in the count (see Note #1); if more than 20% of sperm heads lack tails, the free heads should be counted separately and noted in the laboratory report. 'Pinheads' should be counted separately and commented upon in the report form. Immature germinal cells should not be counted (these will be assessed in the differential morphology count), while round cells and inflammatory cells can be counted separately to determine their respective concentrations.

   c) Only spermatozoa where the head is located on the upper or left limiting lines of a square (marked 'OK' in Figure 3.5B) should be included for that square; do not count spermatozoa located on the lower or right limiting lines (marked 'out' in Figure 3.5B).

(A)   (B)

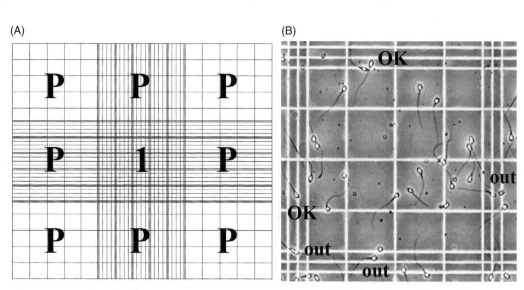

Figure 3.5 (A) Overview of the entire improved Neubauer ruling haemocytometer with the central field (marked '1') surrounded by eight peripheral fields (marked 'P'), each of which is the same size as the central field. (B) Appearance of the central grid of an Improved Neubauer ruling haemocytometer under phase contrast optics. Each chamber consists of the 25 'large squares' (in a 5×5 pattern). Each 'large' square is surrounded by triple rulings and contains 16 small squares. The middle of the three lines limits each large square. Sperm in contact with the upper or left limits are counted ('OK' in the figure) while those in contact with the left and lower limits are not included ('out' in the figure). The small squares facilitate counting when many spermatozoa are present in the large square. Each central grid (25 large squares) measures 1 mm × 1 mm, and has a depth of 0.1 mm, giving a volume of 0.1 mm^3 = 0.1 µl = 100 nl. (Note that the Makler chamber has the same area, but a depth of only 0.01 mm, hence the volume is 0.01 µl = 10 nl, or one tenth of that of the haemocytometer.)

Calculations and Results

The duplicate counts are compared as described in Appendix 5. The total number of assessed spermatozoa (sum) and the difference between the two counts are calculated. An assessment is only accepted if the difference is equal to, or less than, the value obtained in Table App5.3. Otherwise, the counts are discarded and a new haemocytometer preparation made and assessed.

If duplicate dilutions were made then average the two results, provided that they meet the reproducibility criteria for acceptance. If they are not sufficiently close, then repeat the counting procedure for both dilutions.

To get the concentration of spermatozoa in the original semen specimen, the sum of the accepted duplicate counts (total number of spermatozoa in both chambers) is divided by the appropriate factor from Table 3.3, and the result expressed as millions of spermatozoa per ml (×10^6/ml). The total sperm number (×10^6/ejaculate) is obtained by multiplying the ejaculate volume (ml) and sperm concentration. Do not use the incorrect term 'sperm density' when referring to sperm concentration.

Sperm concentration should be expressed as 'millions per millilitre' or ×10^6/ml, and sperm count (total number of spermatozoa in the ejaculate) as 'millions per ejaculate', both with only 1 decimal place. However, for concentration or total count values <1 × 10^6, two significant figures should be used, e.g. 0.094785 × 10^6 could be expressed as 95,000 (per ml or ejaculate).

If reporting a result of 'no spermatozoa', it is preferred that the result is not presented as 0.0 × 10^6/ml, but that an asterisk (*) is written in the place for concentration and total sperm number. A comment should be made if no, or perhaps just occasional motile or immotile, spermatozoa have been observed in an ejaculate or in a centrifuged pellet.

Interpretation Guidelines

Besides incomplete specimen collection and varying abstinence time, there are many other external factors that can influence the total number of spermatozoa in the ejaculate, e.g. fever, genital tract

Table 3.3 Conversion factors for use in calculating the results for sperm concentration determined using haemocytometry. Divide the total number of spermatozoa counted in the two haemocytometer chambers by the appropriate factor to give the concentration of spermatozoa in the original semen specimen in millions of spermatozoa per milliliter (i.e. $\times 10^6$/ml)

Table 3.3A Factors for use when only the central grid (5×5 large squares) have been assessed

Dilution	Number of counted squares per chamber		
	25	10	5
1 + 1	100	40	20
1 + 4	40	16	8
1 + 9	20	8	4
1 + 19	10	4	2
1 + 49	4	1.6	0.8

Table 3.3B Factors for use when at least one more field of 25 large squares than the central grid has been assessed

Dilution	Number of 25-squares fields counted							
	2	3	4	5	6	7	8	9
1 + 1	200	300	400	500	600	700	800	900
1 + 4	80	120	160	200	240	280	320	360
1 + 9	40	60	80	100	120	140	160	180

infection, some drugs and occupational exposure. Interpretation of sperm concentration and total number of spermatozoa in the ejaculate is the responsibility of the requesting physician.

Notes

1. The WHO manuals say not to count free sperm heads, but this will create problems for specimens from subjects with the decapitated sperm defect, or specimens where sperm heads and tails have been separated artefactually, e.g. by over vigorous mixing of the semen specimen or by contaminating detergent: in extreme cases this can result in a false diagnosis of azoospermia.
2. Disposable haemocytometers are commercially available but must be validated and verified before introduction [20]. If counting chambers not made of glass are used, it is essential to ascertain that the optical properties of the material do not make the spermatozoa difficult to observe [20].
3. Direct counting chambers that do not require dilution of the semen are not recommended. Sperm concentration assessments made using the Makler chamber have considerably greater measurement bias, and disposable chambers such as the Kova and Vetriplast chambers should not be used [21]. See Chapter 6 on *Computer-Aided Sperm Analysis* for discussion of the limitations of disposable fixed-depth chambers that fill by capillary action.

Sperm Vitality

Sperm vitality assessments in routine semen analysis are used to establish whether the immotile spermatozoa are live or dead. In most routine situations this means that sperm vitality only needs to be assessed in specimens with <40% motile spermatozoa.

Principle

An intact cell plasma membrane hinders the uptake of the red stain Eosin Y, while a dead cell (i.e. with damaged cell membrane) takes up the stain. Nigrosin is a purple background stain that provides contrast for the unstained (white) live cells, allowing simple assessment using bright field microscopy.

Specimen

- An aliquot of liquefied, well-mixed semen, ideally at 30 (maximum 60) min after ejaculation

Equipment and Disposable Materials

- Microscope with 100× oil immersion objective, bright field not phase contrast (see Appendix 2)
- Microscope slides
- Coverslips, 22 × 50 mm or 24 × 50 mm, #1 thickness

Reagents

- *Eosin-nigrosin stain:*

  0.67 g   eosin Y (C.I. 45380, Europe M 15935),

  10.00 g   nigrosin (C.I. 50420, Europe M 15924)

  0.90 g   sodium chloride

  100 ml   distilled water

  1. Dissolve the eosin Y and sodium chloride in 100 ml distilled water with gentle heating
  2. Add the nigrosin
  3. Bring the solution to boil and allow it to cool to room temperature
  4. Filter the solution through filter paper (e.g. Munktell Class II or Whatman 113V)
  5. Store in a sealed glass bottle
  6. The staining solution should be at room temperature when used

  Note: An equivalent stain is available commercially (Sperm VitalStain, Nidacon International AB, Mölndal, Sweden).

- *Mounting medium:* Use Merck Entellan mountant or other equivalent medium for quick and permanent mounting of slides with coverslips. This is strongly recommended to preserve the slides and to avoid contaminating the objective.

  Note: If an eosin-nigrosin smear gets cold, and then re-warms in a humid (e.g. indoor) environment, condensation can form on the surface of the smear, re-mobilizing the eosin stain and allowing it to enter all the (now dead) spermatozoa in the smear.

Quality Control

For novices: repeated training with experienced staff and using archive material with known results.

For all staff members: Internal Quality Control (IQC) monitoring of the variation between staff members and over time (imprecision).

For the laboratory as one unit: External Quality Assessment (EQA) monitoring of the laboratory's performance in relation to other laboratories (accuracy).

Procedure

1. Mix 50 µl of well-mixed, undiluted, liquefied semen with 50 µl of eosin-nigrosin stain and incubate for 30 s.
2. Place 12–15 µl of the mixture on a clean microscope slide and make a smear.
3. Let the smear air dry and examine it directly or, preferably, mount it permanently the same day and examine after the mountant has dried (e.g. overnight). Mounted smears can be stored at room temperature.
4. Assess at least 200 spermatozoa at 1000× (or 1250×) magnification under oil immersion with a high-resolution 100× bright field non-phase contrast objective. Use properly adjusted bright field optics (Köhler illumination), not phase contrast optics. White (unstained) sperm heads are classified as 'live' and those with any pink or red stain are classified as 'dead' (Figure 3.6), with

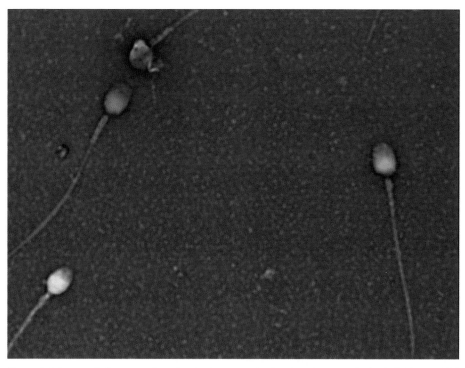

Figure 3.6 A sperm vitality preparation using the one-step eosin-nigrosin stain seen under bright field optics (Köhler illumination) showing three dead (red) spermatozoa and one live (white) spermatozoon with a 'leaky neck' (see also Figure 3.7).

the exception of spermatozoa that show only a slight pink staining in the neck region ('leaky necks'), this is not considered a sign of cell death (Figure 3.7).

5. Although WHO5 recommended duplicate counting for sperm vitality assessments, a recent study has established that this is not necessary for the simple purpose of establishing whether the immotile spermatozoa in a specimen are live or dead [22]. However, if it is done for research purposes, where greater accuracy is needed, then duplicates should be compared in the same way as for motility and morphology (see Appendix 5).

Calculations and Results

The proportion of live spermatozoa is calculated by dividing the number of live spermatozoa counted by the total number of spermatozoa assessed.

The proportion of live spermatozoa is given as an integer percentage (i.e. without decimal points).

Interpretation Guidelines

Sperm vitality measured with a staining method is clinically important when very few or no spermatozoa are motile. Ciliary dyskinesia (immotile cilia syndrome or Kartagener syndrome) is a rare genetic disorder due to defects in the ciliary structure, affecting all cilia in the body of the affected individual, including the sperm tail. In addition to having live but totally immotile spermatozoa, chronic respiratory infections and situs inversus are not uncommon findings in these men.

If the immotile spermatozoa are dead, then cytotoxic anti-sperm antibodies or other negative effects of active inflammatory reactions can be suspected.

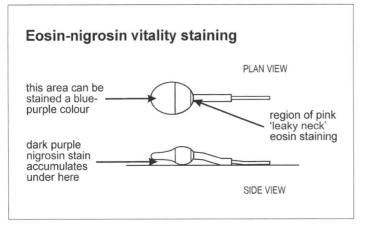

Figure 3.7 Explanatory figures illustrating the two common problems encountered when reading eosin-nigrosin sperm vitality slides.

Notes

1. The proportion of live spermatozoa is usually slightly higher than the proportion of motile spermatozoa in the sample.
2. The WHO5 recommendations for vitality staining [11] can cause spermatozoa to die due to too low osmolarity [23]; the present method has been established not to do that [24].
3. Eosin-nigrosin assessment of sperm vitality does not work well on spermatozoa that have been exposed to glycerol (e.g. cryopreserved spermatozoa), since the glycerol renders their cell membranes permeable to eosin.

Sperm Morphology

Introduction

The importance of sperm morphology in the determination of potential fertility was recognized in the early 1900s and was introduced into routine semen analysis by some researchers. But even a century ago the role and importance of sperm morphology was already controversial [25–28]. Hühner stated in 1921 that 'If many active moving spermatozoa per microscopic field are present, sperm morphology is of no importance and the presence of many abnormal spermatozoa will have no influence on the outcome of the post coital test' [25]. But this statement was contradicted by Cary in 1930, who stated that 'morphology of human spermatozoa bears a definite relation to the success of their migration through cervical mucus' [26], and in 1934 Cary and Hotchkiss repeated this and added that 'Abnormal forms may possess motility but are rarely if ever found in the upper levels of cervical mucus and we must consider them ineffectual for fertilization' [27]. In 1932 Moench and Holt stated that 'Morphology of the sperm head seems to be the most reliable indicator of (the) fertilizing power of these (sperm) cells' [28].

Observations of the morphological appearance of human spermatozoa after migration within periovulatory cervical mucus revealed an improved homogeneous picture in contrast to the very heterogeneous picture seen in contemporaneous semen samples (Figure 3.8) [29]. While the full gamut of mechanisms by which the selection for morphological normality within cervical mucus likely still remains to be elucidated, it is clear that a major selective effector is the innate motility of the spermatozoa [30]. According to Mortimer, the apparent selection for spermatozoa with normal head shape is a concomitant of the higher prevalence of coexisting midpiece and/or tail defects in spermatozoa with abnormal head shape; spermatozoa with midpiece and/or tail defects being less able, or unable, to penetrate cervical mucus due to their inherently dysfunctional motility [31]. Other mechanisms might also exist, and certainly a variety of hypotheses for sperm selection within the higher reaches of the female reproductive tract – the uterus and

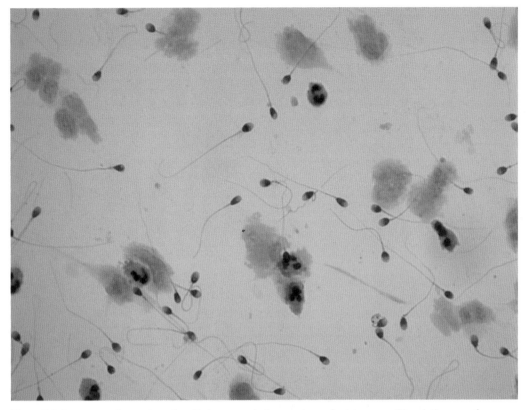

Figure 3.8 Appearance of spermatozoa found in human cervical mucus drawn after intercourse. Although there are a few polymorphonuclear leucocytes and some unidentified material visible, the smooth contours and clear acrosome/post-acrosomal staining are evident. Spermatozoa showing a slight elongation at the posterior head region are regarded as normal/ideal according to Strict Criteria. Micrograph courtesy of Susanne Hollenstein MSc (fiore LAB AG, St Gallen, Switzerland).

oviducts – have been proposed [32–34]. Interestingly, in bovine spermatozoa, the expression of several proteins associated with critical sperm functions, such as sperm cytoskeletal structure, capacitation and sperm-egg interaction, were decreased in pyriform spermatozoa, whereas proteins regulating antioxidant activity, apoptosis and metabolism were increased in morphologically normal spermatozoa [35].

Of key importance to modern andrology is that it was the improved sperm morphology within cervical mucus which led Menkveld to use the more uniform features of these spermatozoa to better describe a morphologically normal human spermatozoon, an approach that became known as the Tygerberg Strict Criteria [36,37]. With the acceptance of (Tygerberg) Strict Criteria for assessing human sperm morphology the importance of the early observations on the biology of morphologically normal spermatozoa became even more evident [36–38], confirming the great importance of careful assessment of sperm morphology characteristics in the complete evaluation of a semen sample. But even though it has been established that certain morphological sperm abnormalities are associated with specific sperm functional defects, it must still be remembered that a morphologically normal appearance at the light microscope level does not necessarily equate to a functionally normal spermatozoon [31,37].

Sperm morphology evaluation within the semen analysis can be divided into two equally important areas: (a) all aspects of the preparation of the stained smears for the morphological evaluation of spermatozoa, and (b) the evaluation process itself for the assessment of sperm morphology and semen cytology. Accurate evaluations of sperm morphology can only be done if the following, very basic, principles and steps are followed as described below.

Sperm Morphology: Preparation of Smears

Equipment
See also Appendix 2.
- Air displacement pipetter, 0–20 µl

Disposable Materials
- Microscope slides with frosted ends
- Coverslips, 22 × 50 mm or 24 × 50 mm, #1 thickness

Notes: 1. The slides for the morphology smears must be clear from any debris or grease; if not, they must be thoroughly cleaned before use, first by washing in a detergent, rinsed in clean water and then rinsed in alcohol and dried. This is to ensure that the semen smear will stick to the glass slide.

2. Coverslips must also be washed with alcohol if indicated [39].

Procedure
1. Smears are prepared either by the 'feathering' or 'apposed slides' techniques. The latter technique is especially useful for semen with increased viscosity (Figure 3.9).
2. Place a small drop of well-mixed, liquefied semen (see Notes), on the slide, using either a positive displacement or an air displacement pipetter. A small drop of semen must be used so that a very thin smear is prepared, and so that no more than 5–10 spermatozoa will be present per microscope field of view at 1000–1250× magnification. For the feathering technique, locate the drop near the frosted end of the slide, for the apposed slides technique, locate the elongated drop near the centre of the slide.
3. Smears are left to air dry before fixing (see below).

Notes
1. Thin smears are essential so that each spermatozoon can be visualized separately, and that all spermatozoa will be in the same focal plane so their true form can be observed.
2. The thickness of the smear and thus the number of sperm per visual field can be controlled by altering the size of the semen drop and by adjusting the angle and speed of the slide used to make the smear.
3. With a high sperm concentration, a small drop of semen (but not <6 µl) should be used.

Feathering technique

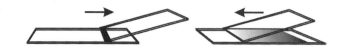

Apposed slides technique

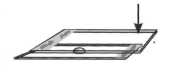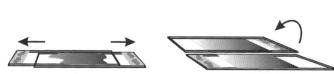

Figure 3.9 Diagram illustrating two alternative techniques for making smears for sperm morphology assessment.

4. With a lower sperm concentration, the size of the drop is increased, but to no more than 15 μl.

5. Changing the angle between the two slides and/or the speed at which the 'feathering' is performed will change the thickness of the smear.

6. When 'feathering', it is important that the semen drop should be pulled across the semen smear slide; pushing the drop can cause artefacts such as lose heads and broken or bent tails.

7. If the sperm concentration is very low ($<2 \times 10^6$/ml) an aliquot of the semen specimen can be centrifuged (maximum 1000 g) and the pellet resuspended in a small amount of clean seminal plasma (i.e. the supernatant) to make the morphology smear.

8. With viscous samples, it may be difficult to prepare good, thin smears unless alternative methods are used. For example:
   - Treatment of the sample with alpha-amylase or chymotrypsin [39]
   - An aliquot of the semen specimen can be diluted with 170 mM NaCl solution (approximately isotonic with liquefied semen) and used to make the smears [1].

9. Semen smears should always be prepared at least in duplicate, so that slides can be stored for later reference purposes, for other studies, or in case the first staining was not successful.

Sperm Morphology: Fixation of Smears

Specimen
- Semen smears that have been left to air dry (see above)

Equipment
See also Appendix 2.
- Staining dishes or Coplin jars

Materials
The fixation procedure will depend on the staining method used; for the Papanicolaou staining method, use analytical grade absolute ethanol or methanol.

Procedure
The fixation procedure will depend on the staining method used. For the Papanicolaou staining procedure, the best technique is to leave the smears until they appear to be just air-dried, i.e. only a few minutes, and then fix them immediately by immersion in analytical grade ethanol or methanol for at least 10 to 15 min.

Notes
1. The smears can be kept in the fixative for longer periods of time if needed, up to several days – but avoid allowing the fixative to evaporate completely.
2. Fixed smears can be stained directly or taken out of the fixative and stored for staining later.
3. If smears are specially prepared for cytological evaluation, they can be fixed immediately using a 50:50 mixture of ethanol and diethyl ether (caution: highly flammable).

Sperm Morphology: Staining of Smears

Background
For routine work, a staining method such as the Papanicolaou procedure [11–13,40] is recommended. This method gives good staining of both spermatozoa and the so-called 'round' cells, such as the precursors or germinal epithelium cells and the various types of leucocytes. The Papanicolaou stain is

a basophilic/acidophilic composition stain. Hence the nucleus of the spermatozoa and other cells stains an intense blue, while the sperm acrosome appears light blue, due to the effect of the haematoxylin under acid conditions. The sperm tails stain blue or, if staining conditions are very good, even red, while the midpiece can also stain red but mostly blue/green. Cytoplasmic residues at the head/neck junction will usually stain blue-green, or sometimes red. Papanicolaou staining also gives a very good staining and definition of non-spermatozoal cells present in semen, due to the fact that Papanicolaou modified the Shorr stain method, which was specially developed for the staining of vaginal epithelium cells [40].

For special procedures, rapid staining methods such as the *Diff-Quik*® or *Hemacolor*® can be used [11,12,39]. Over-staining of the spermatozoa with the rapid staining methods and intense background staining of the dried and fixed seminal plasma are negative aspects of this method, as well as the fact that the spermatozoa undergo swelling, altering their morphological appearance (see Figure 3.10 Plates 1A and 1B). The background effect can be overcome by making very thin smears or by washing the semen samples before making the smears, but washing can lead to additional morphological changes or the presence of severely altered or decondensed spermatozoa.

Spermac® has the advantage of a short staining procedure, and also provides detailed differential staining of the acrosome, post-acrosomal region and tail [41]. *Spermac*® stains the tails and intact acrosomes green and the visual part of the sperm head nucleus red. Due to its intense staining it can also be very useful for photomicrography (Figure 3.10 Plate 1C).

Overall, these rapid staining methods are not advised for routine morphology evaluation, due to their possible negative staining effects. While some laboratories still use the Shorr staining method, it is not recommended for routine morphology evaluations for reasons of better standardization in the sperm morphology evaluation process. Although a staining effect very similar to Papanicolaou staining is observed, the Shorr stain does not always provide good results because the outlines of spermatozoa can appear a little fuzzy, and deep staining of the acrosome can occur with loss of definition, especially if the smears are overstained [42].

SpermBlue® is a relatively new staining process for human and certain animal spermatozoa [43]. The kit contains the *SpermBlue*® fixative and *SpermBlue*® stain, both of which are iso-osmotic in relation to semen. Fixation and staining of air-dried smears takes only 25 min. This technique stains human spermatozoa different hues or intensities of blue, allowing clear distinction of the acrosome, sperm head, midpiece, principal piece of the tail, and even the terminal segment. It has the advantage that, due to the iso-osmotic properties, the sperm head measurements are very similar to those of the spermatozoa in the original seminal plasma [43,44]. To date, no studies have been published comparing this staining method for manual morphology evaluations with either *in-vivo* fertility or *in-vitro* fertilization outcomes.

Equipment

See also Appendix 2.

- Staining dishes (glass)
- Stainless steel racks for staining slides

Disposable Materials

- Analytical grade ethanol
- Ethanol 95%, 80%, 70%, 50% (v/v)
- Harris haematoxylin (Papanicolaou solution 1a, Merck 9253)
- Orange G solution (OG6, Papanicolaou solution 2a, Merck 6888)
- Polychrome solution (EA50, Papanicolaou solution 3b, Merck 9272)
- Absolute 1-propanol
- Xylene substitute
- DPX or other suitable mountant

The Modified Papanicolaou Staining Procedure

1. Allow smears to air dry.
2. Fix for at least 10 to 15 min in analytic grade absolute ethanol.
3. Transfer one slide to the staining rack and the other to the slide filing box or cabinet. Slides should be stored in the dark at room temperature.
4. If all slides are collected, or if a staining rack is full, proceed to staining by taking the rack through the sequential solutions and dyes as below.
5. Staining dishes should be adequately filled so that the whole slide will be immersed. For this reason, it is recommended that staining racks where slides can be placed horizontally on their sides should be used. Up to 20 slides can be placed back-to-back in each staining rack.
6. Proceed with staining according to the procedure in Table 3.4; a 'dip' corresponds to an immersion of about 1 s.
7. Mount the stained slides immediately (see below), and leave them overnight for the mountant to set, or place in a low temperature, dry oven to enhance the drying process.

Sperm Morphology: Mounting of Stained Smears

Procedure

1. Place a thin line of mountant on the middle line over the length of the coverslip, starting and ending about 5 mm from the ends of the coverslip.
2. Take the semen smear slide directly from the last xylene substitute dish and place it smear-side down, directly onto the mountant.
3. Leave for a period of time, so that the weight of the slide spreads the mountant to the sides of the coverslip.
4. Carefully press out any air bubbles with the aid of a pair of forceps and centre the coverslip so that its edge is about 5 mm away from the end of the slide. This will allow for the back-to-back storage of two slides in one slot of a storage box.

Notes

1. If a smear is technically difficult to read, then it might be that the smear was made too thick, or that the staining solutions were old or over-used. In such situations the reserve smear should be stained with fresh solutions and assessed.
2. If the smear was dislodged during the staining process, then either the smear was too thick or the slide was not clean enough.
3. Small, black-blue, fern-like crystals on the stained smears indicate that the haematoxylin solution is old or needs to be filtered.

Sperm Morphology: Evaluation

Background

For the evaluation of sperm morphology, the whole spermatozoon must be considered. A spermatozoon without any morphological defects was previously considered as morphologically 'normal', although it is now recommended that the term 'normal' should not be used to describe those rare spermatozoa, but rather to describe them as 'ideal' forms. The definition for a morphologically ideal spermatozoon is based on the modal form seen after spermatozoa have migrated through good peri-ovulatory cervical mucus either *in vivo* (PCT) or *in vitro* (Figure 3.8) The spermatozoa seen in such a population, and also those bound to the human zona pellucida *in vitro*, are very homogeneous and were used by Menkveld [36] and Menkveld et al. [37] to describe the 'typical' form, a principle that was first adopted in the 1992 WHO

Table 3.4 Sequence of steps for Papanicolaou sperm morphology staining, with explanations

Step	Reagent	Exposure	Comment
1	80% ethyl alcohol	10 dips	Slides transferred directly from the ethanol fixation without drying must pass through at least one container with 50% ethanol.
2	70% ethyl alcohol	10 dips	Air-dried smears that have been kept dry for several days require
3	50% ethyl alcohol	10 dips	longer rehydration time (2–3 min in 50% ethanol).
4	Distilled water	10 dips	
5	Harris' haematoxylin[a]	5 min	If the nuclear staining is weak, a new stain solution should be prepared or exposure time increased
6	Rinse in running water	3 min	To remove unbound haematoxylin
7	0.5% HCl[b]	2 dips	This step can be checked in the microscope, unspecific staining should be removed
8	Rinse in running water	5 min	To readjust pH after acid treatment, sperm nuclei becoming blue (instead of reddish)
9	Scott's water[c]	1 min	This step is essential when the pH of the water is too acidic (pH 4–5)
10	Rinse in running water	1–5 min	
11	50% ethyl alcohol	10 dips	To prepare for cytoplasmic staining with the ethanol soluble stains Orange G6 and EA 50 (or 65) water is removed by passing through
12	70% ethyl alcohol	10 dips	a series of increasing ethanol concentration steps.
13	80% ethyl alcohol	10 dips	The ethanol step after each staining step is to remove excess stain.
14	95% ethyl alcohol	10 dips	
15	Orange G6	5 min	
16	95% ethyl alcohol	5 dips	
17	95% ethyl alcohol	5 dips	
18	EA 50 or 65	5 min	
19	95% ethyl alcohol	5 dips	
20	95% ethyl alcohol	5 dips	
21	95% ethyl alcohol	5 dips	
22	Absolute 1-propanol[e]	5 dips	These steps remove the ethanol in order to be able to use a mountant that is not soluble in ethanol. For alternatives to xylol (xylene) see
23	1-propanol and xylol (1:1)[d,e,]	5 dips	footnote 'e'.
24	Xylol[e]	10 dips	
25	Xylol[e]	10 dips	
26	Xylol[e]	10–20 min	

(Modified from Eliasson, 1974; personal communication).

[a] Harris haematoxylin can be replaced with Mayer's haematoxylin.

[b] 1.0 ml concentrated HCl in 200 ml H_2O.

[c] Dissolve 20.0 g $MgSO_4 \cdot 7H_2O$ and 2.0 g $NaHCO_3$ in 1000 ml H_2O; a small crystal of thymol can be added to avoid microbial growth.

[d] The function of xylol (or xylene) series is to withdraw (dehydrate) all the water from the semen smears. If the xylol becomes milky, due to the presence of the water, replace it immediately with fresh xylol.

[e] **Important note:** since xylene is toxic, especially for lungs due to the fixation of cilia, a fume hood or extraction cabinet must be used when performing the staining procedure. Some health and safety regulations might require that xylene is not used, in which case alternatives include propanol or Neo-Clear® (Merck KGaA, Germany). Steps 22–26 are necessary to replace the ethanol with another solvent for mountants that are insoluble in ethanol (e.g. DPX). These steps can be omitted if ethanol soluble mountants are used. Ethanol soluble mountants can be applied before the smears have air-dried after the last ethanol dip at step 21.

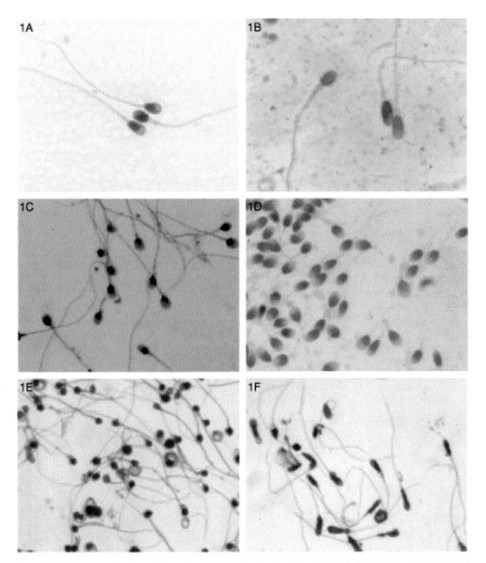

Figure 3.10 Sperm morphology, Plate 1: Sperm staining methods and sperm morphology patterns. (1A) Papanicolaou staining of elongated spermatozoa. (1B) *Hemacolor®* (Merck) rapid staining; same patient as in 1A. Note slight swelling of spermatozoa, leading to rounder and larger forms, as well as background staining. (1C) *Spermac®* staining; acrosomes and tail stain green and nucleus stains red. (1D) Normal morphology pattern of spermatozoa bound to the zona pellucida of a hemizona assay. (1E) Globozoospermia, Spermac® staining. Note small round heads only with red staining, indicating the absence of the acrosomes. (1F) 'Stress pattern' (*Spermac®* staining); all the spermatozoa are elongated. This condition can return to normal if the cause of stress can be removed.

manual, third edition [45], and confirmed as the standard method in the 1999 WHO manual, fourth edition [11]. The comparability of the two approaches (WHO3, 1992, and strict criteria) has been established by direct expert comparison [46].

However, such 'typical' or morphologically normal spermatozoa are now seen at a very low prevalence in semen due to several factors, such as the application of over critical or too strict criteria and adverse environmental influences [47]. This indicates that while 'morphologically normal' spermatozoa are not, per se, functionally normal, there must be some types of morphologically 'abnormal'

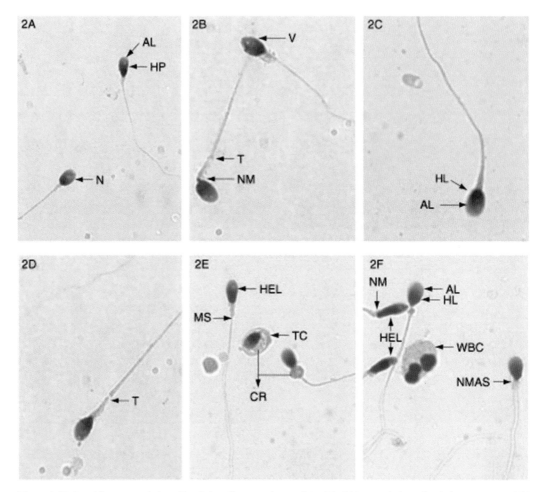

Figure 3.10 (cont.) Sperm morphology, Plate 2: Specific sperm abnormalities. (2A–F) N = morphologically ideal spermatozoon; NM = neck/midpiece defect; T = tail defect; CR = cytoplasmic residue defect; V = vacuole(s). (2A) AL = large acrosome; HP = pyriform head. (2C) HL = head large. (2E) MS = mitochondria shifted towards the head; TC = coiled tail (DAG defect). (2F) HEL = head medium elongated; WBC = polymorphonuclear white blood cell; NMAS = asymmetrical implantation of the neck.

spermatozoa that are capable of fertilizing oocytes, at least *in vitro* [47]. Understanding this will reduce confusion when reading reports of '0% normal forms', and is why this revised edition recommends using the term 'ideal' to describe spermatozoa that do not exhibit any recognizable defects (as does ISO 23162 [13]).

Definition of the 'Ideal' Sperm Morphology

According to the Tygerberg strict criteria [11,12,36,37], an ideal human spermatozoon is defined as one having an oval form with a smooth contour and a clearly visible and well-defined acrosome with homogeneous paler blue staining compared to the darker stained nucleus in the posterior region of the head (Figure 3.10 Plate 2A). The tail should be centrally inserted at the base of the head without any abnormalities of the neck/midpiece and tail region, and no cytoplasmic residues. Ideally the acrosome should cover 30% to 60% of the anterior part of the sperm head. The ideal sized sperm head will measure between 3.0–5.0 μm in length and 2.0–3.0 μm in width depending on the staining used. Papanicolaou and SpermBlue staining results in smaller sperm head measurements [43]. The midpiece should not be longer than 1.5× the length of an ideal head and be about 1 μm

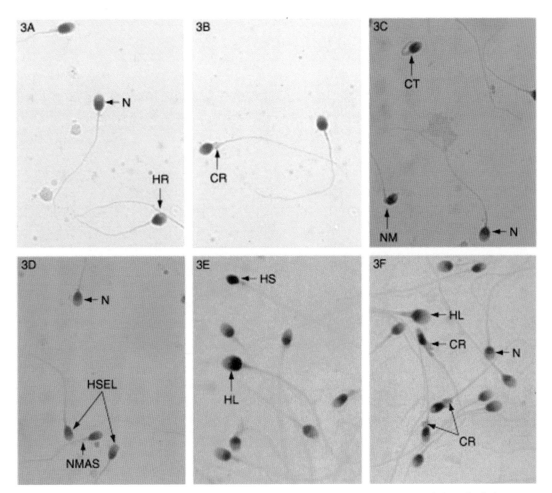

Figure 3.10 (cont.) Sperm morphology, Plate 3: Specific sperm abnormities continued. (3A–F) N = morphologically ideal spermatozoon; NM = neck/midpiece defect; T = tail defect; CR = cytoplasmic residue defect. (3A) HR = round head. (3C) CT = coiled tail. (3D) HSEL = slightly elongated head; NMAS = asymmetric implantation of the neck. (3E) Heterogeneous picture with small- and large-headed spermatozoa. HS = small head; HL = large head. (3F) HL = large head.

thick. The tail should be about 45–50 µm long and without any sharp bends. No residual cytoplasmic material should be present at the head/neck junction or along any part of the tail. For a spermatozoon to be classified as morphologically ideal, the whole spermatozoon must be ideal; borderline or slightly atypical spermatozoa are considered to be non-ideal [36,37].

Identification of Morphologically Atypical Spermatozoa

Non-ideal spermatozoa are those that deviate from the defined criteria for morphologically ideal spermatozoa due to differences in size, structure, or shape. This assessment relates only to the main regions of the spermatozoon. For routine evaluations, differentiation between different abnormalities within the head, or between different types of tail defects, is not performed. If a specific abnormality or non-ideal form is dominant, or even common (e.g. affecting at least 20% of the spermatozoa in the sample), this should be mentioned in the report form.

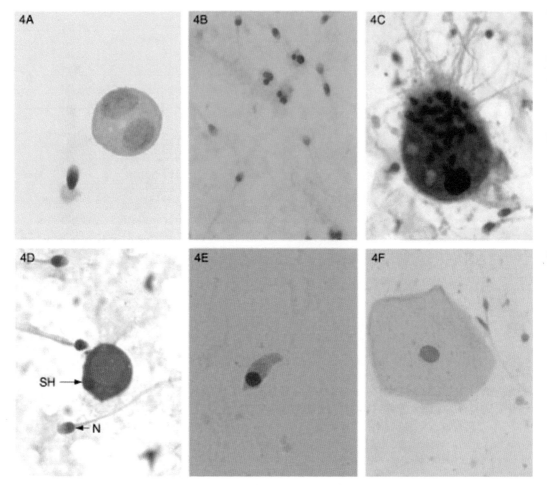

Figure 3.10 (cont.) Sperm morphology, Plate 4: Semen cytology, non-spermatozoal cells that might be seen in semen. (4A) Secondary spermatocyte. (4B) Polymorphonuclear white blood cells. (4C) Macrophage with phagocytosed spermatozoon. (4D) Monocyte with phagocytosed sperm head (SH). (4E) Prostate cell. (4F) Epithelial cell.

Many morphological abnormalities of human spermatozoa at the light microscope level under-lie sperm dysfunction and reflect abnormal sperm ultrastructure, although some ultrastructural anomalies that cause abnormal sperm function also exist in otherwise apparently normal spermatozoa [48].

There are four main classes of defects: (see Figure 3.11)

1. *Head defects*: These include abnormalities due to size and/or form and/or structure:
   a) 'Size', where the sperm head is too small or too large. This is considered as the primary criterion for abnormality, as long as the spermatozoa approximate the oval form.
   b) 'Shape' includes spermatozoa with an elongated or tapering form. The term tapering, i.e. spermatozoa having a narrowed head form due to flattening of the sides, might lead to confusion because it could be visualized by many investigators as a spear-point like spermatozoon. This is only one of the forms that can be included under the category of tapered. A more appropriate term would be elongated spermatozoa, since the so-called 'pear-shaped' or pyriform spermatozoa can also be included in this category.

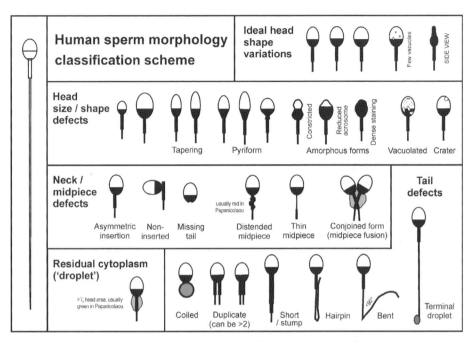

Figure 3.11 Schematic drawings showing the appearance of ideal (previously 'normal') spermatozoa and an illustrative range of morphological defects.

c) 'Structure' includes acrosome defects due to size, i.e. too large (>60% of ideal head size), or too small (<30% of ideal head size). Acrosome defects can also include staining defects of the acrosomes, including acrosomes showing vacuoles or cysts. In some patients a very special defect has been observed where a cyst protrudes from the anterior acrosome area outside of the acrosome, forming a nipple-like structure (hence called a 'nipple defect') which was originally described in the bull. In humans it is regarded as a severe sperm morphology defect [49].

d) 'Duplications', where two or more spermatozoa are joined together at any location of the neck, midpiece or tail by cytoplasmic material, but not covering the sperm head itself.

e) 'Amorphous' includes all spermatozoa with head abnormalities that do not fall in any of the previously mentioned groups; this includes those spermatozoa with slight abnormalities.

2. *Neck/midpiece defects*: This category includes bent necks (i.e. the neck and tail forms an angle of >90° with the sperm head). Thickened necks and midpieces are also included, as well as irregular or bent midpieces, asymmetrical tail insertions, or abnormally thin midpieces (i.e. where the mitochondria have shifted either to the neck region – not to be confused with the presence of cytoplasmic material or residues – or towards the principal piece of the tail). Different combinations of these aberrations can also be present.

3. *Tail defects*: This category includes tails bent at >90° at any part of the tail. A bend at the midpiece/tail junction is considered as a tail defect and not a neck/midpiece defect. Other abnormalities are short tails, coiled tails or irregular tails, or combinations of these. A prevalence of >20% coiled tails should be noted on the report from. In most cases, coiled tails will not be due to artefacts, such as hypo-osmotic stress or ageing, but due to a definite abnormality where the bends of the tail are actually covered by one membrane [48,49]. In the bull this abnormality is known as the DAG defect, named after the bull in which it was first described.

69

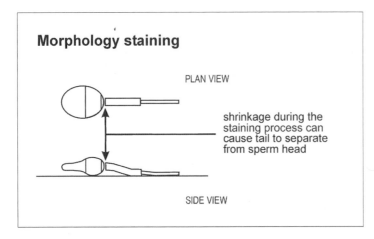

Figure 3.12 Illustration of how shrinkage during the staining process can cause the sperm tail to separate from the sperm head. This is considered an artefact rather than a morphological defect.

Note: During air-drying, fixation and staining it is possible that the tail might appear to become slightly separated from the head. This is considered to be an artefact of the processing and not a morphological defect on the spermatozoon (see Figure 3.12).

4. *Cytoplasmic residues*: Cytoplasmic droplets are better referred to as cytoplasmic residues, which can persist either protruding behind the sperm head at or around the neck/midpiece connection or on the tail itself. There is currently controversy as to whether the presence of cytoplasmic residues or cytoplasmic droplets can be regarded as a normal phenomenon [50], but because they are seldom seen in stained semen smears they are regarded as abnormalities for sperm morphology evaluation. Although no cytoplasmic material should be present, a smooth droplet/residue <30% of the ideal sized sperm head is still regarded as normal. The presence of cytoplasmic residues on spermatozoa is associated with sperm immaturity and the production of excessive reactive oxygen species (ROS) [39,48].

Other Categories

- 'Loose heads' or 'free heads' are not counted as an abnormality. The presence of >20 loose heads per 100 spermatozoa should be noted on the report form.
- 'Unknown cells' are all cells that cannot be positively identified as either sperm precursors or inflammatory cells, and can also be mentioned on the report form.
- 'Pinhead forms' are not included in the sperm morphology evaluation since they are essentially loose or free tails; they typically do not contain any DNA or head structures (some might contain a small amount of condensed chromatin). Again, a high prevalence, >20% relative to the sperm population, should be noted separately.

Teratozoospermia Index

Each morphologically abnormal spermatozoon will have at least one of the four types of abnormalities described above – or any combination of two to all four abnormalities. To reflect this, the Teratozoospermia Index (TZI) was introduced as an indication of the mean number of abnormalities (actually, defective regions) per abnormal spermatozoon [11–13,39,45,46].

Sterilizing Defects

In some men, persistent sperm morphology abnormalities are present as a consequence of genetic factors, such as the failure of the acrosome to develop causing the 'small round-head defect' or 'globozoospermia' defect (Figure 3.10 Plate 1E) [48,49]. These men are considered to be sterile as far as normal *in-vivo* conception is concerned. The condition can be overcome by using ICSI, but success rates are very low. Another example are men with the so-called 'short tail syndrome'. When observed, these conditions must be clearly noted on the report form.

Equipment and Disposable Materials

See also Appendix 2.

- Microscope with bright field illumination and at least three magnification options: a low power magnification (an objective of 10×, 15× or 20×); a higher power magnification option with a 40× objective, and a 100× oil immersion objective. The oil immersion 100× objective should be the highest quality plane-corrected objective available. Eyepieces should be 10×, 12.5× or 15× with wide field magnification.
- Eyepiece with a built-in micrometer (or eyepiece reticle)
- Tally counter, minimum of five channels
- Immersion oil
- Lens cleaning paper

Quality Control

In order to be able to use reference limits obtained from published studies, it is essential that each analyst is properly trained, that the laboratory perform regular Internal Quality Control, and that the laboratory participates in an EQC or EQA programme employing the same criteria, methods and standards as the centres that published the original data.

Sperm Morphology Evaluation Procedure

1. Scan the smear with a low power objective to observe the spreading of the spermatozoa in the smear, the staining quality, and the presence of round cells. If round cells are observed, move to the 40× objective to identify the type of round cells present.
2. Identify suitable areas for the performance of the sperm morphology evaluation.
3. When a suitable area is identified under low power, a small drop of immersion oil is placed on the slide where the light is shining through it, without removing the slide from the microscope stage.
4. Bring the oil immersion objective into place.
5. Sperm morphology evaluation should ideally be performed in more than one area to increase the accuracy of the evaluation. Experience has shown that in some cases a non-random distribution of sperm abnormalities can be present, and an unrepresentative evaluation might be obtained if this is not done.
6. Assess at least 200 spermatozoa [13]. Although it is preferable to count 200 spermatozoa twice to reduce counting error and variability, this may not always be practicable due to the quality of the smear or time constraints. According to WHO5 [51], when the diagnosis and treatment of the patient crucially depends on the percentage of morphological normal spermatozoa present, 200 spermatozoa should be assessed twice to increase the precision.
7. Record the morphological appearance of each spermatozoon as ideal or abnormal. Assign four buttons on the counter for each of the four types of defects (head, neck/midpiece, tail, and the presence of cytoplasmic residues). When a defect is counted, its button is pressed; if more than one defect is present, the buttons for each defect are pressed simultaneously. In this way all the defects of the spermatozoon will be tallied, but the abnormal spermatozoon will only be counted once.
8. If there is any uncertainty about the size of a spermatozoon (especially as too large) it should be measured with the aid of a micrometer eyepiece.

Calculations and Results

- The proportion of ideal spermatozoa is calculated by dividing the number of spermatozoa assessed as ideal by the total number of spermatozoa assessed. The result is given as an integer percentage (no decimal places).
- Concerning the abnormalities seen, while the total of ideal and abnormal cells will add up to the total number of spermatozoa assessed, the sum of all the defects will usually be greater than the total number of spermatozoa that were assessed.
- To calculate the TZI, the sum of all recorded defective regions is divided by the total number of abnormal spermatozoa in which they were counted (i.e. the total number of spermatozoa assessed – number of ideal spermatozoa). By convention, the TZI is reported to two decimal places, and since any given spermatozoon can have between one and four defective regions, the TZI result will always be between 1.00 and 4.00.

Interpretation of Results

The obtained results of the percentage of morphologically ideal (a.k.a. 'normal') spermatozoa, expressed as % ideal, can be used to classify the sperm morphology in the semen sample as being either 'normal' or 'abnormal' based on the lower reference limits as per the 2010 WHO manual, fifth edition ('WHO5') [51], with a lower reference limit of ≥4% morphological normal/ideal spermatozoa when the sperm morphology evaluation was performed according to the (Tygerberg) strict criteria. However, the recent WHO6 manual [12] urged shifting focus towards using 'decision limits' rather than reference ranges for interpreting semen analysis results, as discussed in Appendix 1 of this book.

This WHO5 value supersedes the previously defined poor, good and normal prognosis groups with cut-off values of ≤4%, 5–14% and ≥15%, respectively [47]. Without the aid of these prognostic groups this new, very low, lower reference limit for sperm morphology might not provide as strong a predictive value for fertility potential as originally reported when the (Tygerberg) strict criteria were introduced [47,52].

To still be able to obtain a strong prognosis based on the percentage of morphological ideal/normal spermatozoa, it is of the upmost importance that the holistic approach to sperm morphology assessment described above be followed. Furthermore, when a result falls below the WHO5 low cut-off limit value (<4% ideal normal) it can be of significant clinical importance to provide physicians with more detailed information on abnormal sperm patterns or abnormalities, allowing more informed decisions regarding ART treatment strategies [47].

Notes

1. Since the TZI is considered an important measure of human sperm morphology, it is recommended that standard sperm morphology assessments include recording of the four basic types of defects. For some reason the 1999 WHO Manual [11] used only three of the four abnormal categories to calculate the TZI, as cytoplasmic residues were excluded. The ESHRE manual [1] states that this is a wrong interpretation of the TZI, and recommended that the original TZI score be calculated according to the standard protocol as described in the 1992 WHO manual [45], with a clear indication that this earlier, correct definition has been used. Subsequent editions of the WHO manual [11,12], as well as ISO 23162 [13], all use the correct definition and calculation.

2. For evaluating sperm morphology, a microscope with good quality optics should be used, equipped with bright field Köhler illumination and a 100× oil immersion, non-phase contrast objective, giving a total magnification of at least 1000× but preferably 1250×.

3. The use of the highest possible magnification is important; if this is not used, only the most obvious abnormalities will be observed.

4. The objectives should be arranged on the microscope nosepiece in such a way that the low power objective is between the 40× objective and the 100× oil immersion objective. This allows for alternating between the different magnifications when scanning the smear and reduces the risk of accidentally turning the 40× objective into a drop of immersion oil.

5. If, for screening purposes, spermatozoa are only scored as ideal or abnormal, only two channels of the laboratory counter are used.

6. A brief overview of the possible future application of automated sperm morphology assessment using artificial intelligence (AI)-enhanced software is included towards the end of Chapter 6, *Computer-Aided Sperm Analysis*.

Semen Cytology from Stained Smears

Background

The evaluation of semen cytology is an important part of a semen analysis and is performed using the fixed and stained smear used for sperm morphology evaluation.

Principle

The Papanicolaou stain adapted for spermatozoa is also useful to identify round cells as leucocytes or immature germ cells.

Specimen

- The same stained and mounted slides as for sperm morphology assessment

Equipment

See also Appendix 2.

- Microscope with 10×, 40× and 100× objectives
- Coplin jar for fixation of smears
- Coplin jars or staining dishes for staining slides
- Staining dishes and racks, if required for the chosen staining method

Disposable Materials

- Microscope slides with frosted ends
- Coverslips, either 22 × 50 mm or 24 × 50 mm, #1 thickness
- Fixative (as per intended method), e.g. freshly-mixed 1:1 ethanol:diethyl ether (e.g. in a stoppered measuring cylinder)
- Stain(s) as per the intended method

Procedure

1. For the evaluation of semen cytology, i.e. the investigation for the presence of round cells, such as leucocytes, germinal epithelium cells (precursors), as well as micro-organisms, a thicker smear can be prepared.

2. A small drop of egg albumin can be added to the semen drop to assure a better adherence of the cellular matter to the slides or use poly-L-lysine coated slides.

3. The smears are fixed immediately in a 1:1 mixture of ethanol:diethyl ether and stained alongside the slides for sperm morphology evaluations.

4. The slides are screened at a low magnification (10× or 20× objective).

5. If any cells or organisms are observed, turn to the 40× objective to make a better identification.

6. Polymorphonuclear leucocytes (PMNs) are especially important. The importance of precursors or germinal epithelium cells in semen is not clear, although it might indicate an early stage spermatogenic dysfunction, presence of a varicocele, or any other type of testicular stress. The presence of these two types of round cells is recorded separately as the estimated number of cells per high power (40× objective) field.

Note: If one or more of these cells are observed per 40× objective (high power) field, a leucocyte peroxidase test should be performed.

Calculations and Results

- The presence of leucocytes (polymorphonuclear neutrophils) is expressed as number of cells/100 spermatozoa and, with help of the sperm concentration, as a concentration ($\times 10^6$/ml in semen).
- The presence of precursors (germinal epithelium cells) is expressed in the same way.

Interpretation of Results

While the presence of $\geq 1 \times 10^6$/ml white blood cells has been regarded by the WHO as leucocytospermia [11], the position taken in WHO6 [12] is that there is currently no evidence-based reference ranges for peroxidase-positive cells in semen from fertile men. However, pending additional evidence, the consensus value of 1×10^6 peroxidase-positive cells per ml has been retained as a threshold value for clinical significance. Although values greater than or equal to this value are considered abnormal, there is no known cut-off indicating when medical treatment of an infection is necessary. See also the section below on interpretation guidelines for identification of peroxidase-positive cells.

Identification of Peroxidase-Positive Cells

Principle

Inflammatory cells in semen, i.e. neutrophil, basophil and eosinophil granulocytes, can be identified cytochemically due to their containing peroxidase. This method uses a traditional histochemical procedure (the Endtz test) to identify the peroxidase enzyme that characterizes polymorphonuclear granulocytes [53]. However, it does not detect activated polymorphs which have released their granules or other types of leucocytes that do not contain peroxidase activity (e.g. lymphocytes). While this peroxidase cytochemical technique is the one most commonly used, the immunocytochemical approach (see Chapter 4) can provide more information. Only cells that contain peroxidase activity will stain brown, all other cells will counterstain pink (Figure 3.13).

Specimen

- Fresh, liquefied and well-mixed semen, ideally within 30–60 min after ejaculation

Equipment

See also Appendix 2.
- Microscope with 20× and 40× objective (bright field or phase contrast optics)
- Positive displacement pipetter, 0–50 µl or 0–100 µl, for taking the semen aliquot
- Air displacement pipetter 0–50 µl or 0–100 µl
- 75 × 25 mm (3" × 1") microscope slides and 22 × 22 mm coverslips
- Makler chamber

Disposable Materials

- Tips to match the air displacement pipetter
- Tips for the positive displacement pipetter
- Eppendorf tubes 1.5 ml

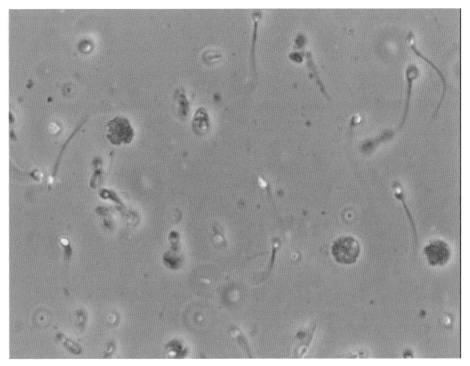

Figure 3.13 Appearance of brown stained peroxidase-positive cell (inflammatory cell) in semen under phase contrast optics (40× objective).

Reagents

Stock Solution
- Dissolve 125 mg benzidine in 50 ml of 96% (v/v) methanol
- Dissolve 150 mg cyanosine (phloxine) in 50 ml of distilled water
- Mix the benzidine and cyanosine solutions in a dark glass bottle
- Store at +4°C for up to six months

Working Solution
- Add 50 μl of hydrogen peroxide (6% or 20 volumes) to 1.0 ml of the stock solution
- Keep at ambient temperature
- Discard at the end of the workday

Calibration
No specific calibration is required.

Quality Control
If there is any doubt about the results, prepare a fresh working solution. Stock solution accidentally left out of the refrigerator or in bright light should be discarded.

Procedure

1. Mix 10 μl of liquefied semen and 10 μl of the working solution on a clean slide and cover with a 22 × 22 mm #1½ coverslip.
2. Examine under a 20× objective (use 1.5× intermediate magnification if available) using bright field optics. If more than one brown (peroxidase-positive) cell is seen per five fields, then proceed according to steps #3 to #5 below; if not, then discard the preparation and enter a value of zero on the Laboratory Report Form.
3. Mix 10 μl of liquefied semen and 10 μl of the working solution in a small Eppendorf tube.
4. Transfer 4.5 μl of the mixture onto a Makler chamber and position the cover glass carefully over the grid area, pressing down and rotating slightly so that inference fringes can be seen between the apposed glass surfaces at the four support pillars.
5. Examine the preparation under a 20× objective using bright-field optics. Count the number of peroxidase-positive (brown) cells in the entire ruled-grid area.

Calculations and Results

Divide the number of peroxidase-positive cells counted over the Makler chamber grid area by five to get their concentration in the original semen sample in millions/ml. Report the result with no more than one decimal place.

As per WHO recommendations, $\geq 1 \times 10^6$/ml peroxidase-positive cells is considered abnormal [11,12,51]. Recent studies indicate that even lower concentrations of leucocytes, between 0.2 and 0.5 × 10^6/ml, might be important markers for inflammatory disorders that can be significant in regard to a man's fertility potential [39,54–56], although other studies have found no relationship between leucocytes in semen and either other semen parameters or clinical signs of inflammatory disorders [57].

Notes

1. A benzidine-cyanosine stain is commercially available as the LeucoScreen™ kit from FertiPro (Beernem, Belgium).

Examination of Semen after Vasectomy

Introduction

After vasectomy, it is important to establish whether the surgical procedure has been successful, i.e. that the communication between the testis and the urethra has been completely severed. This is done by examining the ejaculate for the presence of spermatozoa. Since it takes some time to empty the male reproductive tract of spermatozoa, it is essential to wait and not start the semen investigation until three to four months after the surgery [58,59]. It is believed that it is important that the subject has regular ejaculations during the period before the investigation [60].

Specimen

- Fresh ejaculate (examination starting ideally 30 min after ejaculation)

Equipment

See also Appendix 2.
- As for general sperm concentration assessment
- Centrifuge
- Air displacement pipetter, 0–100 μl

Disposable Materials
- Centrifuge tubes, 15 ml, conical bottom, non-toxic to spermatozoa
- Tips for air displacement pipetter
- Microscope slides
- Coverslips, 22 × 22 mm, #1½ or #2 thickness

Calibration

No specific calibration is required except for the same microscope adjustments as for examining a wet preparation.

Quality Control

The method is semi-quantitative only, aimed at establishing whether any spermatozoa are present in the ejaculate; no quality control is needed beyond the training required for working with wet preparations and the assessment of sperm concentration.

Procedure
1. Make a wet preparation and scan through the entire area of the coverslip.
2. If no spermatozoa are detected in the wet preparation, the entire semen sample should be centrifuged at approximately 1000 g for 20 min.
3. After centrifugation, most of the supernatant seminal plasma is removed and the sperm pellet is re-suspended in the remaining minimum volume of seminal plasma supernatant.
4. A new wet preparation is made from the resuspended pellet and covered with a 22 × 22 mm coverslip.
5. Scan through the entire area of the coverslip (at least 400 fields) using phase contrast optics at a magnification of 400×.

Calculations and Results

If motile or immotile spermatozoa are identified when the whole area of a coverslip (at least 400 fields under a 22 × 22 mm coverslip) has been scanned, the numbers of motile and immotile spermatozoa are recorded on the semen specimen report form.

Interpretation Guidelines
1. In general, it is required that a subject produce two or three consecutive complete ejaculates without any detectable spermatozoa to be pronounced as 'clear'. The persistent presence of spermatozoa months after vasectomy, combined with regular ejaculations can, in some cases, be due to partial surgical failure or possible re-canalization [61]. Reappearance of spermatozoa after repeated absence might be due to re-canalization of the vas deferens [62].
2. Another, sperm-independent, analysis for vasectomy success can be the assessment of epididymis-specific neutral alpha-glucosidase (NAG) [63]. Consequently, the examination of one ejaculate at least three months post-vasectomy with findings of no (motile) spermatozoa and an insignificant level of NAG would constitute two independent signs of blocked passage, and may be sufficient to conclude that the vasectomy has been successful.

Notes

Morphology staining of the smeared pellet is not suitable due to the small, but in these cases significant, risk of contamination with spermatozoa from the staining solutions.

References

1. Kvist U, Björndahl L, eds. *Manual on Basic Semen Analysis*. Oxford: Oxford University Press, 2002.

2. Mortimer D. *Practical Laboratory Andrology*. Oxford: Oxford University Press, 1994.

3. Pound N, Javed MH, Ruberto C, et al. Duration of sexual arousal predicts semen parameters for masturbatory ejaculates. *Physiol Behav* 2002; **76**: 685–9.

4. Zavos PM, Goodpasture JC. Clinical improvements of specific seminal deficiencies via intercourse with a seminal collection device versus masturbation. *Fertil Steril* 1989; **51**: 190–3.

5. Kamischke A, Nieschlag E. Treatment of retrograde ejaculation and anejaculation. *Hum Reprod Update* 1999; **5**: 448–74.

6. MacLeod J, Gold RZ. The male factor in fertility and infertility. V. Effect of continence on semen quality. *Fertil Steril* 1952; **3**: 297–315.

7. Carlsen E, Andersson AM, Petersen JH, Skakkebaek NE. History of febrile illness and variation in semen quality. *Hum Reprod* 2003; **18**: 2089–92.

8. Cooper TG, Brazil C, Swan SH, Overstreet JW. Ejaculate volume is seriously underestimated when semen is pipetted or decanted into cylinders from the collection vessel. *J Androl* 2007; **28**: 1–4.

9. Björndahl L, Kvist U. Sequence of ejaculation affects the spermatozoon as a carrier and its message. *Reprod Biomed Online* 2003; 7: 440–8.

10. MacLeod J, Gold RZ. The male factor in fertility and infertility. III. An analysis of motile activity in the spermatozoa of 1000 fertile men and 1000 men in infertile marriage. *Fertil Steril* 1951; **2**: 187–204.

11. World Health Organization. *WHO Laboratory Manual for the Examination of Human Semen and Sperm-Cervical Mucus Interactions*, 4th edn. Cambridge: Cambridge University Press, 1999.

12. World Health Organization. *WHO Laboratory Manual for the Examination and Processing of Human Semen*, 6th edn. Geneva: World Health Organization, 2021.

13. International Organization for Standardization. *ISO 23162:2021 Basic Semen Examination – Specification and Test Methods*. Geneva: International Organization for Standardization, 2021.

14. Mortimer D. Laboratory standards in routine clinical andrology. *Reprod Med Review* 1994; **3**: 97–111.

15. Sifer C, Sasportes T, Barraud V, et al. World Health Organization grade 'a' motility and zona-binding test accurately predict IVF outcome for mild male factor and unexplained infertilities. *Hum Reprod* 2005; **20**: 2769–75.

16. Verheyen G, Tournaye H, Staessen C, et al. Controlled comparison of conventional in-vitro fertilization and intracytoplasmic sperm injection in patients with asthenozoospermia. *Hum Reprod* 1999; **14**: 2313–19.

17. Barratt CLR, Björndahl L, Menkveld R, Mortimer D. The ESHRE Special Interest Group for Andrology Basic Semen Analysis Course: a continued focus on accuracy, quality, efficiency and clinical relevance. *Hum Reprod* 2011; **26**: 3207–12.

18. Mortimer D, Shu MA, Tan R. Standardization and quality control of sperm concentration and sperm motility counts in semen analysis. *Hum Reprod* 1986; **1**: 299–303.

19. Mortimer D, Shu MA, Tan R, Mortimer ST. A technical note on diluting semen for the haemocytometric determination of sperm concentration. *Hum Reprod* 1989; **4**: 166–8.

20. Kirkman Brown J, Björndahl L. Evaluation of a disposable plastic Neubauer counting chamber for semen analysis. *Fertil Steril* 2009; **91**: 627–31.

21. Zuvela E, Matson P. Performance of four chambers to measure sperm concentration: results from an external quality assurance programme. *Reprod Biomed Online* 2020; **41**: 671–8.

22. Mortimer D. A technical note on the assessment of human sperm vitality using eosin-nigrosin staining. *Reprod Biomed Online* 2020; **40**: 851–5.

23. Björndahl L, Söderlund I, Johansson S, et al. Why the WHO recommendations for eosin-nigrosin staining techniques for human sperm vitality assessment must change. *J Androl* 2004; **25**: 671–8.

24. Björndahl L, Söderlund I, Kvist U. Evaluation of the one-step eosin-nigrosin staining technique for human sperm vitality assessment. *Hum Reprod* 2003; **18**: 813–16.

25. Hühner M. Methods of examining for spermatozoa in the diagnosis and treatment of sterility. *Int J Surg* 1921; **34**: 91–100.

26. Cary WH. Sterility diagnosis: The study of sperm cell migration in female secretion and interpretation of findings. *NY State J Med* 1930; **30**: 131–6.

27. Cary WH, Hotchkiss RS. Semen appraisal. A differential stain that advances the study of cell morphology. *JAMA* 1934; **102**: 587–90.

28. Moench GL, Holt H. Biometrical studies of head lengths of human spermatozoa. *J Lab Clin Med* 1932; **17**: 297–316.

29. Menkveld R, Van Zyl JA, Kotze T, Joubert G. Possible changes in male fertility over a 15-year period. *Arch Androl* 1986; **17**: 143–4.

30. Mortimer D. Selectivity of sperm transport in the female genital tract. In: Cohen J, Hendry WF, eds. *Spermatozoa, Antibodies and Infertility*. Oxford & London: Blackwell Scientific Publications, 1978.

31. Mortimer D. Sperm form and function: Beauty is in the eye of the beholder. In: van der Horst G, Franken D, Bornman R, et al., eds. *Proceedings of the 9th International Symposium on Spermatology*. Bologna: Monduzzi Editore, 2002.

32. Holt WV, Fazeli A. Do sperm possess a molecular passport? Mechanistic insights into sperm selection in the female reproductive tract. *Mol Hum Reprod* 2015; **21**: 491–501.

33. Kölle S. Transport, distribution and elimination of mammalian sperm following natural mating and insemination. *Reprod Dom Anim* 2015; **50**: 2–6.

34. Miller DJ. The epic journey of sperm through the female reproductive tract. *Animal* 2018; **12 Suppl 1**: S110–20.

35. Shojaei Saadi HA, van Riemsdijk E, Dance AL, et al. Proteins associated with critical sperm functions and sperm head shape are differentially expressed in morphologically abnormal bovine sperm induced by scrotal insulation. *J Proteomics* 2013; **82**: 64–80.

36. Menkveld R. *An investigation of environmental influences on spermatogenesis and semen parameters*. PhD Dissertation, Faculty of Medicine, University of Stellenbosch, South Africa, 1987.

37. Menkveld R, Stander FS, Kotze TJ, et al. The evaluation of morphological characteristics of human spermatozoa according to stricter criteria. *Hum Reprod* 1990; **5**: 586–92.

38. Coetzee K, Kruge TF, Lombard CJ. Predictive value of normal sperm morphology: a structured literature review. *Hum Reprod Update* 1998; **4**: 73–82.

39. Menkveld R. The basic semen analysis. In: Oehninger S, Kruger TF, eds. *Male Infertility*. London: Informa Healthcare, 2007, 141–70.

40. Papanicolaou GN. A new procedure for staining vaginal smears. *Science* 1942; **95**: 438–9.

41. Oettlé EE. Using a new acrosome stain to evaluate sperm morphology. *Vet Med* 1986; **81**: 263–6.

42. Henkel R, Schreiber G, Sturmhoefel A, et al. Comparison of three staining methods for the morphological evaluation of human spermatozoa. *Fertil Steril* 2008; **89**: 449–55.

43. van der Horst, G, Maree L. *SpermBlue*: a new universal stain for human and animal sperm which is also amenable to automated sperm morphology analysis. *Biotech Histochem* 2009; **84**: 299–308.

44. Maree L, du Plessis SS, Menkveld R, van der Horst G. Morphometric dimensions of the human sperm head depend on the staining method used. *Hum Reprod* 2010; **25**: 1369–82.

45. World Health Organization. *WHO Laboratory Manual for the Examination of Human Semen and Sperm-Cervical Mucus Interactions*, 3rd edn. Cambridge: Cambridge University Press, 1992.

46. Mortimer D, Menkveld R. Sperm morphology assessment – Historical perspectives and current opinions. *J Androl* 2001; **22**: 192–205.

47. Menkveld R. Clinical significance of the low normal sperm morphology value as proposed in the fifth edition of the *WHO Laboratory Manual for the Examination and Processing of Human Semen*. *Asian J Androl* 2010; **12**: 47–58.

48. Mortimer D. The functional anatomy of the human spermatozoon: relating ultrastructure and function. *Mol Hum Reprod* 2018; **24**: 567–92.

49. Oettlé EE, Menkveld R, Swanson RJ. Photographs with interpretations. In: Menkveld R, Oettlé EE, Kruger TF, et al., eds. *Atlas of Human Sperm Morphology*. Baltimore: Williams & Wilkins, 1991, 15–65.

50. Cooper TG, Yeung CH, Fetic S, et al. Cytoplasmic droplets are normal structures of human sperm but are not well preserved by routine procedures for assessing sperm morphology. *Hum Reprod* 2004; **19**: 2283–8.

51. World Health Organization. *WHO Laboratory Manual for the Examination and Processing of Human Semen*, 5th edn. Geneva: World Health Organization, 2010.

52. Kruger TF, Menkveld R, Stander FSH, et al. Sperm morphological features as a prognostic factor in in vitro fertilization. *Fertil Steril* 1986; **46**: 1118–23.

53. Endtz AW. A rapid staining method for differentiating granulocytes from 'germinal cells' in Papanicolaou-stained semen. *Acta Cytol* 1974; **18**: 2–7.

54. Wolff H. The biologic significance of white blood cells in semen. *Fertil Steril* 1995; **63**: 1143–57.

55. Lackner J, Schatzl G, Horvath S, et al. Value of counting white blood cells (WBC) in semen samples to predict the presence of bacteria. *Eur Urol* 2006; **49**: 148–52; discussion 52–3.

56. Punab M, Loivukene K, Kermes K, Mandar R. The limit of leucocytospermia from the microbiological viewpoint. *Andrologia* 2003; **35**: 271–8.

57. Rodin DM, Larone D, Goldstein M. Relationship between semen cultures, leukospermia, and semen analysis in men undergoing fertility evaluation. *Fertil Steril* 2003; **79 Suppl 3**: 1555–8.

58. Bedford JM, Zelikovsky G. Viability of spermatozoa in the human ejaculate after vasectomy. *Fertil Steril* 1979; **32**: 460–3.

59. Lewis EL, Brazil CK, Overstreet JW. Human sperm function in the ejaculate following vasectomy. *Fertil Steril* 1984; **42**: 895–8.

60. Jouannet P, David G. Evolution of the properties of semen immediately following vasectomy. *Fertil Steril* 1978; **29**: 435–41.

61. Hancock P, Woodward BJ, Muneer A, Kirkman-Brown JC. 2016 Laboratory guidelines for postvasectomy semen analysis: Association of Biomedical Andrologists, the British Andrology Society and the British Association of Urological Surgeons. *J Clin Pathol* 2016; **69**: 655–60.

62. Breitinger MC, Roszkowski EH, Bauermeister AJ, Rosenthal AA. Duplicate vas deferens encountered during inguinal hernia repair: a case report and literature review. *Case Rep Surg* 2016; **2016**: 8324925.

63. Cooper TG, Yeung CH, Nashan D, Jockenhovel F, Nieschlag E. Improvement in the assessment of human epididymal function by the use of inhibitors in the assay of alpha-glucosidase in seminal plasma. *Int J Androl* 1990; **13**: 297–305.

Chapter 4

Extended Semen Analysis

Antisperm Antibodies

Men (and women) with antisperm antibodies ('ASABs') have reduced fertility [1] and hence testing should be mandatory for all subfertile men [2]. ASABs on spermatozoa will interfere with normal cell function, e.g. penetration into cervical mucus, capacitation, the acrosome reaction and fertilization [3–6]. However, the presence of ASABs is not an absolute indicator of subfertility, since even men with high levels of ASABs can be fertile [7]. Although clinical data are limited, at least 50% of the motile spermatozoa need to be coated with antibodies (assessed using bead-based mixed antiglobulin reaction ('MAR') methodology) before a test is considered to be clinically significant [2]. Recent data has shown a significantly lower natural live birth rate in women whose partners were 100% MAR positive *vs* 50–99% MAR positive [8]. In order to determine if ASABs are interfering with sperm function, the consensus of opinion is that when these tests are positive, additional testing, e.g. sperm-cervical interaction tests, should be done [9] (see Chapter 8).

Although there are correlations between the presence and level of ASABs with specific characteristics of semen, e.g. men with antibodies have reduced sperm motility and higher levels of agglutination, these correlations are relatively weak and as such cannot be used to pre-screen which men should/should not be tested for ASABs [10,11].

There remains considerable controversy surrounding the testing of ASABs and their role in fertility [12–14]. Primarily, this is because there is still no clear information, despite considerable effort, as to the nature and identity of the antigens on the sperm surface that interfere with the reproductive process. Consequently, the testing that is performed detects antibodies on or to spermatozoa, but these antibodies may have no real functional significance. In addition, as a result of the lack of clarity of the nature of the antigens, the testing for ASABs remains in its infancy and hence results need to be interpreted with caution. Historically, testing used agglutination and cytotoxicity assays, but now direct testing of the spermatozoa themselves, most often using the MAR test, is employed.

Antisperm antibodies in semen belong almost exclusively to two immunoglobulin classes: IgA and IgG. There is evidence that IgA antibodies, particularly in the cases of men with vasovasostomy, have greater clinical importance than do IgG antibodies [15], although for subfertile men who have not had a vasectomy there are no clear data to suggest IgA is more significant than IgG. IgM antibodies, because of their large molecular size, are rarely found in semen – but if they are, then they should be treated seriously as possible evidence of trauma within the male tract. The clinical significance of the location of where the antibodies bind to the spermatozoa (i.e. to the head, midpiece or tail) is also unclear, although binding restricted to the tail-tip is not associated with impaired fertility and can be present in fertile men [2,3].

The primary screening test for ASABs is performed on the fresh semen sample using the mixed antiglobulin reaction (MAR) test. For these tests to be valid, at least 200 motile spermatozoa must be available for counting. The results from the different testing reagents do not always agree. Additionally, data from proficiency testing shows some difficulties in classifying a positive *vs* a negative ASAB test [16], even when using the same method, e.g. indirect MAR [17].

Methods for traditional tests for sperm agglutinating antibodies (e.g. the Friberg 'tray agglutination test' or 'TAT') and sperm immobilizing antibodies (e.g. the Isojima 'sperm immobilization test' or 'SIT') have not been provided here. Detailed protocols for these techniques can be found elsewhere [5].

Outline of Testing Methods

Two different types of testing are used: **_direct testing_**, whereby the sperm sample itself is tested, and **_indirect testing_**, where reproductive tract fluids (seminal plasma, follicular fluid, cervical mucus) or serum are tested. In indirect testing, the antibodies in these fluids are adsorbed onto prepared (i.e. seminal plasma free) donor spermatozoa, and these spermatozoa then tested for antibody binding in a direct test format.

In both cases, the beads/particles adhere to the motile and immotile spermatozoa that have surface-bound antibodies (or have adsorbed them), and the percentage of motile spermatozoa with beads bound is recorded.

Direct MAR Test

Principle

In the MAR test a 'bridging' antibody (anti-IgG or -IgA) is used to attach the antibody-coated beads to unwashed seminal spermatozoa bearing surface IgG or IgA. The direct IgG and IgA MAR tests are performed by mixing fresh, untreated semen separately with latex particles (or prepared erythrocytes) coated with human IgG or IgA. To this suspension is added a mono-specific anti-human-IgG or anti-human IgA, and the formation of mixed agglutinates between particles and motile spermatozoa indicates the presence of IgG and IgA antibodies on the spermatozoa. As an internal control, agglutination between beads serves as a positive control for antibody-antigen recognition.

While the protocol uses products from FertiPro (Beernem, Belgium), other, less widely used commercial variants of the MAR test include _MarScreen_® and _Immunospheres_, both of which have IgG, IgA and IgM tests (both products are now owned by Scopescreen Inc, Brighton, MI, USA; see www.scopescreen.com/products/); _MarScreen_® uses coloured latex beads for the different isotypes.

Specimen

Freshly ejaculated human semen which has liquefied.

Equipment

- Microscope (phase contrast optics, maximum total magnification 400×) with 37°C heated stage
- A 37°C temperature-controlled incubator
- Humidity chamber for incubating tests
- Pipettes for 1–20 µl volumes

Disposable Materials

- Clean glass slides 3" × 1" (75 × 25 mm)
- Coverslips 22 × 22 mm, #1½ thickness

Reagents

- _SpermMar_ commercial test kit (FertiPro NV, Beernem, Belgium). Reagents must be stored at 2° to 8°C when not in use and are stable for 12 months from the date of manufacturing; do not freeze. For use, allow the reagents to warm to ambient temperature and mix each vial thoroughly before each test.

Calibration

None required.

Quality Control

Tests should be run with controls. These can include ASAB-positive semen and ASAB-negative semen. This semen can be provided by men with and without ASABs, as detected by previous direct MAR testing. Positive spermatozoa can be produced by incubating washed spermatozoa with seminal plasma known to contain antibodies (see Indirect MAR Test, below). Alternatively, positive and negative controls can be obtained from commercial companies, e.g. FertiPro and Scopescreen Inc (see above).

Procedure

For the IgG Test

1. Place 3.5 µl drops of (a) unwashed fresh semen, (b) IgG-coated latex particles and (c) antiserum to IgG next to each other on a clean microscope slide.
2. Mix the semen and latex particles drops, then mix in the antiserum drop.
3. Apply a 22 × 22 mm coverslip to provide a depth of approximately 20 µm and place the slide in a humid chamber to settle at room temperature (2–3 min).

For the IgA Test

1. Place 3.5 µl drops of (a) unwashed fresh semen and (b) IgA-coated latex particles next to each other on a clean microscope slide.
2. Mix the semen and latex particles drops.
3. Apply a 22 × 22 mm coverslip to provide a depth of approximately 20 µm and place the slide in a humid chamber to settle at room temperature (2–3 min).

For Either Test

4. Examine the wet preparation under a phase contrast microscope at 200–400× magnification (bright field optics can be used with coloured beads). If spermatozoa have antibodies present on their surface, they will have latex beads adhering to them (Figure 4.1).

Calculations and Results

Motile spermatozoa with a few or even a group of particles attached are classed as positive. In the absence of coating antibodies, the spermatozoa will be seen swimming freely between the particles. It is important to score moving spermatozoa as a spermatozoon may be immotile and have beads in close proximity

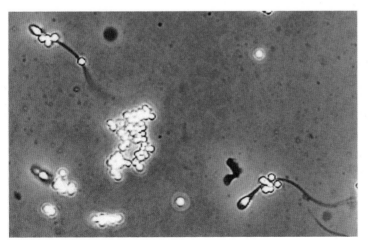

Figure 4.1 Example of beads binding to spermatozoa in an antisperm antibody test.

(false negative). In some circumstances, the motile spermatozoa will have beads attached but not show forward progressive movement; such cells should be regarded as positive binding. At least 200 motile spermatozoa should be counted and the percentage of the motile spermatozoa that have particles attached is calculated. Record the class (IgG or IgA) and the site of binding of the latex particles to the spermatozoa (head, mid-piece, tail).

Interpretation Guidelines

The presence of ASABs is not an absolute indicator of subfertility. At least 50% of the motile spermatozoa need to be coated with antibodies before a test is considered to be clinically significant [2].

Notes

None required.

Indirect MAR Test

Principle

The indirect MAR test is used to detect anti-sperm antibodies in heat-inactivated, sperm-free fluids (serum, seminal plasma or bromelain-solubilized cervical mucus). Antibody-free spermatozoa bind ASABs from the test fluid and are then assessed as in the direct MAR test.

Specimen(s)

- *Cervical mucus:* Must be pre-treated (solubilized) using bromelain. Dilute mucus 1+1 with 10 IU bromelain/ml in sterile water, stir and incubate at 37°C for 10 min. When liquefaction is complete, centrifuge at 2000 *g* for 10 min and use the supernatant.
- Inactivate any complement in the fluid (serum, seminal plasma or cervical mucus) by heating at 56°C for 30–45 min.
- Dilute the heat-inactivated sample to be tested, e.g. 1+15 for the IgG-test and 1+3 for the IgA test in swim-up medium, e.g. HEPES-buffered cultured medium, ideally without albumin (unless verified as ASAB-free) or patient serum.

Equipment

- Microscope (phase contrast optics, maximum total magnification 400×) with 37°C heated stage
- A 37°C temperature-controlled incubator
- Water bath (for inactivating complement)
- Humidity chamber for incubating tests
- Pipettes for 1–200 μl volumes

Disposable Materials

- Clean glass slides 3" × 1" (75 × 25 mm)
- Coverslips 22 × 22 mm, #1½ thickness

Reagents

- *SpermMar* commercial test (FertiPro, Beernem, Belgium). Reagents must be stored at 2° to 8°C when not in use and are stable for 12 months from the date of manufacturing; do not freeze. For use, allow the reagents to warm to ambient temperature and mix each vial thoroughly before each test.
- Bromelain (EC 3.4.22.32) for cervical mucus solubilization

- HEPES-buffered medium for dilutions, e.g. Earle's Balanced Salt Solution ('EBSS': 116.4 mM NaCl, 5.4 mM KCl, 1.8 mM $CaCl_2$, 1 mM $MgCl_2$, 5.5 mM glucose, 19 mM Na lactate, 0.81 mM $MgSO_4$, 10 mM HEPES)
- *ASAB-free donor spermatozoa:* Prepare motile donor spermatozoa from a man lacking ASABs using density gradient centrifugation (see Chapter 9). Adjust the final motile sperm concentration to 20×10^6/ml in a HEPES-buffered medium with a maximum of 10 mg/ml of HSA that is known to be negative for ASABs (not serum).

Quality Control

Tests should be run with controls. These can include ASAB-positive seminal plasma/serum and ASAB-negative seminal plasma/serum. This seminal plasma/serum can be provided by men with and without ASABs, as detected by previous direct MAR testing. Positive spermatozoa can be produced by incubating washed spermatozoa with seminal plasma known to contain antibodies (see Indirect MAR Test, below). Alternatively, positive and negative controls can be obtained from commercial companies, e.g. FertiPro and Scopescreen Inc (see above).

Procedure

1. *Incubation of donor spermatozoa with fluid to be tested*
   a) Mix 100 μl sperm suspension with 100 μl diluted fluid to be tested.
   b) Incubate at 37°C for 1 h.
   c) Wash the spermatozoa by adding 2 ml HEPES-buffered media, mix well and centrifuge for 10 min at 400 *g*.
   d) Remove the supernatant with a pipette.
   e) Repeat the washing step on the pellet.
   f) Remove the supernatant with a pipette and resuspend the sperm pellet in 50 μl medium by gentle pipetting or low speed vortexing.
2. *Procedure for the Indirect MAR Test*
   Perform the test as described for the Direct MAR Test using the pre-incubated donor spermatozoa instead of semen.

Calculations and Results

Motile spermatozoa with a few or even a group of particles attached are classed as positive. In the absence of coating antibodies, the spermatozoa will be seen swimming freely between the particles. It is important to score moving spermatozoa as a spermatozoon may be immotile and have beads in close proximity (false negative). In some circumstances, the motile spermatozoa will have beads attached but not show forward progressive movement; such cells should be regarded as positive binding. At least 200 motile spermatozoa should be counted and the percentage of the motile spermatozoa that have particles attached is calculated. Record the class (IgG or IgA) and the site of binding of the latex particles to the spermatozoa (head, mid-piece, tail).

Interpretation Guidelines

The presence of ASABs is not an absolute indicator of subfertility since cases even with high levels of ASABs can be fertile. At least 50% of the motile spermatozoa need to be coated with antibodies before a test is considered to be clinically significant. In order to determine if the ASABs are interfering with sperm function, the consensus of opinion is that when these tests are positive (>50% sperm binding) additional tests (sperm-cervical mucus contact test, sperm-cervical mucus capillary tube test) should be done (see Chapter 8) [2].

Microbiological Examination of the Semen Sample

Bacterial Infections

There is increasing evidence of a seminal microbiome, the composition resulting from the various parts of the reproductive tract, and the major part of the microbiota may not have any impact on fertility [18,19]. However, bacterial infection of the male reproductive tract can affect spermatogenesis and mature spermatozoa, as well as the secretory function of the accessory glands, and can lead to subfertility [20–22]. The site of infection varies with type of bacteria, and the pathogens can be sexually transmitted.

Recent reviews indicate that there is no difference in the prevalence of *Chlamydia trachomatis* between fertile and infertile men, and it has no significant impact on semen parameters [21,22].

Bacteria that are associated with impairment of semen parameters and/or sperm function include, among others: *Pseudomonas aeruginosa*, *Ureaplasma urealyticum* and species of *Staphylococcus*, *Mycoplasma* and *Enterococcus* and *Prevotella*; evidence regarding pathogenicity of *Escherichia coli* is equivocal, and *Lactobacillus* may have a protective effect [21,22].

The underlying mechanisms are unclear, but proinflammatory cytokines, bacterial toxins, and oxidative stress leading to DNA-damage and induction of apoptosis, may play important roles [23]. The impact of bacterial infections on male infertility is still unclear, and conflicting results might be due to different effects of various bacterial strains, but also to limitations of the studies.

Examination of the Ejaculate

Infections can be asymptomatic, and signs of infection are not always observed by microscopic examination of the ejaculate. However, both macroscopic and microscopic assessment of semen can reveal evidence of infection. Such observations are:

- Brown or reddish colour of semen due to the presence of erythrocytes
- High semen volume
- A strong, putrescent smell
- A large number of microorganisms
- Excessive numbers of leukocytes ($>1 \times 10^6$/ml)
- A high proportion of dead spermatozoa
- Most of the spermatozoa are covered by antisperm antibodies

Biochemical analyses of the ejaculate can also reflect infection. Examples are:

- A decrease in the secretion of markers of accessory gland function
- Excessive generation of reactive oxygen species (ROS) due to a high amount of leukocytes
- Increased levels of various immunoglobulins, cytokines and growth factors

Upon suspicion of inflammation, microbiological evaluation of the semen sample should be performed by a laboratory specialized in the field. The patient must be instructed to wash his hands and penis before masturbation, and the specimen should be collected in a sterile container. Sterile pipettes and pipette tips must be used upon withdrawal of samples or when preparing dilutions. The time before microbiological culturing of the semen specimen should be as short as possible, and not exceed 3 hours.

Viral Infections

Sexually transmitted viruses like human immunodeficiency virus (HIV), cytomegalovirus (CMV), human papillomavirus (HPV), herpes simplex virus (HSV), human herpes virus (HHV) and hepatitis B virus (HBV) have been detected in human semen [24,25]. Furthermore, the presence of Zika virus (ZIKV) and Ebola virus (EBOV) in semen has been reported as well as cases of sexual transmission of these viruses. Chronically infecting DNA viruses and retroviruses may be present in the reproductive tract throughout life, whereas RNA viruses causing an acute infection are usually present in semen for a short period. The negative impact of mumps orthorubulavirus (MuV) infection on sperm parameters and male fertility is well documented, and HSV and HPV are found to be associated with abnormal sperm parameters [26,27]. HIV-1 infection in advanced stage is associated with impaired sperm parameters. The clinical implications of the viral infections for fertility status are, however, not clear. The presence of SARS-CoV-2 in semen has been investigated, and while SARS-CoV-2 was detected in some studies, the reports are conflicting [28–31].

Detection of virus in semen is largely achieved by the use of polymerase-chain-reaction and deep-sequencing approaches.

Details of the microbiology, diagnosis and treatment of infections, as well as the handling and preparation of infectious specimens are described in detail in the monograph by Elder, Baker & Ribes [20].

Notes

1. Lysozymes and zinc in the seminal plasma have antibacterial properties, and a negative bacterial culture does not rule out an infection.
2. Microorganisms in semen can be due to contaminants from the patient's skin or from the air, thus having no clinical relevance.

Leukocytes in Semen

Semen contains a number of different types of non-sperm cells. These can be classed either as leukocytes or non-leukocytes, the latter consisting of primarily germ cells, e.g. spermatids. Leukocytes, predominantly neutrophils, are present in almost all human ejaculates [32–34].

There is a considerable controversy about the role of leukocytes in semen. The initial concept was that leukocytes were a negative factor for fertility and a clear sign of infection. However, several large studies have revealed there to be no significant relationship between either the types or concentration of leukocytes (determined using monoclonal antibody staining) and semen parameters or, more importantly, in-vivo conception [32–34]. A systematic review and metanalysis examining the relationship between leucocytospermia and ART outcome concluded that there was no relationship to fertilization rate or pregnancy rate [35]. However, leukocytes do produce significant amounts of reactive oxygen species which, particularly when limited antioxidant protective mechanisms are available, can be highly detrimental to sperm function [34], e.g. in washed sperm preparations.

Surprisingly, there is no consensus on what is a 'normal' number of leukocytes in semen. There are data on mean levels in infertility clinic patients (390,000/ml ejaculate) [30] but limited information is available from fertile control subjects. The WHO reference limit is set at 1×10^6 leukocytes/ml as the threshold for leukocytospermia [36], but the evidence to support this value is relatively weak, with some authors believing it to be too low while others say it is too high. Historically, men with $>1 \times 10^6$ leukocytes/per ml in semen were thought to have a significant likelihood of a genital infection compared to men with $<1 \times 10^6$ leukocytes/ml of semen [37]. However, with more sophisticated modern methods to detect subclinical genital infections, this cut-off point is of little value [38,39].

Leukocytes can be detected and quantified in stained preparations otherwise made for morphological examination (Papanicolaou staining procedure). In such preparations, leukocytes can be differentiated from spermatids and spermatocytes by differences in staining coloration, as well as by the distinctive nuclear size and shape (Figure 4.2). However, the more accurate way to detect leukocytes is to use specific assays, such as the detection of peroxidase positive cells (see Chapter 3) and the use of monoclonal antibodies against leukocyte-specific antigens [32,40].

Immunocytochemical Staining for the Pan-Leukocyte Antigen CD45

Principle

The principle is that the pan-leukocyte monoclonal antibody recognizes the leukocytes. Visualization is via a secondary antibody. Leukocytes are stained reddish brown.

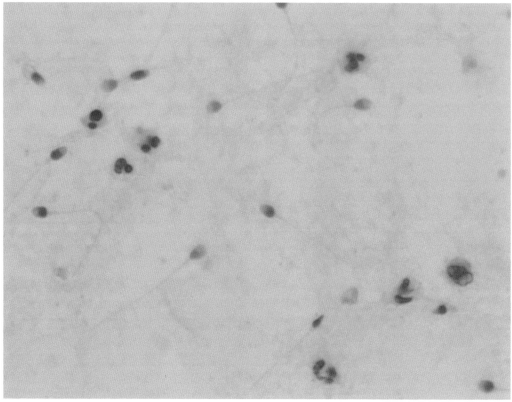

Figure 4.2 Example of leukocytes stained with Papanicolaou.

Specimen
- Prepared semen samples

Equipment
- Bright field microscope (at least 200× total magnification) with built-in eyepiece grid reticle/graticule
- Air displacement pipettes
- Tally counter
- Centrifuge

Disposable Materials
- Clean glass slides 3" × 1" (75 × 25 mm)
- Coverslips 22 × 22 mm, #1½ thickness

Reagents
- Dulbecco phosphate-buffered saline (PBS)
- Tris-buffered saline: Dissolve 60.55g Tris base and 85.20g NaCl in ~800ml reagent water; adjust to pH 8.6 using 1 N HCl and then make up to 1000 ml with reagent water
- Haematoxylin
- Tetramisole (levamisole) 1.0 M: Dissolve 2.4 g (-)-tetramisole.HCl in 10 ml purified water
- Substrate: To 9.7 ml of pH 8.2 Tris buffer add 2 mg naphthol AS-MX phosphate, 0.2 ml dimethylformamide and 0.1 ml of 1.0 M tetramisole; then add 10 mg Fast Red TR salt and filter just before use

- Fixative: Acetone alone or mix 95 ml acetone and 95 ml absolute methanol and add 10 ml 37% (v/v) formaldehyde
- Primary antibody: A mouse monoclonal antibody against the common leukocyte antigen (CD45), widely available commercially (e.g. Santa Cruz Biotechnology Inc; see www.scbt.com/search?Ntt=cd45)
- Secondary antibody: Anti-mouse rabbit immunoglobulins; the dilution used will depend on antibody titre and source (e.g. 1:25 dilution of the Z259 antibody manufactured by DAKO Corp)
- Alkaline phosphatase:anti-alkaline phosphatase complex (APAAP): Widely available commercially (e.g. Sigma Aldrich)

Calibration
The primary calibration is in calculating the final concentration of leukocytes (see below).

Quality Control
For QC purposes, peripheral blood leukocytes can be used. These cells will stain with the pan leukocyte marker. As a negative control the primary antibody can be omitted.

Procedure
1. *Preparing the spermatozoa:*
   a) Mix an aliquot of liquefied semen (approximately 0.5 ml) with 5× the volume of phosphate-buffered saline (PBS) in a centrifuge tube.
   b) Centrifuge at 500 *g* for 5 min at room temperature, remove the supernatant and suspend the sperm pellet in 5× its volume of PBS.
   c) Centrifuge at 500 *g* for 5 min at room temperature.
   d) Repeat this procedure and suspend the pellet in PBS to the original volume of the semen sample.
   e) Dilute the suspension 2–5× further in PBS depending on the concentration of spermatozoa.
2. *Preparing the sperm smears:*
   a) Prepare two smears of 5 µl aliquots of the suspension on clean glass slides and allow to air-dry. These can be fixed and stained immediately or wrapped in foil after fixing and stored at -70°C for later processing (up to several weeks).
   b) Fix the air-dried cells in absolute acetone for 10 min (or the acetone/methanol/formaldehyde fixative for 90 s).
   c) Wash twice with TBS and allow to drain.
3. *Antibody labeling:*
   a) Cover each aliquot of fixed cells with 1 µl primary monoclonal antibody and incubate for 30 min in a humidified chamber at room temperature.
   b) Wash the slides twice with TBS and allow to drain.
   c) Cover the cells on the smear with 10 µl secondary antibody and incubate for 30 min in a humidified chamber at room temperature.
   d) Wash twice with TBS and allow to drain.
   e) Add 10 µl APAAP to each smear.
   f) Incubate for 1 h in a humidified chamber at room temperature.
   g) Wash twice in TBS and allow to drain.
   h) Incubate with 10 µl alkaline phosphatase substrate for 20 min at room temperature.
   i) Counter stain and mount: Wash the slides with TBS and counterstain for a few seconds with haematoxylin; wash in tap water and mount in an aqueous mounting system.

4. *Assessment:* The entire cell suspension is examined and both CD45-positive cells and spermatozoa are counted until 200 CD45-positive cells have been counted.

Calculations and Results

The concentration of CD45-positive cells is calculated relative to that of spermatozoa. If N is the number of CD45-positive cells counted in the same fields as 100 spermatozoa and S is the concentration of sperm in millions/ml, then the concentration (C) of the given cell type in millions/ml can be calculated from the formula $C = S \times (N/100)$.

Interpretation Guidelines

There is no consensus on what is a 'normal' number of leukocytes in semen. There are data on mean levels in infertility clinic patients (390,000/ml) [34], but limited information is available from fertile control subjects.

Assessment of Immature Germ Cells in Semen

These include round spermatids and spermatocytes but rarely spermatogonia. They are often degenerating and, on a wet semen smear, difficult to distinguish from some leukocytes. However, they can be identified in stained semen smears based on differences in staining colouration, as well as by their distinctive nuclear size and shape. Alternatively, the number of immature germ cells in semen can be calculated from the difference between the number of round cells in the semen sample minus the number of leukocytes (examined using monoclonal antibodies). Using the latter method, Aitken and colleagues showed that the median number of germ line cells per ml of semen was 435,000 [34]. Interestingly, although there is limited data, the concentration of immature cells may be negatively associated with fertility [41].

Reactive Oxygen Species Measurement

Introduction

Mammalian spermatozoa have been shown to produce oxygen radicals and to export them to the extracellular medium [42–46]. The main source of oxygen radicals in spermatozoa appears to be the mitochondria, as the result of the monovalent reduction of molecular oxygen during oxidative phosphorylation [43].

Spermatozoa have a relatively high content in polyunsaturated fatty acids in their membrane and, in particular, in docosahexaenoic acid (DHA), which makes them especially vulnerable to lipid peroxidation induced by oxygen radicals [47]. DHA is thought to play a major role in regulating membrane fluidity in spermatozoa, and is the main substrate of lipid peroxidation, accounting for 90% of the overall rate of lipid peroxidation in human spermatozoa [47]. Oxidation of phospholipid-bound DHA has been shown to be the major factor that determines the motile lifespan of spermatozoa *in vitro* [47], as well as membrane damage and DNA oxidation [48,49]. The rate of lipid peroxidation of spermatozoa *in vitro* is determined by (i) oxygen concentration and temperature in the extracellular medium; (ii) ROS production; (iii) the activity of antioxidant enzymes in spermatozoa; and (iv) the content of phospholipid-bound DHA [45,47]. The equilibrium between these factors determines the overall rate of lipid peroxidation and oxidative stress *in vitro*. During the process of sperm maturation, spermatozoa retain a critical level of DHA resulting in: (i) optimal membrane fluidity required to support sperm motility and the early steps of fertilization; and (ii) minimal risk of oxidative damage to the sperm membranes and DNA [50].

Mammalian sperm metabolic strategy is geared towards maximal production of ATP in the flagellum through anaerobic glycolysis rather than maximal efficiency through the Krebs's cycle, thus minimizing the flux of reducing NADH equivalents through the inner mitochondrial membrane and the production of oxygen radicals. Therefore, this metabolic strategy can be considered as an additional antioxidant mechanism in sperm of paramount importance.

Oxygen radicals produced by sperm include the superoxide anion (O_2^-); its conjugated acid, the hydroperoxyl radical ($HO_2^\bullet$); hydrogen peroxide (H_2O_2), produced mostly through the dismutation of the superoxide anion by superoxide dismutase; and the hydroxyl radical ($OH^\bullet$) produced by the reaction of superoxide anion with hydrogen peroxide in the presence of heavy metals [45]. Oxygen radicals, as a group, are currently designated as reactive oxygen species (ROS).

Most ROS found in semen are produced by immature spermatozoa and by leukocytes. Although ROS levels produced by activated leukocytes could be several orders of magnitude higher than those produced by spermatozoa, immature spermatozoa may produce comparable levels of ROS in the presence of proinflammatory factors [51]. In addition to the ROS produced by immature sperm and leukocytes, semen may also contain ROS produced from the epithelial cells of the epididymis [52]. ROS levels in semen derived from all these different sources have been shown to be inversely correlated with normal sperm function and directly correlated with male infertility [53,54].

Reactive oxygen species are measured in semen by chemiluminescence using luminol as a substrate [55,56]. Luminol is a highly sensitive probe that reacts with a variety of ROS at neutral pH. It has the ability to measure both extracellular as well as intracellular ROS. ROS have a very short lifespan and, therefore, must be measured quickly after semen collection. The free-radical combines with luminol to produce photons that are then converted to an electrical signal which is then measured with a luminometer [48]. The levels of ROS produced are measured as counted photons per minute (CPM).

More recently, it has been shown that disruption of the redox state of cells can cause toxic effects resulting in ROS and peroxide production leading to damage of sperm protein lipids and DNA. Oxidation-reduction potential (ORP) has recently been described as an integrated measure of the balance between total oxidants such as oxidized thiols, superoxide radical, hydroxyl radical, hydrogen peroxide, nitric oxide, peroxynitrite, metal transition ions, and total reductants such as reduced thiols, ascorbate, alpha and beta tocopherol, beta-carotene and uric acid [57–61]. A method for measuring semen or seminal plasma ORP, the MiOXSYS test, is described later in this chapter.

Reactive Oxygen Species Measurement Using Luminol Chemiluminescence

Principle
Luminol is extremely sensitive and reacts with a variety of ROS at neutral pH [57]. It can measure extracellular and intracellular ROS. Free radicals combine with luminol to produce a light signal that is converted to an electrical signal (photon) by a luminometer. The number of free radicals produced are measured as relative light units per second per million spermatozoa [58].

Specimen(s)
Liquefied semen collected, ideally, at the laboratory after a three-day period of prior sexual abstinence. A semen analysis should be performed on the specimen.

Equipment
- Air displacement pipettes, 0–10 μl and 100–1000 μl
- Positive displacement pipetter (400 μl) for taking semen aliquots
- Pipette controller
- Vortex mixer
- Luminometer, AutoLumat model LB 953 (Berthold Technologies, Oak Ridge, TN, USA)

Disposable Materials

- Disposable polystyrene tubes with caps, 17 × 20 mm (e.g. Fisher Scientific cat.no. 14-959-491)
- Polystyrene round bottom tubes, 12 × 75 mm (e.g. Falcon #2003)
- Disposable serological pipettes, 1 ml, 2 ml, 10 ml

Reagents

DMSO solution: Sigma D8779. Store at room temperature in the dark until expiration date.

PBS solution: Dulbecco's phosphate-buffered saline solution, (PBS-1X; Catalog # 9235, Irvine Scientific, Santa Ana, CA).

Hydrogen peroxide: 30% (v/v) for positive control.

Luminol stock solution: 100 mM solution: Dissolve 0.177 g of luminol (5-amino-2,3 dehydro-1,4 phthalazinedione; Sigma A8511) in 10 ml of DMSO in a polystyrene tube. Cover the tube in aluminum foil, since luminol is light sensitive. This solution, which is a clear, straw colour when prepared, can be stored at room temperature in the dark for up to six months. Discard if there is any change in colour or turbidity.

Luminol working solution: 5mM solution: Mix 20 μl luminol stock solution with 380 μl DMSO in a foil-covered polystyrene tube. Prepare the solution fresh prior to use and store at room temperature in the dark until needed. Discard at the end of the day.

Calibration

None required.

Quality Control

- Reagent lot numbers and expiry dates are recorded in the assay QC log.
- Criteria for rejecting a result: no spermatozoa are present in the specimen.

Procedure

Note: Create an appropriate file structure on the PC or network where the data are to be stored, e.g. a folder called 'ROS Data' with suitably named sub-folders, e.g. 'Clinical ROS' for the Excel spreadsheets and 'Measurement Files' for the Berthold measurement data.

A. Luminometer setup

Note: It is important that the instrument settings are in place before adding the reagents to the tube and loading the samples.

1. Switch on the luminometer and attached computer; allow to warm-up for 10–15 min.
2. On the computer's desktop, click on the 'Berthold tube master' icon to start the programme.
3. From the 'Setup Menu', select 'Measurement Definition' and then 'New Measurement'; the software prompts with 'Measurement Name'. Enter as operator initials, date, and analyte +assayID (e.g. AB 20210313 ROSXX); copy and click 'OK'.
4. The software will show 'Measurement Definition' on the Toolbar, displaying the information just entered.
5. Under 'Luminometer Measurement Protocol', select 'Rep. Assay' from the drop-down menu and define each of the 'Parameters' as follows:

   Read time: 1 s
   Background read time: 0 s
   Total time: 900 s

Table 4.1 Example of tube setup for the measurement of reactive oxygen species by chemiluminescence

Tubes	Label	PBS (µl)	Test sample (µl)	H₂O₂ (30%) (µl)	Luminol (µl)
1–3	Blank	400			
4–6	Negative control	400			10
7–9	Patient specimen A		400		10
10–12	Patient specimen B		400		10
13–15	Patient specimen C		400		10
16–18	Positive control	400		50	10

Cycle time: 30 s

Delay 'Inj M read': 0 s

Injector M (µL): 0 s

Temperature (°C): 37

Temperature control (0=OFF): 1= ON

Click to save.

B. Running the assay

Note: Patient specimens are analysed in triplicate.

1. Prepare sufficient 6-ml polystyrene tubes (12 × 75 mm) as indicated in Table 4.1.
2. Add reagents to the bottom of the tubes and not to the side. Vortex mix to ensure that the luminol mixes with the rest of the reagent/sample mixture.
   - Change the pipette tip when adding the reagent/sample mixture to each tube.
   - Gently vortex the tubes to mix the aliquots uniformly but avoid creating bubbles.
3. Place all the labelled tubes in the luminometer in numerical sequence.
4. From the Setup Menu select 'Assay Definition' and then 'New Assay'.
   a) Go to 'Sample Type' in the menu and select 'Normal'. Then press 'OK'.
   b) Go to file, click 'New', click 'Workload' and press 'OK'.
   c) Go to 'Save As' and save in an appropriate folder such as the 'Clinical ROS' folder.
   d) Save your 'Workload' (initials, date, analyte and measurement, patient initials) in the 'Clinical ROS' 'Workload' file.
   e) After saving the 'Workload', the name of the file will show in the 'Title Bar'. The samples are ready to be analysed.
5. Wait 3–5 min to make sure everything is working fine.

C. Saving and printing the results

1. After finishing the measurement, the computer will ask you to 'Save' the Excel spreadsheet in the 'Clinical ROS' sub-folder.
2. Save Berthold measurement in the 'Measurement Files' sub-folder e.g. using the same name, e.g. RK 20210313 ROS XX.
3. Print spreadsheet as the 'chart 1' and the Berthold sheet.
4. Close the Excel spreadsheet. Print the 'Workload' sheet.
5. Make sure that all three sheets are printed before saving and closing the file.

Calculations and Results

1. Calculate the average RLU value for the negative control, each analysis sample, and the positive control.
2. For each analysis sample, calculate its ROS value:

   Sample ROS = (sample average RLU value) – (average RLU value for negative control)

3. Correct the sample ROS by dividing it by the sperm concentration in M/ml.

Interpretation Guidelines

Normal range: <93 RLU/s/10^6 spermatozoa/ml
Critical value: ≥93: RLU/s/10^6 spermatozoa/ml

Notes

1. Factors that can affect ROS measurements:
   a) The luminometer instrument, its calibration, determination of sensitivity, dynamic range and units used.
   b) The concentration and type of probe used.
   c) The concentration and volume of the semen sample, reagents and temperature of the luminometer.
   d) Variations in the time between semen collection and ROS measurement.
   e) Viscous samples and incomplete liquefaction may interfere with chemiluminescent signals.
   f) Centrifugation of semen can result in an artificial increase in the chemiluminescent signal due to the shear force generated during centrifugation.
   g) Presence of serum albumin: the use of a medium that contains bovine serum albumin can generate spurious signals in the presence of human seminal plasma.
   h) Medium pH: luminol is sensitive to pH changes.
   i) Non-specific interferences.

2. Troubleshooting:
   a) Clean the interior of the instrument with antistatic spray, especially the chain belt. Keep a container filled with distilled water inside the instrument at all times to maintain humidity and reduce static.
   b) Check the instrument background reading from the 'rate meter'. It should not be ≥20 RLU. If it is ≥20 RLU then contact the vendor.
   c) Check the reagents for contamination. First, check the PBS buffer. Does this resolve the problem? If not, go to the next step.
   d) Check the luminol solution. Prepare a fresh luminol solution. Does this resolve the problem? If not, go to the next step.
   e) Prepare luminol in fresh DMSO.
   f) Test multiple runs in triplicate for blank, negative control and positive control.

Seminal Plasma Redox State: The MiOXSYS Test

Background

It has been shown that disruption of the reduction-oxidation or 'redox' status of cells can cause toxic effects resulting in ROS and peroxide production leading to damage of sperm proteins, lipids and DNA. Oxidation-reduction potential (ORP) has recently been described as an integrated measure of the balance between total oxidants such as oxidized thiols, superoxide radical, hydroxyl radical, hydrogen peroxide, nitric oxide, peroxynitrite, metal transition ions, and total reductants such as reduced thiols, ascorbate, alpha and beta tocopherol, beta-carotene and uric acid [62,63].

Principle

The MiOXSYS system measures the amount of oxidative and reductive stress (redox balance) in semen or seminal plasma by measuring ORP [64–66]. The biological sample is applied to the MiOXSYS analyzer sensor and inserted into a galvanostat-based reader. The test starts when the sample fills the reference electrode, thus completing the electrochemical circuit. The static ORP is a snapshot of current redox balance, and correlates with disease, severity of injury and mortality: a higher static ORP reading is indicative of oxidative stress.

Specimen

Liquefied semen collected as described in Chapter 3. The sample used for ORP analysis can be either fresh or frozen-thawed semen or seminal plasma.

Equipment

- MiOXSYS analyzer instrument (Ayto BioScience, Englewood, CO, USA)
- MiOXSYS analyzer Calibration Verification Key (CVK)
- Positive displacement pipetter for 30 µl aliquots

Disposable Materials

- Tips for pipetter

Reagents

- MiOXSYS Sensor

Quality Control

- Good laboratory practice recommends the use of the control materials; users should follow the appropriate regulations and accreditation guidelines concerning the running of external controls.
- Each new lot or shipment of MiOXSYS sensors need to be verified upon receipt and before use. Testing of external controls should be performed in accordance with appropriate regulations and accreditation guidelines. A separate sensor must be used for each external control test. MiOXSYS external control solution kits are supplied separately by the vendor.
- Calibration verification testing should be performed using the CVK at installation and at monthly intervals thereafter to verify that the analyzer is still within calibration.
  a) Turn on the MiOXSYS analyzer instrument.
  b) Insert the CVK into the sensor slot with the A-side facing up; the analyzer will indicate that a calibration check is being performed on the A-side.
  c) When complete, the results will be displayed as: Side A: ORP = ##.# mV • ICell = -##.# nA
  d) Before removing the CVK, record the date, time, and ORP and ICell results in the equipment log for the instrument.
  e) Repeat the procedure for the B-side of the CVK.
  f) Verify that the results for both sides A and B are within the Acceptance Limits shown on the CVK card.
  g) If the MiOXSYS analyzer is out of calibration discontinue its use and contact the vendor.

Procedure

1. *MiOXSYS analyzer setup*
   a) Press the power button on the MiOXSYS analyzer; the green power LED will illuminate.
   b) MiOXSYS analyzer and the date and time will appear on the display screen during 3 s.
   c) When the analyzer is ready the message 'Insert Sensor' will appear on the display screen.
2. *Analyzing the sample*
   a) Unwrap a MiOXSYS analyzer sensor. Hold it by the edges, shiny side up, with the electrodes towards the analyzer, then insert it fully into the analyzer. Once the sensor is inserted properly 'Waiting for Sample' will appear on the display screen, and a 2 min sample detection countdown timer will begin.

b) Using a pipetter, apply 30 μl of the specimen into the sample application port of the inserted sensor; make sure that the entire port is covered.

c) Testing begins automatically when the sample reaches the reference cell of the sensor; proper execution of the test is also indicated by the blinking of the blue testing LED. Once the test has been initiated the display screen will show 'Processing Sample' and the time remaining to complete the test. Do not press any buttons or remove the sensor while testing is in progress.

Note: If an error occurs during testing, an error code will appear on the display screen and the red alert LED will illuminate. Note the error reading and follow the instructions on the screen to clear the error.

d) Audible beeps will indicate the completion of the test: results will appear on the display screen in the following order: date, time and static ORP in millivolts or mV.

e) Remove the sensor immediately after recording the results. Dispose of the used sensor as biohazardous waste.

f) Once the used MiOXSYS sensor is removed, 'Insert Sensor' will appear on the display screen and the analyzer is ready to perform the next test.

Calculations and Results

1. If the test was performed in replicate, calculate the average ORP for the specimen.

2. Calculate the *standardized ORP (sORP)* result for the specimen by dividing the (average) ORP value by the sperm concentration in M/ml: sORP = X.XX mV/10^6 spermatozoa/ml

3. Figure 4.3 shows a representative Receiver Operating Characteristics curve for whole semen predicting abnormal semen quality: AUC = area under the curve; PPV = positive predictive value; NPV = negative predictive value.

   Using a cut-off of 1.36 mV/10^6 spermatozoa/ml the Sensitivity is 68.6%, the Specificity 83.1% and the Accuracy 75.2%. The reference value is <1.36 mV/10^6 spermatozoa/ml.

Notes

1. The time between sample collection and ORP measurement can affect the test result.

2. Sample viscosity or incomplete liquefaction can interfere with sample flow, affecting it reaching the reference cell of the sensor.

3. Prior centrifugation of the specimen can lead to an artificial increase in ORP because of the shearing forces generated by centrifugation.

Biochemical Test – Prostate: Assessment of Zinc in Seminal Fluid

Background

Zinc ions are secreted by the human prostate into the prostatic fluid. The secretion is androgen dependent. Zinc in semen is used as a marker for the prostatic fluid contribution to the ejaculate. Zinc contributes to the stabilization of the sperm nucleus.

Principle

A commercially available colorimetric assay for determination of zinc was validated for seminal fluid by Johnson and Eliasson [67]. The reagent, 2-(5-bromo-2-pyridylazo)-5-(N-propyl-N-sulfopropylamino)-phenol (5-Br- PAPS), binds a zinc ion and turns into a blue-violet colour, absorbing light at the wavelength of 560 nm. However, this kit is no longer available, and the described method has been validated and verified for human semen from a method applied for determination of trace zinc in various biological circumstances [68].

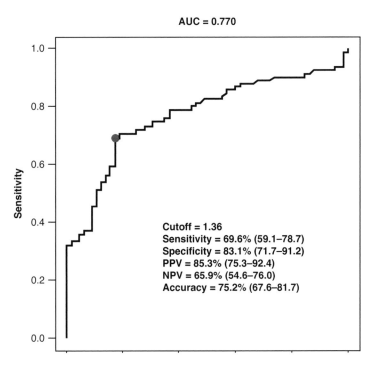

AUC = 0.770

Cutoff = 1.36
Sensitivity = 69.6% (59.1–78.7)
Specificity = 83.1% (71.7–91.2)
PPV = 85.3% (75.3–92.4)
NPV = 65.9% (54.6–76.0)
Accuracy = 75.2% (67.6–81.7)

Figure 4.3 A representative ROC curve for whole semen predicting abnormal semen quality: AUC = area under the curve; NPV = negative predictive value; PPV = positive predictive value.

Specimen

Sperm-free seminal plasma obtained from liquefied whole semen by centrifugation (3000 g × 20 min); supernatant decanted and stored at -20°C up to 12 months.

Equipment

- Microtiterplate reader (spectrophotometry)
- Vortex mixer
- Balance, 0.1 mg accuracy
- Pipetters for 5–50 µl, 50–200 µl, 30–300 µl and 200–1000 µl
- Multi-stepper pipetter for 100 µl and 1000µl
- Test tube racks
- Measurement flasks 100 ml
- Magnetic stirrer
- Large flask (500–1000 ml)

Disposable Materials

- Polystyrene 'Ellermann' test tubes (10 × 75 mm; 3 ml) with stoppers
- Microtiter plates, 96 wells, flat bottom
- Tips for pipetters 0.5–300 µl
- Tips for pipetters 200–1000 µl
- Gloves

Reagents

Stock solutions

1. *Double distilled H_2O*, a total of 400 ml is required for preparations described.
2. *Standard solution: 50 μM zinc calibrator:*
   a) Dissolve 288 mg of $ZnSO_4 \cdot 7H_2O$ in 100 ml double-distilled water.
   b) Dilute further (×200) by taking 500 μl of the above solution and adding it to 99.5 ml double-distilled water to get a standard concentration of 50 μM; store at -20°C, or at +4° to +8°C for up to six months.
3. Carbonate bicarbonate buffer, pH 9.8, 200 mM:
   a) Dissolve 13 capsules of Sigma-Aldrich C3041 in 325 ml of purified water.
   b) Store at +4°C for at least three months.
4. *Sodium citrate, 850 mM*, e.g. Sigma-Aldrich C3674 (MW 258.1):
   a) Dissolve 11.0 g in 50 ml of carbonate bicarbonate buffer.
   b) Can be stored at +4°C for at least three months.
5. *5-Br-PAPS, 0.7 mM*, e.g. Sigma-Aldrich 180017 (MW 537.3):
   a) Dissolve 19 mg in 50 ml of carbonate bicarbonate buffer.
   b) Can be stored at +4°C for at least three months.
6. *Deferoxamine mesylate, 205 mM*, e.g. Sigma-Aldrich D9533 (MW 656.8):
   a) Dissolve 96 mg in 60 ml of carbonate bicarbonate buffer.
   b) Can be stored at +4°C for at least three months.
7. *Salicylaldoxime, 29 mM*, e.g. Sigma-Aldrich 84172 (MW 137.1):
   a) Dissolve 239 mg in 60 ml of double-distilled water.
   b) Can be stored at +4°C for at least three months.

Working solutions (prepare on the day for the assessment)
1. *Zinc standard for calibration:* Dilute the 50 μM with double-distilled water to get four standards and a blank as shown in Table 4.2 to obtain 1 ml of each.
2. *Staining solution A:* Mix together in a first step
   - 7.0 ml carbonate bicarbonate buffer
   - 7.0 ml 5-Br-PAPS stock solution
   - 4.0 ml sodium citrate stock solution
   - 5.0 ml deferoxamin mesylate stock solution
3. *Final working solution:* Mix together
   - 20 ml of staining solution A
   - 5.0 ml salicylaldoxime stock solution

Table 4.2 Preparation of the calibration solutions for the measurement of zinc in seminal plasma

Calibrator concentration (μmol/l)	50 μmol/l zinc standard (ml to take for dilution)	Double-distilled water (ml to use for the dilution)	Corresponding to seminal zinc concentration (mmol/l)
40	0.8	0.2	8
20	0.4	0.6	4
10	0.2	0.8	2
5	0.1	0.9	1
0	0	1.0	0

Calibration

Achieved using the calibration standards prepared at 'Working Solutions' #2.

Quality Control

Use internal QC samples with known target results and acceptable range of variability to verify each run of assessments. It is practical to prepare a further diluted (1:1) QC, to also have a low control with half the target value of the ordinary QC. A further 1:1 diluted QC sample can be extremely helpful for verification of each assay run.

- *Internal quality control samples (QC):* Make a pool of sperm-free seminal plasma from 100–300 patient specimens (see Specimen above); thaw individual stored aliquots and mix together in a 500–1000 ml flask with a magnetic stirrer. Label sealable test tubes with IQC batch ID and date; pipette 50–100 µl of the well-mixed specimen into each tube, cap tightly and store at -20°C until use.
- Determine zinc concentration in 10 replicates at 5 different occasions. Calculate the 95% confidence interval for zinc concentration. The mean results of the QC samples should be within the 95% interval in order to approve a series of analyses.

Procedure

Precautions: All material (calibrators, samples, QC samples and reagents) must be handled according to safety rules. Personal protective equipment (clothes, latex gloves) shall be used during all work. All disposables shall be handled according to rules.

Note: All procedures are carried out at 'ambient' temperature, i.e. 15–35°C.

1. Thaw seminal fluid samples and one internal QC sample, mix well with vortex.
2. Dilute samples and QC-samples in total 1:200 in duplicates. Use a positive displacement pipette for seminal plasma. Make two serial dilutions to minimize deviations, for instance: add 900 µl water and 100 µl seminal plasma or 100 µl QC-sample to test tubes in duplicates and mix thoroughly with vortex. In the second step, take 50 µl of this dilution to a new Ellermann tube and add 950 µl water.

   If performing a series of fructose determinations, the first serial dilution can be retained. If low semen volume does not allow this dilution scheme it is essential to note that in the report form. In cases of low ejaculate volume, you could use 5 µl semen and add 995 µl water in a test tube. Note that the uncertainty in the final result increases when starting with small volumes.
3. Preparation of calibrators: Prepare the series of five zinc calibration solutions as per Table 4.3.
4. Add in duplicate, 40 µl of each calibrator, diluted seminal plasma and diluted QC-samples, into the wells of a 96-well plate. Note that every sample should be well mixed by vortex before pipetting.
5. Add 200 µl of the fresh chromogen reagent to each well. Avoid the formation of bubbles. Use reverse technique for pipetting (before filling the pipette, press the pipette knob into bottom level and then fill. When pushing out into the well – stop at the *first* 'stop' of the pipetter).
6. Mix 5 min on a 96-well plate shaker.
7. Read the plate at 560 nm wavelength.

Table 4.3 Preparation of zinc calibration solutions

Calibrator	Molarity (µM)	µl of zinc 50 µM	µl of water
S_1	0	0	1000
S_2	5	100	900
S_3	10	200	800
S_4	20	400	600
S_5	40	800	200

Calculations and Results

1. Read the zinc concentration in mmol/l for each sample from the standard curve.
2. Samples with values higher than the highest standard should be reanalysed at higher dilution.
3. Check that the mean of the QC-samples is within the decided interval to approve this series of results.
4. Multiply all values with the dilution factor (200) to get the zinc concentration in undiluted seminal plasma. Use one decimal place: 1.461 is given as 1.5 mmol/l.
5. Multiply the ejaculate volume (in ml to one decimal place) and the zinc concentration to give the total amount of secreted zinc in the ejaculate in μmoles. Use one decimal place, e.g. semen volume 3.2 ml × 1.461 = 4.675 is reported as 4.7 μmol/ejaculate.

Interpretation Guidelines

- A total content of 2.4 μmol zinc or more in the ejaculate indicates a normal prostatic contribution to the ejaculate.
- Values below 2.4 μmol indicate low contribution of the androgen-dependent prostatic fluid to the ejaculate. This can be seen after a short time of abstinence, particularly in hypogonadal men, men treated with for instance finasteride, and men with prostatic inflammation. The latter may also cause an increased concentration of inflammatory cells. Furthermore, incomplete collection of the ejaculate, for instance missing the first ejaculate portion, often results in a combination of few spermatozoa and low zinc.
- The zinc concentration is also used in split-ejaculate fractions together with fructose concentration to determine the relative contribution from the prostatic and the seminal vesicles, respectively, to the different fractions.

Notes

1. Make sure that no air bubbles are present in the wells. To empty a bubble, insert a pipette tip (20–200 μl) into the bubble.

Biochemical Test – Seminal Vesicles: Quantitative Assessment of Fructose in Seminal Fluid

Background

Fructose in semen emanates mainly from the seminal vesicles with a minor contribution from the corresponding secretory epithelium in the ampullary part of the vas deferens. The secretion is androgen dependent. Fructose in semen is used as a marker for the secretory contribution of the seminal vesicles to the ejaculate or to characterize the origin of split ejaculate fractions. A normal secretory contribution of fructose means that these parts of the Wolffian ducts (seminal vesicles and ampulla) are intact and display an androgen-dependent secretion that is emptied at emission/ejaculation [36,69,70].

Principle

Fructose reacts, in the presence of hydrochloric acid under heat, with indol and produces a coloured complex that can be measured at the wavelength of 470 nm.

Specimen

Sperm-free seminal plasma obtained from liquefied whole semen by centrifugation (3000 g × 20 min). The supernatant is decanted and can be stored at -20°C up to 12 months.

Equipment

- Microtiter-plate reader
- Micropipetters for 5–50 μl, 50–200 μl, 30–300 μl and 200–1000 μl ranges

- Multi-stepper pipetter for 50–1000 µl
- Vortex mixer
- Balance, 0.1 mg accuracy
- Water-bath (set at 50°C)
- Thermometer, precision ±1°C
- 1 stopwatch, precision ±1 min/h
- Measurement flask or cylinder 100 ml
- Test tube racks

Disposable Material

- Ice
- Eppendorf tubes 1.5 ml
- Polystyrene 'Ellermann' test tubes (10 × 75 mm; 3 ml) with stoppers
- Parafilm
- Microtiter-plate, 96 wells, flat bottom
- Pipetter tips 0.5–300 µl, 5–200 µl and 200–1000 µl

Reagents

1. Two *deproteinizing solutions*:
   a) 63 mM $ZnSO_4 \cdot 7H_2O$: dissolve 1.8 g in 100 ml water
   b) 0.1 M NaOH; dissolve 0.4 g NaOH in 100 ml water
2. *Colour reaction solution:* 2 µM indole reagent + 16 µM benzoic acid. Dissolve 200 mg benzoic acid in 90 ml water shaking in a water bath at 60°C, then dissolve 0.025 g indole in this solution and make up to 100 ml. Store at +4°C.
3. *Fructose stock solution* (22.4 mM) for calibrators: Dissolve 0.403 g fructose in 100 ml pure water. Stable for six months at +4 to +8°C.
4. *Concentrated hydrochloric acid:* concentrated HCl is 37% (v/v)
5. *Water:* Reagent grade water

Calibration

See Table 4.4. Dilute the stock solution 1/10 to get highest calibrator (2.24 mmol/l). Dilute serially 1:2 (1+1) with water to achieve the additional calibrators of 1.12, 0.56, 0.28 and 0.14 mmol/l, respectively, and use water as standard 0.0 mmol/l.

Quality Control

Use internal QC samples with known target results and acceptable range of variability to verify each run of assessments. It is practical to prepare a further diluted (1:1) QC, to also have a low control with half the target value of the ordinary QC. A further 1:1 diluted QC sample can be extremely helpful for verification of each assay run.

- *Internal quality control samples* (QC): Make a pool of sperm-free seminal plasma from 100–300 patient specimens (see Specimen above). Thaw individually stored samples or groups of samples and mix together in a 500–1,000 ml flask with a magnetic stirrer. Label sealable Ellermann tubes with the IQC batch ID and date and then pipette 50–100 µl of the well-mixed seminal plasma into each tube, cap tightly and store at –20°C until use.
- Determine the fructose concentration in 10 replicates at 5 different occasions. Calculate the 95% confidence interval for each fructose concentration. The mean results of the IQC samples should be within the 95% interval in order to approve an analysis series.

Table 4.4 Preparation of fructose calibration solutions

Calibrator	Molarity (mM)	Fructose solution	Water
S_1	0.00	—	0.5 ml
S_2	0.14	0.5 ml of 0.28 mM (S_3)	0.5 ml
S_3	0.28	0.5 ml of 0.56 mM (S_4)	0.5 ml
S_4	0.56	0.5 ml of 1.12 mM (S_5)	0.5 ml
S_5	1.12	0.5 ml of 2.24 mM (S_6)	0.5 ml
S_6	2.24	0.1 ml of fructose stock solution (22.4 mM)	0.9 ml

Procedure

Precautions: All material (calibrators, samples, QC samples and reagents) must be handled according to safety rules. Personal protection (clothes, latex gloves) shall be used during all work. All disposables shall be handled according to rules.

Note: Check that the water-bath is at 50°C.

1. Thaw the seminal fluid samples and one IQC sample and use the vortex mixer to ensure each sample is well mixed.
2. Dilute each of the seminal fluid and IQC samples ×40. Use a positive displacement pipette to add 25 µl of each sample to 975 µl of water in separate Ellermann tubes and mix on the vortex mixer.
    Notes: a) If dilutions have been done for zinc assessment, use the first, 1:10 dilution of seminal plasma and dilute this 1:4. To 300 µl of water add 100 µl of the 1:10 diluted seminal plasma.
            b) When low semen volume: Make a 1:40 dilution by adding 7 µl of seminal fluid to 273 µl of water in an Ellermann tube. Note that the measurement uncertainty increases when starting with small volumes. Always make careful notes of non-standard dilutions.
3. Add 50 µl $ZnSO_4$ and 50 µl NaOH to Eppendorf tubes. The number of tubes is calculated as 2× the total number of seminal plasma and IQC samples.
4. Transfer duplicate 200 µl aliquots of diluted seminal fluid samples, diluted IQC sample, and each calibrator (0–2.24 mM) to Eppendorf tubes, close their lids, vortex mix each sample and incubate for 15 min at ambient temperature.
5. Centrifuge all Eppendorf tubes at 7000 g × 5 min.
6. Take off 100 µl of each supernatant and transfer to acid-proof test tubes.
7. Add 100 µl indole reagent to each tube and mix. Then add 1 ml of concentrated HCl to each tube. Seal all tubes using acid-proof stoppers.
8. Incubate for 20 min in a water bath heated to +50°C, and cool in ice water for 15 min.
9. Inside a fume hood: Transfer 250 µl of all seminal plasma samples, QC samples and calibrators to a 96-well plate.
10. Cover the top of the plate with acid-proof transparent plastic film (to avoid corrosion of the spectrophotometer).
11. Read the plate in the 96-well plate reader at 470 nm.
12. Remove the plate *immediately* after reading and leave the spectrophotometer open for 10 min to allow the HCl fumes to disperse.

Calculations and Results

1. Read the fructose concentration in mmol/l for each sample from the calibration curve.
2. Note that samples with values higher than the highest standard should be reanalysed using a higher dilution.
3. Check that the mean of the IQC samples is within the established acceptable range to approve this series of results.

4. Multiply values by the dilution factor of 40 to get the fructose concentration in undiluted seminal plasma. Use one decimal place, e.g. 11.5 mmol/l.
5. Multiply by the ejaculate volume in ml with one decimal, to give the total amount of secreted fructose in the ejaculate in µmol. Use one decimal place, e.g. volume 3.2 ml × 11.5 mmol/l = 36.8 µmol/ejaculate.

Interpretation Guidelines

- A content of 13.0 µmol fructose or more per ejaculate indicates normal secretory contribution from the seminal vesicles to the ejaculate [36].
- A content of <13.0 µmol indicates a low androgen specific contribution of vesicular fluid to the ejaculate. This can be seen after a short time of abstinence, in partially hypogonadal men, and in men where emission or ejaculation of fluid is impaired. Emission can be hindered by neuromuscular disease, surgical treatment, drugs, an obstruction in the ejaculatory ducts, or temporarily by an inflammation of the seminal vesicles or prostate.
- Very low content of fructose, in combination with low semen volume and azoospermia, could be due to a total obstruction of the Wolffian ducts, as can be seen in agenesis of the Wolffian ducts.
- The fructose concentration is also used in split ejaculate fractions together with zinc concentration to determine the relative origin of the fractions.

Qualitative Assessment of Fructose in Semen

Background
See previous section on quantitative assessment of fructose in seminal plasma.

Principle
The assay is a simple, semi-quantitative colourimetric test for any keto-hexose [71].

Specimen
Well-mixed liquefied semen.

Equipment
- Electric hotplate, to be used at 55°C
- Porcelain spotting plate
- Air displacement pipetter 10–100 µl

Disposable Materials
- Pipetter tips, 10–100 µl

Reagents

Test Reagent: Dissolve 0.4 g of p-methyl-aminophenol sulphate ('metol') and 8.0 g of urea in 20 ml of 40% sulphuric acid. Store in a brown glass bottle covered with aluminium foil to minimize photo-oxidation. Keep at +4°C when not in use. Stable for two to three months. Discard if there are any signs of contamination or sedimentation.
Note: The urea was omitted in error from the method described in the original publication [71].

Fructose Standard: *Stock solution* = 2.7 mg of fructose dissolved in 100 ml of reagent water (i.e. 27 µg/ml, equivalent to 15 mmol fructose/l, an average seminal plasma value). This stock is kept at +4°C when not in use and discarded if there are any signs of contamination or sedimentation. *Working solution* is a 100× dilution of the stock solution, made using reagent water. It is prepared daily and any unused portion discarded at the end of the day.

Calibration and Quality Control

None required as this is a qualitative test only. If the working fructose standard fails to show a blue colour in the test, then both it and the reagent should be discarded and fresh solutions prepared.

Procedure

1. Pre-heat a white porcelain spotting plate to 55°C on an electric hotplate.
2. Dilute the test sample 1:100 with reagent water.
3. a) Place 20 µl and 50 µl aliquots of the test sample in separate wells on the spotting plate.
   b) In another well place 50 µl of reagent water as a blank, and 50 µl of the working fructose standard in another.
4. Allow all wells to evaporate to dryness.
5. Add one drop (about 50 µl) of the reagent solution to each well.
6. Heat for 10 min.
7. Examine each well for the development of a distinct blue colouration or a blue ring, indicative of the presence of fructose (or any other keto-hexose).

Calculations and Results

The intensity of the blue colouration is proportional to the keto-hexose (fructose) concentration; aldohexoses such as glucose do not react. Positive reactions in the 20 and 50 µl test sample wells correspond to semen fructose concentration of ≥ 1080 and ≥ 2700 µg/ml respectively (i.e. ≥ 6 and ≥ 15 mmol/l, respectively).

Interpretation Guidelines

See previous section on the quantitative assessment of fructose in seminal plasma.

Biochemical Test – Epididymis: Assessment of Neutral α-Glucosidase in Seminal Fluid

Background

Neutral iso-enzyme α-glucosidase is an androgen-dependent enzyme secreted from the epididymis. The total activity of *neutral* α-glucosidase in semen is an indicator of the amount of excretion from the cauda epididymis emitted at ejaculation. However, in seminal plasma there is also significant amounts of an acidic iso-enzyme, originating from the prostate [72].

Principle

The prostatic iso-enzyme is inhibited with the detergent sodium dodecyl sulphate (SDS) whereafter selective measurement of the epididymal form is possible. The enzymatic action of α-glucosidase is assessed by measuring the cleavage of p-nitrophenol part of α-D-glucopyranoside. The chromogen p-nitrophenol is yellow and its yellow colour is augmented by the addition of sodium carbonate. Castanospermine inhibits all α-glucosidase activity and is used as a control for non-specific degradation of the substrate [36,73].

Specimen

Sperm-free seminal plasma obtained from liquefied whole semen (preferably within 60 min after ejaculation) by centrifugation (3000 *g* × 20 min). The supernatant is decanted and can be stored at -20°C for up to 12 months.

Equipment

- Microtiterplate reader, 405 nm (spectrophotometry)
- Vortex mixer
- Balance, precision 0.001 g
- Pipetters for 5–50 µl, 50–200 µl, 30–300 µl and 200–1000 µl
- Multi-stepper pipetter for 100 µl and 1000 µl
- Test tube racks
- Measurement flasks 100 ml
- Magnetic mixer on heated stage
- Water bath
- Thermometer, precision ±1°C
- Stopwatch, precision ±1 min/h
- Measuring cylinders 100 ml

Disposable Materials

- Eppendorf tubes 1.5 ml
- Polystyrene 'Ellermann' test tubes (10 × 75 mm; 3 ml) with stoppers
- Microtiter plates, 96 wells, flat bottom
- Pipetter tips 0.5–300 µl, 200–1000 µl and 1–10 ml
- Gloves

Reagents

- *0.1 M phosphate buffer, pH 6.8:* Prepare 0.1 M K_2HPO_4 (8.7 g in 500 ml reagent water) and 0.1 M KH_2PO_4 (dissolve 6.8 g in 500 ml reagent water). Mix equal volumes of each and then adjust the pH to 6.8: to increase the pH add K_2HPO_4, to decrease the pH add KH_2PO_4.
- *0.1 M phosphate buffer pH 6.8 with 1% sodium dodecyl sulphate (SDS):* Add 1.0 g SDS to 100 ml of the 0.1 M phosphate buffer pH 6.8. Note that the solution precipitates at low temperature but dissolves upon mild warming.
- *5 mM P-nitrophenol (stock solution):* Dissolve 0.139 g PNP (Sigma 1048) in 100 ml pure water. Warm up to 60°C to dissolve. Store in light protected vessel at 4°C. Make a fresh solution every three months.
- *0.1 M Na_2CO_3 solution – Colour reagent 1:* Dissolve 5.3 g Na_2CO_3 in 500 ml reagent water.
- *0.1 M Na_2CO_3 solution with 0.1% SDS:* Add 0.5 g SDS to 500 ml of 0.1 M Na_2CO_3 solution.
- *16.6 mM 4-Nitrophenyl α-D-glucopyranoside (PNPG) in 1% SDS:* Dissolve 0.1 g PNPG (Sigma N-1377) in 20 ml 0.1 M phosphate buffer pH 6.8 with 1% SDS, cover the vessel with a lid and warm up on a hot magnetic stirring plate, stir the solution at, but not above, 50°C for 10 min. Some crystals may remain undissolved. Keep at 50°C before use within 30 min and at 37°C (not below) when in use.
- *Castanospermine 1 mM:* Add 5.3 ml reagent water to a vial of 1 mg castanospermine (Sigma C-3784). Freeze in aliquots at -20°C.

Calibration

The calibration solutions are prepared just before the incubation is stopped.

1. Prepare solutions A and B:
   - Solution A: Add 200 µl of 5 mM p-nitrophenol to 9.8 ml Na_2CO_3 solution with 0.1% SDS.
   - Solution B: This is the 0.1 M Na_2CO_3 solution with 0.1% SDS.
2. Prepare dilutions to obtain calibrators C_0 to C_5 as per Table 4.5.

Table 4.5 Preparation of α-glucosidase calibration solutions

Calibrator	Activity in U/l (μmol product formed)	Solution A (μl)	Solution B (μl)
C_0	0 (0)	0	1000
C_1	12.4 (20)	200	800
C_2	24.8 (40)	400	600
C_3	37.2 (60)	600	400
C_4	49.6 (80)	800	200
C_5	61.9 (100)	1000	0

Quality Control

Use internal QC samples with known target results and acceptable range of variability to verify each run of assessments. It is practical to prepare a further diluted (1:1) QC, to also have a low control with half the target value of the ordinary QC. A further 1:1 diluted QC sample can be extremely helpful for verification of each assay run.

Internal quality control samples (QC): Make a pool of seminal plasma and freeze in 50–100 μl aliquots. Determine the α-glucosidase activity in 10 replicates at 5 different occasions. Calculate the 95% confidence interval for the assessed α-glucosidase activity. The mean results of the QC samples in each batch should be within the 95% confidence interval in order to approve an analysis series.

Procedure

Precautions: All material (calibrators, samples, QC-samples and reagents) should be handled according to laboratory safety rules. Personal protection (clothes, latex gloves) shall be used during the work. All used material (disposable) shall be handled according to local safety regulations.

1. Make sure that the PNPG-solution is kept at 50°C.
2. Thaw the seminal plasma samples, one internal QC sample and an aliquot of the inhibitor castanospermine using a water bath at 37°C.
3. Vortex each tube with seminal plasma and withdraw in duplicate 15 μl with a positive displacement pipette and place it in new 1.5 ml Eppendorf tubes. Also shake the tubes containing the internal control and inhibitor. Add 15 μl of well-mixed QC sample into duplicate tubes labelled (a) QC and (b) castanospermine blank.
4. Add 8 μl of the 1 mM castanospermine solution to the 'castanospermine blank' tubes and vortex.
5. Add 100 μl of the PNPG solution to all tubes and apply the tube stoppers. Note that the PNPG should be warm otherwise it will precipitate and needs to be rewarmed up to 50°C in order to prevent it cooling below 37°C. Vortex all assay tubes.
6. Incubate at 37°C for 120 min in a water bath. Control the temperature and time.
7. Prepare the calibrators and make ready just before the incubation is stopped.
8. Add 1000 μl of 0.1 M Na_2CO_3 solution to stop the reaction and augment the yellow colour.
9. Pipette 250 μl of the calibrators and samples into a 96-well plate and read the plate at the wavelength of 405 nm.

Notes

Make sure that no air bubbles are present in the wells. To empty a bubble, insert a pipette tip (20–200 μl) into the bubble.

Calculations and Results

1. Plot the results for the calibrators. On the X-axis plot μmoles of p-nitrophenol and the corresponding activity (see Calibration above) and the absorbance on the Y-axis. Note that the activity

corresponding to a given amount of product formed is only valid when the method is performed as described here. Since 1 unit (U) of glucosidase-activity equals the formation of 1 μM product (p-nitrophenol) per min at 37°C, the correction factor for 15 μl seminal plasma in a total volume of 1115 μl incubated for 120 min is 1115/15/120 = 0.6194. Hence 100 μmol formed multiplied by the factor 0.6194 corresponds to 61.9 U/l.

2. Samples with values higher than the highest calibrator should be reanalysed at higher dilution.
3. Subtract the mean value for the castanospermine tubes from each mean activity value from seminal plasma and QC samples. This eliminates product not caused by the α-glucosidase activity.
4. Check that the mean of the QC samples is within the decided interval to approve this series of results.
5. Report the neutral α-glucosidase activity with one decimal place e.g. 12.47 is given as 12.5 U/l, or as 12.5 mU/ml since seminal plasma is measured in ml.
6. Multiply by the ejaculate volume in ml with one decimal, which will give the total amount of secreted α-glucosidase activity in the ejaculate in milli Units (mU). Use one decimal place, e.g. volume 3.2 ml × 12.47 = 39.904 is given as 39.9 mU/ejaculate.

Interpretation Guidelines

- Values above 20 mU per ejaculate means a 95% probability for normal passage through the epididymis (meaning no obstruction). A combination of normal levels of zinc, fructose and neutral α-glucosidase indicates a representative ejaculate with secretory contributions from all major sources to the ejaculate.
- Values below 20 mU/ejaculate indicate disturbed emission of fluid through the Wolffian ducts (vas deferens – ejaculatory ducts) which can be caused by neuromuscular impairment or obstructions.
- Azoospermia with low values for neutral α-glucosidase and low values for fructose indicates a high obstruction in the ejaculatory ducts or agenesis of the Wolffian ducts.
- A low value for neutral α-glucosidase combined with normal values for zinc and fructose indicates a representative ejaculate delivered after successful vasectomy.
- Contrastingly, absence of spermatozoa combined with low neutral α-glucosidase activity and low fructose level does not primarily indicate a successful vasectomy but an obstruction between the seminal vesicles and the urethra. Thus, such an ejaculate is not indicative of vasectomy success.

Sequence of Ejaculation

Introduction

Ejaculation is a sequential emptying of epididymal and vas deferens contents (sperm) and secretions from the prostate and seminal vesicles. Normally, spermatozoa are expelled first together with prostatic fluid, while the later ⅔ of the ejaculate volume is dominated by seminal vesicular fluid [74–77].

Pathological changes in the sequence of ejaculation can occur. Spermatozoa exposed to abnormal amounts of seminal vesicular fluid have poorer motility, die faster, and their chromatin is less stable.

Principle

The man is instructed to collect the individual fractions of the ejaculate in the order they are expelled and in separate containers (Figure 4.4). If the man empties more fractions than vials provided in the collection device, all the last fractions are collected in the last vial.

In the separately collected fractions, semen volume, sperm concentration and biochemical markers for prostatic secretion (zinc), seminal vesicular fluid (fructose), and epididymis (α-glucosidase) can be assessed.

Specimen

Ejaculate fractions collected at the laboratory after, ideally, a three-day period of prior sexual abstinence.

Equipment

- Device with four to six specimen containers linked together, e.g. mounted in a row on a plastic ruler, or held in a disposable holder made of corrugated cardboard (see Figure 4.4) [78].

Disposable Materials

- Semen specimen collection containers
- Disposable specimen collection container holder, if available

Calibration

None required.

Quality Control

No specific quality control besides those required for sperm counting and biochemistry.

Procedure

1. Number the specimen containers in sequential order in addition to the usual specimen ID labelling.
2. Have the subject collect the sequential ejaculate fractions.
3. Confirm the correct order of the ejaculate fractions collected into the specimen containers with the subject.

(A)

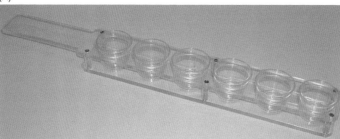

(B)

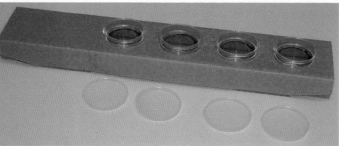

Figure 4.4 Examples of (A) a six-vial plastic reusable device, and (B) a four-vial corrugated cardboard disposable device, for the collection of split ejaculates.

4. Analyse each of the fractions separately for the usual semen characteristics as well as seminal plasma biochemistry assays.

Note: Coagulum formation will not occur in fractions dominated by prostatic fluid. For those fractions, investigations can start immediately (5–10 min warming in the incubator if motility is to be assessed). For coagulated fractions, incubation for 30 min at 37°C usually dissolves the coagulum, with exceptions for fractions with an extreme composition (lack of proteases of prostatic origin).

Calculations and Results

1. For each fraction, calculate concentrations and total amount of spermatozoa, zinc and fructose, as well as the zinc:fructose molar ratio.
2. Calculate the relative distribution of spermatozoa, zinc and fructose: add up the total numbers for each parameter, and calculate the percentage found in each fraction. See Figure 4.5.

Example: The number of spermatozoa in each of the fractions was 75, 40, 14, 8 and 2×10^6. The total number of spermatozoa in the ejaculate was therefore 139×10^6 and the first fraction contained 75/139 = 54%, the second fraction contained 29%, etc. If possible, use graphic presentations (3D histograms) to present data in addition to tabulated results (see also Appendix 4).

Interpretation Guidelines

The first ⅓ of the ejaculate should contain the main bulk of spermatozoa and also the dominant part of the prostatic secretion (see Figure 4.5). A high admixture of seminal vesicular fluid in the fractions containing high proportions of the spermatozoa could provide a reasonable explanation for poor motility in an earlier specimen with isolated motility problems: either a high concentration of fructose in the first, sperm-rich fractions, or that most spermatozoa are expelled in the later ejaculate fractions.

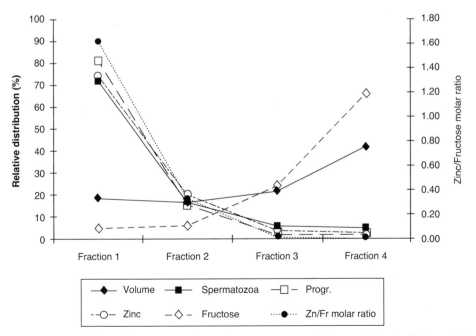

Figure 4.5 Example graph showing the distribution of spermatozoa, zinc and fructose within a four-fraction split ejaculate.

109

Notes

Subjects might benefit from practicing the split ejaculate collection technique.

References

1. Chamley LW, Clarke GN. Antisperm antibodies and conception. *Semin Immunopathol* 2007; **29**: 169–84.

2. Rowe PJ, Comhaire FH, Hargreave TB, Mahmoud AMA. *WHO Manual of the Standardized Investigation, Diagnosis and Management of the Infertile Male.* Cambridge: Cambridge University Press, 2000.

3. Chiu WW, Chamley LW. Clinical associations and mechanisms of action of antisperm antibodies. *Fertil Steril* 2004; **82**: 529–35.

4. Lombardo F, Gandini L, Lenzi A, Dondero F. Antisperm immunity in assisted reproduction. *J Reprod Immunol* 2004; **62**: 101–9.

5. Mortimer D. *Practical Laboratory Andrology.* New York: Oxford University Press, 1994.

6. Bronson RA, Cooper GW, Rosenfeld DL. Sperm-specific isoantibodies and autoantibodies inhibit the binding of human sperm to the human zona pellucida. *Fertil Steril* 1982; **38**: 724–9.

7. Leushuis E, et al. Immunoglobulin G antisperm antibodies and prediction of spontaneous pregnancy. *Fertil Steril* 2009; **92**: 1659–65.

8. Barbonetti A, et al. Relationship between natural and intrauterine insemination-assisted live births and the degree of sperm autoimmunisation. *Hum Reprod* 2020; **35**: 1288–95.

9. Barbonetti A, et al. Prevalence of anti-sperm antibodies and relationship of degree of sperm auto-immunization to semen parameters and post-coital test outcome: a retrospective analysis of over 10 000 men. *Hum Reprod* 2019; **34**: 834–41.

10. Barratt CL, Dunphy BC, McLeod I, Cooke ID. The poor prognostic value of low to moderate levels of sperm surface-bound antibodies. *Hum Reprod* 1992; **7**: 95–8.

11. Verón GL, et al. Incidence of sperm surface autoantibodies and relationship with routine semen parameters and sperm kinematics. *Am J Reprod Immunol* 2016; **76**: 59–69.

12. Helmerhorst FM, Finken MJ, Erwich JJ. Antisperm antibodies: detection assays for antisperm antibodies: what do they test? *Hum Reprod* 1999; **14**: 1669–71.

13. Hjort T. Antisperm antibodies and infertility: an unsolvable question? *Hum Reprod* 1999; **14**: 2423–6.

14. Mahmoud A, Comhaire F. Antisperm antibodies: use of the mixed agglutination reaction (MAR) test using latex beads. *Hum Reprod* 2000; **15**: 231–3.

15. Meinertz H, Linnet L, Fogh-Andersen P, Hjort T. Antisperm antibodies and fertility after vasovasostomy: a follow-up study of 216 men. *Fertil Steril* 1990; **54**: 315–21.

16. Matson PL. External quality assessment for semen analysis and sperm antibody detection: results of a pilot scheme. *Hum Reprod* 1995; **10**: 620–5.

17. Bohring C, Krause W. Interlaboratory variability of the indirect mixed antiglobulin reaction in the assessment of antisperm antibodies. *Fertil Steril* 2002; **78**: 1336–8.

18. Altmäe S, Franasiak JM, Mändar R. The seminal microbiome in health and disease. *Nat Rev Urol* 2019; **16**: 703–21. https://doi.org/10.1038/s41585-019-0250-y

19. Koedooder R, Mackens S, Budding A, et al. Identification and evaluation of the microbiome in the female and male reproductive tracts. *Hum Reprod Update* 2019; **25**: 298–325. https://doi.org/10.1093/humupd/dmy048

20. Elder K, Baker D, Ribes J. *Infections, Infertility and Assisted Reproduction.* Cambridge: Cambridge University Press, 2005.

21. Farahani L, Tharakan T, Yap T, et al. The semen microbiome and its impact on sperm function and male fertility: a systematic review and meta-analysis. *Andrology* 2020. https://doi.org/10.1111/andr.12886

22. Baud D, Pattaroni C, Vulliemoz N, et al. Sperm microbiota and its impact on semen parameters. *Front Microbiol* 2019; **10**: 234. https://doi.org/10.3389/fmicb.2019.00234

23. Oghbaei H, Rastgar Rezaei Y, Nikanfar S, et al. Effects of bacteria on male fertility: spermatogenesis and sperm function. *Life Sci* 2020; **256**: 117891. https://doi.org/10.1016/j.lfs.2020.117891

24. van der Kuyl AC, Berkhout B. Viruses in the reproductive tract: on their way to the germ line? *Virus Res* 2020; **286**: 198101. https://doi.org/10.1016/j.virusres.2020.198101

25. Williamson DA, Chen MY. Emerging and reemerging sexually transmitted infections. *N Engl J Med* 2020; **382**: 2023–32.

26. Kurscheidt FA, Damke E, Bento JC, et al. Effects of herpes simplex virus infections on seminal parameters in male partners of infertile couples. *Urology* 2018; **113**: 52–8. https://doi.org/10.1016/j.urology.2017.11.050

27. Weinberg M, Sar-Shalom Nahshon C, Feferkorn I, et al. Evaluation of human papilloma virus in semen as a risk factor for low sperm quality and poor in vitro fertilization outcomes: a systematic review and meta-analysis. *Fertil Steril* 2020; **113**: 955–69. https://doi.org/10.1016/j.fertnstert.2020.01.010

28. Pan F, Xiao X, Guo J, et al. No evidence of severe acute respiratory syndrome-coronavirus 2 in semen of males recovering from coronavirus disease 2019. *Fertil Steril* 2020; **113**: 1135–9.

29. Li D, Jin M, Bao P, et al. Clinical characteristics and results of semen tests among men with coronavirus disease 2019. *JAMA Network Open* 2020; **3**: e208292.

30. Holtmann N, Edimiris P, Andree M, et al. Assessment of SARS-CoV-2 in human semen: a cohort study. *Fertil Steril* 2020; **114**: 234–9.

31. Aitken RJ. COVID-19 and human spermatozoa: potential risks for infertility and sexual transmission? *Andrology* 2020. https://doi.org/10.1111/andr.12859

32. Tomlinson MJ, Barratt CL, Cooke ID. Prospective study of leukocytes and leukocyte subpopulations in semen suggests they are not a cause of male infertility. *Fertil Steril* 1993; **60**: 1069–75.

33. Aitken RJ, Buckingham D, West K, et al. Differential contribution of leukocytes and spermatozoa to the generation of reactive oxygen species in the ejaculates of oligozoospermic patients and fertile donors. *J Reprod Fertil* 1992; **94**: 451–62.

34. Aitken RJ, West K, Buckingham D. Leukocytic infiltration into the human ejaculate and its association with semen quality, oxidative stress, and sperm function. *J Androl* 1994; **15**: 343–52.

35. Castellini C, et al. Relationship between leukocytospermia, reproductive potential after assisted reproductive technology, and sperm parameters: a systematic review and meta-analysis of case-control studies. *Andrology* 2020; **8**: 125–35.

36. World Health Organization. *WHO Laboratory Manual for the Examination and Processing of Human Semen*, 5th edn. Geneva: World Health Organization, 2010.

37. Comhaire F, Verschraegen G, Vermeulen L. Diagnosis of accessory gland infection and its possible role in male infertility. *Int J Androl* 1980; **3**: 32–45.

38. Eggert-Kruse W, Zimmermann K, Geißler W, et al. Clinical relevance of polymorphonuclear (PMN-) elastase determination in semen and serum during infertility investigation. *Int J Androl* 2008; **32**: 317–29.

39. Henkel R, Offor U, Fisher D. The role of infections and leukocytes in male infertility. *Andrologia* 2020; **21**: e13743.

40. Nahoum CR, Cardozo D. Staining for volumetric count of leukocytes in semen and prostrate-vesicular fluid. *Fertil Steril* 1980; **34**: 68–9.

41. Tomlinson MJ, Barratt CL, Bolton AE, et al. Round cells and sperm fertilizing capacity: the presence of immature germ cells but not seminal leukocytes are associated with reduced success of in vitro fertilization. *Fertil Steril* 1992; **58**: 1257–9.

42. Alvarez JG, Storey BT. Spontaneous lipid peroxidation in rabbit epididymal spermatozoa. *Biol Reprod* 1982; **27**: 1102–8.

43. Holland MK, Alvarez JG, Storey BT. Production of superoxide and activity of superoxide dismutase in rabbit epididymal spermatozoa. *Biol Reprod* 1982; **27**: 1109–18.

44. Alvarez JG, Storey BT. Lipid peroxidation and the reactions of superoxide and hydrogen peroxide in mouse spermatozoa. *Biol Reprod* 1984; **30**: 833–41.

45. Alvarez JG, Touchstone JC, Blasco, L, Storey BT. Spontaneous lipid peroxidation and production of hydrogen peroxide and superoxide in human spermatozoa. Superoxide dismutase as major enzyme protectant against oxygen toxicity. *J Androl* 1987; **8**: 338–48.

46. Aitken RJ, Clarkson JS. Cellular basis of defective sperm function and its association with the genesis of reactive oxygen species by human spermatozoa. *J Reprod Fertil* 1987; **81**: 459–69.

47. Alvarez JG, Storey BT. Differential incorporation of fatty acids into and peroxidative loss of fatty acids from phospholipids of human spermatozoa. *Mol Reprod Dev* 1995; **42**: 334–46.

48. Fraga CG, Motchnik PA, Shigenaga MK, et al. Ascorbic acid protects against endogenous oxidative DNA damage in human sperm. *Proc Natl Acad Sci USA* 1991; **88**: 11003–6.

49. Fraga CG, Motchnik PA, Wyrobek AJ, et al. Smoking and low antioxidant levels increase oxidative damage to sperm DNA. *Mutat Res* 1996; **351**: 199–203.

50. Ollero M, Guzman-Gi E, Lopez MC, et al. Characterization of subsets of human spermatozoa at different stages of maturation: implications in the diagnosis and treatment of male infertility. *Hum Reprod* 2001; **16**: 1912–21.

51. Saleh RA, Agarwal A, Kandirali E, et al. Leukocytospermia is associated with increased reactive oxygen species production by human spermatozoa. *Fertil Steril* 2002; **78**: 1215–24.

52. Drevet JR. The antioxidant glutathione peroxidase family and spermatozoa: a complex story. *Mol Cell Endocrinol* 2006; **250**: 70–9.

53. Aitken RJ, Gordon E, Harkiss D, et al. Relative impact of oxidative stress on the functional competence and genomic integrity of human spermatozoa. *Biol Reprod* 1998; **59**: 1037–46.

54. Agarwal A, Makker K, Sharma R. Clinical relevance of oxidative stress in male factor infertility: an update. *Am J Reprod Immunol* 2008; **59**: 2–11.

55. Shekarriz M, Thomas AJ Jr, Agarwal A. Incidence and level of seminal reactive oxygen species in normal men. *Urology* 1995; **45**: 103–7.

56. Allamaneni SSR, Agarwal A, Nallela KP, et al. Characterization of oxidative stress status by a simple clinical test: evaluation of reactive oxygen species levels in whole semen and isolated spermatozoa. *Fertil Steril* 2005; **83**: 800–3.

57. Benjamin D, Sharma RK, Moazzam A, Agarwal A. Methods for the detection of ROS in human sperm samples. In: Agarwal A, Aitken RJ, Alvarez JG, eds. *Studies on Men´s Health and Fertility*. New York: Springer Science + Business Media, 2012, 257–73.

58. Sharma RK, Agarwal A. Reactive oxygen species and male infertility (review). *Urology* 1996; **48**: 835–50.

59. Shapiro HM. Redox balance in the body: an approach to quantitation. *J Surg Res* 1972; **13**: 138–52.

60. Bar-Or D, Bar-Or R, Rael LT, et al. Heterogeneity and oxidation status of commercial human albumin preparations in clinical use. *Crit Care Med* 2005; **33**: 1638–41.

61. Stagos D, Goutzourelas N, Bar-Or D, et al. Application of a new oxidation-reduction potential assessment method in strenuous exercise-induced oxidative stress. *Redox Rep* 2015; **20**: 154–62.

62. Robert KA, Sharma R, Henkel R, Agarwal A. An update on the techniques used to measure oxidative stress in seminal plasma. *Andrologia* 2020: e13726. https://doi.org/10.1111/and.13726

63. Douglas C, Parekh N, Kahn LG, et al. A novel approach to improving the reliability of manual semen analysis: a paradigm shift in the workup of infertile men. *World J Mens Health* 2019. https://doi.org/10.5534/wjmh.190088

64. Agarwal A, Arafa M, Chandrakumar R, et al. A multicenter study to evaluate oxidative stress by oxidation-reduction potential, a reliable and reproducible method. *Andrology* 2017; **5**: 939–45.

65. Agarwal A, Panner Selvam MK, Arafa M, et al. Multi-center evaluation of oxidation-reduction potential by the MiOXSYS in males with abnormal semen. *Asian J Androl* 2019; **21**: 565–9.

66. Vassiliou A, Martin CH, Homa ST, et al. Redox potential in human semen: validation and qualification of the MiOXSYS assay. *Andrologia* 2020; e13938.

67. Johnsson Ø, Eliasson R. Evaluation of a commercially available kit for the colorimetric determination of zinc in human seminal plasma. *Int J Androl* 1987; **10**: 435–40.

68. Wang J, Niu Y, Zhang C, Chen Y. A micro-plate colorimetric assay for rapid determination of trace zinc in animal feed, pet food and drinking water by ion masking and statistical partitioning correction. *Food Chem* 2018; **245**: 337–45.

69. Cooper TG, Weidner W, Nieschlag E. The influence of inflammation of the human male genital tract on secretion of the seminal markers α-glucosidase, glycerophosphocholine, carnitine, fructose and citric acid. *Int J Androl* 1990; **13**: 329–36.

70. Dreden P, Richard P, Gonzales J. Fructose and proteins in human semen. *Andrologia* 1989; **21**: 576–9.

71. Jungreis E, Nechama M, Paz G, Homonai T. A simple spot test for the detection of fructose deficiency in semen. *Int J Androl* 1989; **12**: 195–8.

72. Paquin R, Chapdelaine R, Dube JY, Tremblay RR. Similar biochemical properties of human seminal plasma and epididymal α-1,4-glucosidase. *J Androl* 1984; **5**: 277–82.

73. Cooper TG, Yeung CH, Nashan D, et al. Improvement in the assessment of human epididymal function by the use of inhibitors in the assay of α-glucosidase in seminal plasma. *Int J Androl* 1990; **13**: 297–305.

74. MacLeod J, Gold RZ. The male factor in fertility and infertility. III. An analysis of motile activity in the spermatozoa of

1000 fertile men and 1000 men in infertile marriage. *Fertil Steril* 1951; **2**: 187–204.

75. Lindholmer C. Survival of human spermatozoa in different fractions of split ejaculate. *Fertil Steril* 1973; **24**: 521–6.

76. Björndahl L, Kjellberg S, Kvist U. Ejaculatory sequence in men with low sperm chromatin-zinc. *Int J Androl* 1991; **14**: 174–8.

77. Björndahl L, Kvist U. Influence of seminal vesicular fluid on the zinc content of human sperm chromatin. *Int J Androl* 1990; **13**: 232–7.

78. Björndahl L, Kvist U. Sequence of ejaculation affects the spermatozoon as a carrier and its message. *Reprod Biomed Online* 2003; **7**: 440–8.

Sperm DNA

Introduction

The integrity of the paternal genome is of paramount importance in the initiation and maintenance of a viable pregnancy, whether *in vivo* or *in vitro*. The presence in the embryonic genome of DNA strand breaks and/or modifications at the level of DNA nucleotides coming from the paternal genome, that were not repaired by the oocyte or the embryo after fertilization, is incompatible with normal embryo and fetal development [1–4].

DNA damage in spermatozoa can affect both mitochondrial and nuclear DNA, and can be induced by six main mechanisms [5]:

- Apoptosis during the process of spermatogenesis
- DNA strand breaks produced during the remodelling of sperm chromatin during the process of spermiogenesis
- Post-testicular DNA fragmentation induced mainly by oxygen radicals, including the hydroxyl radical and nitric oxide, during sperm transport through the seminiferous tubules and epididymis
- DNA fragmentation induced by endogenous endonucleases
- DNA damage induced by radio and chemotherapy
- Damage induced by environmental toxicants

Of these six mechanisms, post-testicular damage during sperm transport through the epididymis appears to play the major role in causing sperm DNA fragmentation. This is supported by several reports which demonstrate that DNA fragmentation is higher in epididymal [6] and ejaculated [7–9] spermatozoa compared to testicular spermatozoa [10].

DNA fragmentation induced by the hydroxyl radical results in the formation of 8-OH-guanine and 8-OH-2′-deoxyguanosine in a first stage followed by double-stranded DNA fragmentation thereafter [11]. While DNA damage of the first type could be repaired – to some extent – by the oocyte, double-stranded DNA damage is virtually irreversible and incompatible with the development of a viable pregnancy. Sperm DNA fragmentation values in ejaculated human spermatozoa above 20%, as assessed by TUNEL [12], above 30%, as assessed by the SCSA test [13], ≥15% by the Halosperm sperm chromatin dispersion test [14,15], or above 60% double-strand breaks for ICSI by the COMET Test [16] are associated with low pregnancy rates. While it might be considered that the remaining spermatozoa with no DNA damage could fertilize the egg and result in a viable pregnancy, a significant proportion of these spermatozoa could have DNA base modifications of the 8-OH-guanine and 8-OH-2′-deoxyguanosine type. Therefore, the probability that a spermatozoon with normal DNA would fertilize the egg would be much lower than that expected in the presence of a DNA fragmentation value of 20% or 30%, respectively. That is, in addition to the measurable 20% and 30% of spermatozoa with DNA fragmentation, the remainder of the spermatozoa would have some type of DNA damage that is not compatible with the development of a term pregnancy. This concept has been designated as the 'iceberg effect' [4,13]. If, on the other hand, DNA damage is related to acid- or alkali-labile sites or single-strand DNA breaks, like those produced during the process of chromatin remodelling, this type of damage would not usually be expressed after fertilization, since it would require dissociation of both DNA strands during sperm decondensation.

Tests like the SCSA, DBD-FISH [17], SCD test [14,15], Chromomycin A3 staining [18] or COMET assay [19,20] require an initial denaturation step in order to detect measurable DNA fragments or potential breaks in the DNA backbone. In contrast, TUNEL [18], *in situ*-nick translation (ISNT) [18,21], or COMET under neutral pH conditions [16,19], do not require a denaturation step and measure actual single- (ISNT, TUNEL and COMET) and double-stranded (TUNEL and COMET) DNA breaks.

Since the intracellular pH of the oocyte is around 7.0, the susceptibility to DNA fragmentation measured by the first group of tests would be of little or no consequence for pronuclei formation or embryo development, since under neutral pH the sperm DNA strands will not dissociate. In addition, this type of DNA damage could be easily repaired by the oocyte. In contrast, fertilization of an oocyte by a spermatozoon with significant double-stranded DNA damage could severely compromise the implantation and pregnancy potential of the resulting embryo, since this type of damage is virtually unrepairable. Therefore, tests that measure DNA damage affecting critical sequences of sperm DNA should have a higher predictive value in ART than tests that measure 'potential' DNA damage. This is supported by numerous reports [8,22–24]. In contrast, tests that measure 'potential' DNA damage generally have a very low predictive value in ART [25].

The results reported by Borini et al. [24], and Duran et al. [22], provide strong evidence for the high predictive value of the TUNEL test. This is even more striking in the report by Duran et al., in which the predictive value of TUNEL was applied to IUI cycles, where a limited number of oocytes is usually available compared to IVF [22]. That is, while in IVF the probability that a mature oocyte be fertilized by a spermatozoon with intact DNA or that a spermatozoon with damaged DNA fertilizes an oocyte with a high DNA repair capacity is relatively high, given the high number of oocytes usually obtained after oocyte retrieval, this probability is much lower in IUI, where usually only one or two oocytes are available. It should be noted that although the TUNEL test is frequently used to determine apoptosis in cells, TUNEL positivity is not always synonymous with apoptosis, since hydroxyl radical-induced DNA damage also results in double-stranded DNA fragmentation that can be detected by the TUNEL test [26]. Also of importance is that since more than 90% of DNA is comprised by non-protein-coding regions or introns, the probability that DNA damage will affect protein-coding regions (exons) is very low. This would also explain, at least in part, why spermatozoa carrying some type of DNA damage could result in a viable pregnancy.

Despite the predictive value issues indicated above, the SCSA is still the test for which the most clinical data are available [4,27,28]. In fact, many of the current indications for sperm DNA fragmentation testing have been derived from the results obtained with the SCSA. Using the SCSA, Wyrobek et al. demonstrated a statistically significant increase in sperm DNA fragmentation in men above 45 years of age [29]. Another study found that men who are homozygous null for glutathione-S-transferase M1 are less likely to detoxify metabolites of carcinogenic polycyclic aromatic hydrocarbons found in air pollution, making them more susceptible to the effects of air pollution on sperm chromatin [5]. This could explain, at least partially, why sperm DNA fragmentation can occur episodically without an apparent cause [30]. It has also been reported that a significant proportion of patients with varicocele have pathological levels of sperm DNA fragmentation, as measured by the SCSA, and that a significant decrease in DNA fragmentation was observed after varicocele repair [31,32]. In one study, 65% of patients with abnormal sperm DNA fragmentation levels returned to normal levels after the varicocelectomy [32].

More recently, it has become apparent that tests such as the Halosperm and COMET tests provide a relatively high predictive value in terms of reproductive outcome [33]. Particularly, constitutive double-strand breaks of sperm DNA that occur during meiosis I, when present above a threshold of 60% as measured by the COMET test at neutral pH, appear to correlate with failed embryo development beyond Day 3, implantation failure and recurrent miscarriage [34,35].

In conclusion, the presence of acid- or alkali-labile DNA breaks in the paternal genome above a critical threshold may not necessarily lead to failed pregnancy after ART. Although the presence of extensive double-strand DNA breaks and high levels of 8-OH-guanine and 8-OH-2′-deoxyguanosine, like those produced after hydroxyl radical-induced damage during sperm transport through the seminiferous tubules and the epididymis, could severely compromise embryo development.

115

However, even if there is significant DNA damage, the probability that a viable pregnancy will ensue is going to depend on:

- The proportion of spermatozoa with damaged DNA
- The extent of DNA fragmentation per cell
- The level of 8-OH-guanine and 8-OH-2'-deoxyguanosine in sperm DNA
- The type of DNA regions that are damaged (i.e., introns vs. exons)
- The ability of the fertilized oocyte and the embryo to repair this DNA damage
- The number of oocytes available
- The methodology used for the processing of the sperm samples for ART, which should always follow the basic principle of *primum non nocere*
- The type of test used to measure DNA fragmentation [36]

Some of these factors cannot be measured, for example whether the DNA damage affects exons or introns, or whether the sperm DNA damage has been repaired by the oocyte and/or the embryo. Consequently, the predictive value of sperm DNA fragmentation tests will always have DNA region, oocyte- and embryo-derived uncertainty factors and hence cannot have a 100% negative predictive value, as was originally suggested by the 'iceberg effect' model proposed by Evenson [13]. The concomitant determination of DNA fragmentation and nucleotide modifications of the 8-OH-guanine and 8-OH-2'-deoxyguanosine type in sperm DNA, could significantly improve the predictive value of tests that measure DNA fragmentation, especially those that measure double-stranded DNA breaks. However, tests that measure 8-OH-guanine and 8-OH-2'-deoxyguanosine are not yet available for application in a clinical setting.

Indications for Sperm DNA Fragmentation Testing

The main indications for sperm DNA fragmentation testing are:

- Idiopathic infertility
- Repeated pregnancy failure in IVF without an apparent cause
- Day 3 *et seq* embryo block
- Recurrent miscarriage
- Previous treatment with chemo- and/or radiotherapy
- Recent episode of high fever
- Clinical varicocele (grades 2 and 3)
- Male age above 45 years

The tests currently recommended to measure sperm DNA fragmentation, given their high predictive value and commercial availability, are the COMET at alkaline and neutral pH, the TUNEL and Halosperm tests.

While current clinical practice guidelines do not recommend routine testing of all male partners for sperm DNA damage [1,3], physicians need to be cognizant of the issue and pursue testing and potential causative factors in pertinent cases [2].

TUNEL Assay

Principle

The TUNEL assay method relies on the enzyme terminal deoxynucleotide transferase (TdT), which attaches deoxynucleotides to the 3'-hydroxyl terminus of DNA breaks. TdT is expressed in certain immune cells and acts during V(D)J recombination.

Specimen

Ejaculates collected by masturbation into sterile containers (see Chapter 3).

Equipment

- Eppendorf pipetters (5 μl, 10 μl)
- Shaker
- Eppendorf microcentrifuge
- Fluorescence microscope
- Flow cytometer

Materials

- Disposable Falcon tubes with caps (15 ml)
- Tips for Eppendorf pipetters (5 μl, 10 μl)
- Pipettes (1 ml, 2 ml, 10 ml)
- Eppendorf tubes

Reagents

Pre-labelling:	Washing solution: Dulbecco's phosphate-buffered saline (PBS).
Fixation solution:	Paraformaldehyde, 4% in PBS, pH 7.4, freshly prepared.
Permeabilization solution:	0.1% Triton X-100 in 0.1% sodium citrate, freshly prepared.
PBS:	Dulbecco's Phosphate Buffered Saline Solution, (PBS-1X; Cat# 9235, Irvine Scientific, Santa Ana, CA).
Labelling solutions:	TUNEL Enzyme Solution (TUNEL enzyme kit from Roche; Cat# 1168479910). TUNEL Label Solution (TUNEL enzyme kit from Roche; Cat# 1168479910).
Positive control reagent:	DNAase I solution (Roche, Cat# 09536282001).
Anti-fluorescein antibody:	Fab fragment from sheep conjugated with horseradish peroxidase (Roche, Cat# 1684817).
Diaminobenzidine substrate:	DAB substrate (Roche, Cat# 1718096).

Procedures – Flow Cytometry

1. Wash the test sample two times in PBS and adjust volume to obtain a total of 10×10^6 spermatozoa.
2. Transfer aliquot of sperm suspension to Eppendorf tube.
3. Add two volumes of PBS and mix thoroughly.
4. Centrifuge in Eppendorf microcentrifuge at 300 $g \times 2$ min.
5. Discard supernatant.
6. Add 200 μl of PBS to the resulting pellet and resuspend.
7. Add 200 μl of PBS of 4% paraformaldehyde (final concentration of paraformaldehyde = 2%).
8. After incubation, add 200 μl of PBS to stop fixation process. At this point, the sample can be stored at +4°C until further analysis.
9. Divide fixed sample in three aliquots and transfer one aliquot to three different Eppendorf tubes:
   a) Test sample
   b) Positive control
   c) Negative control
10. Centrifuge at 300 $g \times 2$ min.
11. Discard supernatant.

12. Add 200 μl of PBS and centrifuge two times at 300 g × 2 min.
13. Discard supernatant.
14. Add 100 μl of permeabilization solution to pellet.
15. Incubate at +4°C during 2 min.
16. Add 300 μl of PBS and centrifuge at 300 g × 2 min.
17. For the positive control tube, add 100 μl of DNAase I and incubate at 15–25°C during 10 min.
18. Prepare the TUNEL Reaction Mixture by adding 5 μl of TUNEL Enzyme Solution to 45 μl of TUNEL Label Solution, one 50 μl aliquot for each of the test sample and positive control tubes.
19. Add 50 μl of the TUNEL Reaction Mixture to the test sample, and 50 μl to the positive control tube.
20. Add 50 μl of TUNEL Label Solution only to the negative control tube.
21. Incubate at 37°C during 60 min in the dark (e.g. inside an incubator at 37°C).
22. Add 300 μl of PBS to each tube and centrifuge at 300 g × 2 min.
23. Repeat step #22 one more time.
24. Discard supernatant and add 500 μl of PBS.
25. Keep at +4°C in the dark until analysis by flow cytometry.
26. Sperm DNA fragmentation is monitored with a FACScan flow cytometer.
    Note: The flow cytometry parameters depend on the instrument utilized. The parameters provided here correspond to a Becton Dickinson FACScan instrument (Becton Dickinson, San Jose, CA, USA) equipped with a 15 mW argon-ion laser for excitation. A minimum of 10,000 spermatozoa are quantified. Light scattering and fluorescence data are obtained at a fixed gain setting in logarithmic mode. Green fluorescence from FITC is detected in the FL1 sensor through a 550-nm dichroic long-pass filter and a 525-nm band-pass filter.

Procedure – Fluorescence Microscopy

Perform steps 1 to 23 as per the flow cytometry protocol.

24. Discard the supernatant and add 50 μl of PBS.
25. Keep at +4°C in the dark until analysis.
26. Smear on slide and place coverslip on top.
27. Adjust fluorescence microscope to an excitation wavelength in the range of 450 to 500 nm (e.g. 488) and detection wavelength in the range of 515 to 565 nm.
28. For each preparation, assess between 200 and 500 spermatozoa. Count the total number of spermatozoa under phase contrast, and the number of spermatozoa showing green fluorescence; see Calculations and Results.

Note: Alternatively, another fluorochrome such as propidium iodide (PI) can be used as a general DNA stain to label all sperm nuclei in the preparation being assessed, requiring dual band fluorescence (see Figure 5.2).

Procedure – Brightfield Microscopy

Perform steps 1 to 23 as per the flow cytometry protocol.

24. Discard the supernatant and add 50 μl of PBS.
25. Smear onto a microscope slide and air dry for 10 min.
26. Add 50 μl of anti-fluorescein antibody solution.
27. Incubate in a humidified chamber for 30 min at 37°C.
28. Rinse with 100 μl of PBS.
29. Repeat step #28 twice.
30. Add 50 μl of DAB substrate.
31. Wait 2 min.
32. Place a coverslip on top.
33. For each preparation assess between 200 and 500 DAB-stained spermatozoa by brightfield microscopy; see Calculations and Results.

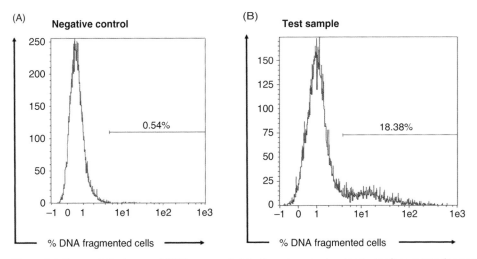

Figure 5.1 Representative images of TUNEL assay analysis by flow cytometry showing the % of sperm DNA fragmentation. (A) = negative control (without TDT enzyme); (B) = test sample. Images courtesy of Dr Alberto Pacheco Castro, Andrology Laboratory Director, IVI Madrid, Madrid, Spain.

Calculations and Results

Flow cytometry: All fluorescence signals of labeled spermatozoa are analyzed by flow cytometry. About 10,000 spermatozoa are examined for each assay at a flow rate of less than 100 cells/s. The excitation wavelength is 488 nm supplied by an argon laser at 15 mW. Green fluorescence (480–530 nm) is measured in the FL-1 channel and red fluorescence (580–630 nm) in the FL-2 channel.

The negative control is the test sample not incubated with the terminal deoxynucleotidyl transferase enzyme (TdT) and the positive control is the test sample incubated with DNase. The percentage of positive cells (green fluorescence) in the test sample is calculated on a 1023-channel scale using the flow cytometer software FlowJo Mac version 8.2.4 (FlowJo LLC, Ashland, OR). The percentage of TUNEL positive spermatozoa (DFI) in the test sample is calculated by subtracting spermatozoa with green fluorescence in the negative control (GFNC) from spermatozoa with green fluorescence in the test sample (GFTS) divided by total spermatozoa with green fluorescence in the positive control (GFPC):

$$DFI = [(GFTS - GFNC)]/(GFPC)$$

Fluorescence microscopy: Assess between 200 and 500 spermatozoa for each test sample and also for the positive and negative controls. Calculate the ratio of spermatozoa showing green fluorescence compared to the total number of spermatozoa assessed under phase contrast. Use the percentage of fluorescent spermatozoa in the test sample minus the percentage of fluorescent spermatozoa in the negative control to calculate the final result.

Brightfield microscopy: Assess between 200 and 500 spermatozoa for each test sample and the positive and negative controls. Subtract DAB-stained spermatozoa in the negative control and obtain the ratio of stained to total spermatozoa counted by brightfield and phase-contrast microscopy, respectively.

Reference Limits

Normal range: <20%

Abnormal values: ≥20%

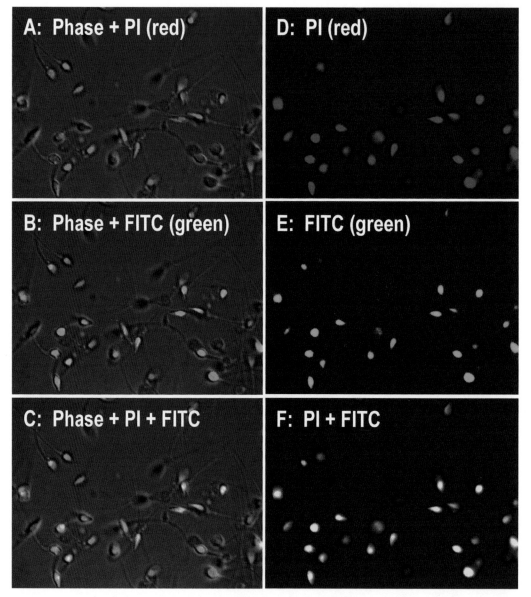

Figure 5.2 Sperm chromatin assessment by TUNEL using fluorescence microscopy. All images are of the same field of spermatozoa: matching images of propidium iodide ('PI' as a general DNA stain; red), FITC (green), and PI+FITC fluorescence, with and without concurrent phase contrast optics, are shown in the left- and right-hand columns, respectively. See text for further explanation of the TUNEL assay. However, it is clear that some spermatozoa are not labeled by either fluorochrome, indicating the origin of possible artifact in this test. Images courtesy of Madelaine From Björk, Andrology Laboratory, Karolinska University Hospital, Huddinge, Sweden.

Quality Control

- For internal quality control, run duplicates of each sample (test sample, positive and negative control). Replicate values should be within 5% for flow cytometry and 10% for fluorescence and brightfield microscopy.
- For external quality control, send aliquots of fixed samples to a reference laboratory for analysis by TUNEL/flow cytometry. Values should be within 10% for flow cytometry and 15% for fluorescence and brightfield microscopy.

Comet Assay

Principle

The Comet test run under neutral and alkaline pH conditions permits analysis of single- and double-strand sperm DNA fragmentation based on the migration of sperm DNA fragments after cell lysis and protamine extraction in an agarose matrix as a consequence of an applied electric field.

The protocol below was generously provided by Dr Agustín García-Peiró of the Barcelona Male Infertility Center ('CIMAB') at the Universitat Autònoma de Barcelona, Barcelona, Spain.

Specimen

Fresh, cryopreserved or frozen semen samples.

Equipment

- Rack for 1.5 ml Eppendorf tubes
- Rack for 200 µl Eppendorf tubes
- Freezing block
- Automatic pipetters, 2–20 µl and 50–200 µl
- Refrigerator
- Fume adsorber cabinet (with carbon filter)
- Electrophoresis equipment
- Phase contrast microscope
- Fluorescence microscope
- Centrifuge
- Microwave oven
- Metal plate
- Heating plate
- Tweezers
- Scissors

Materials

- Sterile 50 ml urine containers
- Eppendorf tubes: 1.5 ml and 200 µl
- Pasteur pipettes
- Tips for automatic pipetters
- Agarose-treated slides
- 20 × 20 mm #1½ weight coverslips
- 22 × 50 or 24 × 50 mm #1 weight coverslips

Reagents and Solutions

As described in Table 5.1. Note that the lysis solutions are formulated for use with several samples (formulations for single-use lysis solutions would contain only 0.1 g of DTT per 100 ml in LS1 and 0.05 g per 100 ml in LS2).

Procedure

1. Thaw the sample at room temperature.
2. Add PBS 1× to fill the 1.5-ml Eppendorf tube. Centrifuge the thawed sample at 300 g × 2 min. Discard supernatant. Repeat the process twice.

Table 5.1 Preparation of reagents and solutions for the COMET assay. Reagent water is water purified at least by reverse osmosis, but ideally using a Milli-Q® Type 1 ultrapure water system (Millipore Sigma, see www.emdmillipore.com)

Reagent	Quantity to prepare	Preparation and quantity to measure		Supplier	Catalogue #
Agarose-treated slides	50 slides	Agarose, low melting temperature	1.0 g	Sigma-Aldrich	A9414
		Reagent water	100 ml		
Agarose aliquots	50 ml	Agarose	0.5 g	Sigma-Aldrich	A9414
		Reagent water	50 ml		
TBE 10× solution	1000 ml $pH_o = 8.3$	Trizma® base	108.0 g	Sigma-Aldrich	T6066
		Boric acid	27.5 g	Sigma-Aldrich	B6768
		0.5 M EDTA	63.6 ml	Life Technologies	AM9262
		Reagent water	936.4 ml		
TBE solution for neutral electrophoresis and washes	1000 ml $pH_o = 8.5$	TBE 10×	100 ml		
		Reagent water	900 ml		
0.9% NaCl solution	1000 ml $pH_o = 5-6$	NaCl	9.0 g	Sigma-Aldrich	S7653
		Reagent water	1000 ml		
Cold alkaline solution	1000 ml $pH_o = 12.0$	NaOH	1.2 g	Sigma-Aldrich	S5881
		NaCl	58.44 g	Sigma-Aldrich	S7653
		Reagent water	1000 ml		
Alkaline electrophoresis solution	1000 ml $pH_o = 12.2$	NaOH	1.2 g	Sigma-Aldrich	S5881
		Reagent water	1000 ml		
Neutralization solution	1000 ml $pH_o = 10.0$ $pH_f = 7.5$	Trizma® base	48.44 g	Sigma-Aldrich	T6066
		Reagent water	1000 ml		
Ethanol 70%	1000 ml	Ethanol	700 ml	Merck	1009835000
		Reagent water	300 ml		
Ethanol 90%	1000 ml	Ethanol	900 ml	Merck	1009835000
		Reagent water	100 ml		
Ethanol 100%	1000 ml	Ethanol	1000 ml	Merck	1009835000
Lysis Solution 1	75 ml $pH = 7.5$	DTT	9.26 g	Thermo-Fisher	R0862
		Trizma® base	3.64 g	Sigma-Aldrich	T6066
		SDS 10%	7.5 ml	Sigma-Aldrich	71736L
		Reagent water	67.5 ml		
Lysis Solution 2	75 ml $pH_f = 7.5$	Trizma® base	3.64 g	Sigma-Aldrich	T6066
		DTT	4.63 g	Thermo-Fisher	R0862
		NaCl	8.7 6 g	Sigma-Aldrich	S7653
		EDTA 0.5 M	7.5 ml	Life Technologies	AM9261
		Reagent water	67.5 ml		
PBS 10×	1000 ml $pH_o = 6.9$ $pH_f = 7.5$	NaCl	80.0 g	Sigma-Aldrich	S7653
		KCl	2.0 g	Sigma-Aldrich	P9333
		Na_2HPO_4	14.4 g	Sigma-Aldrich	S5136
		KH_2PO_4	2.4 g	Sigma-Aldrich	P5655

Table 5.1 (cont.)

Reagent	Quantity to prepare	Preparation and quantity to measure		Supplier	Catalogue #
		Reagent water	1000 ml		
DAPI		SlowFade® Gold antifade mountant with DAPI		Life Technologies	S36938

3. Check the concentration of the sample by placing 3 μl on a normal slide and adjust it to observe about 10 spermatozoa per field of view under the 20× objective.

4. Boil water in the microwave oven. Liquefy an aliquot of gelled agarose for 1–2 min. Shake the tube to homogenize the agarose.

5. Add 50 μl of agarose with 25 μl of sample and pipette to homogenize.

6. Quickly place 25 μl of the agarose-sample mixture onto each of two agarose-treated slides and cover the drop with a 20 × 20 mm coverslip. One of the slides will be assigned to the Neutral Comet and the other to the Alkaline Comet.

7. Allow the two slides (Alkaline and Neutral) to gel for 5 min on a metal plate in a refrigerator.

8. Remove the coverslips very gently, avoiding breaking the gels.

9. Immerse the slides in Lysis 1 solution for 30 min at ambient temperature. Slightly tilt the slides to remove excess solution.

10. Immerse slides in Lysis 2 solution for 30 min at ambient temperature. Slightly tilt the slides to remove excess solution.

11. Wash the slides in TBE: 2 min for the Neutral Comet slide and 2 min for the Alkaline Comet.

12. *Slide intended for Neutral Comet:*
    a) Perform an electrophoresis of the slide destined for Neutral Comet at 1 V/cm for 12.5 min, using TBE (neutral electrophoresis solution) as buffer.
    b) Immerse the slide in 0.9% NaCl for 2 min.
    c) Remove the neutral electrophoresis solution, gently wash the cell with water and Milli-Q water and fill the cell with the alkaline electrophoresis solution.

13. *Slide intended for Alkaline Comet:*
    a) Immerse the slide intended for the Alkaline Comet in the cold alkaline solution in the refrigerator for 2.5 min.
    b) Perform the electrophoresis of this slide at 1 V/cm for 4 min using the alkaline electrophoresis solution as a buffer.
    c) Remove the alkaline electrophoresis solution and wash the cuvette with tap water and Milli-QQ water.

Both types of slides:

12. Incubate in the neutralization solution for 5 min.

13. Inside the fume adsorber cabinet, cover the slides with 70%, 90% and 100% ethanol, sequentially, for 2 min each. Remove each ethanol by slightly tilting the slide.

14. Let the slides dry horizontally inside the cabinet.

17. *Analysis:*
    a) Add 2 drops of SlowFade® Gold antifade mountant with DAPI and cover with a 22 × 50 or 24 × 50 coverslip.
    b) Evaluate under a fluorescence microscope, classifying 100 spermatozoa as either fragmented or non-fragmented.

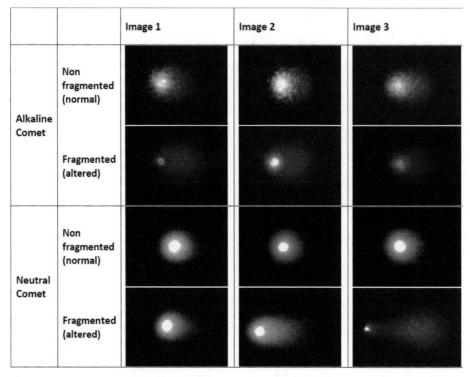

		Image 1	Image 2	Image 3
Alkaline Comet	Non fragmented (normal)			
	Fragmented (altered)			
Neutral Comet	Non fragmented (normal)			
	Fragmented (altered)			

Figure 5.3 Microscopic images (40× objective, DAPI staining) showing non-fragmented (normal) and fragmented (altered) spermatozoa obtained by the Alkaline Comet Assay for the detection of single-strand breaks and the Neutral Comet Assay for the detection of double-strand breaks. Figure courtesy of Dr Agustín García Peiró, Barcelona Male Infertility Center CIMAB, Spain.

Results

The test samples and the internal control samples are evaluated under a fluorescence microscope (manually or using a specific software), classifying 100 spermatozoa between fragmented and non-fragmented according to the criteria shown in Figure 5.3.

Reference Limits

Alkaline COMET: Values of >45% of spermatozoa with single-strand DNA fragmentation are considered abnormal.

Neutral COMET: Values of >60% of spermatozoa with double-strand DNA fragmentation are considered abnormal.

Sperm Chromatin Dispersion Test (SCD Test/Halosperm Test)

Principle

The Halosperm Test is a variant method of the Sperm Chromatin Dispersion (SCD) assay and determines the vulnerability of sperm DNA to acid denaturation following the principle that induced condensation is directly related to sperm DNA fragmentation. Spermatozoa are suspended in an agarose micro gel before being placed on an agarose pre-treated slide, effectively achieving a 'suspension-like environment' on the slide [15].

An acid solution is then applied to denature the sperm chromatin and followed by treatment with a lysis buffer to lyse the sperm membranes and remove nuclear proteins. As a result, a halo of dispersed

DNA loops surrounds the central core of the sperm nucleus and this can be viewed under brightfield microscopy after suitable staining.

Spermatozoa with intact DNA will have large halos while those with increasing levels of DNA fragmentation will produce decreasing sized halos, even to the extent of a very small halo or perhaps even no halo at all.

The protocol below was generously provided by Dr Jaime Gosàlvez of the Universidad Autónoma de Madrid (UAM), Madrid, Spain.

Specimen
Semen samples collected by masturbation into a sterile container (see Chapter 3).

Equipment
- Eppendorf pipetters (5 µl, 10 µl)
- Water-bath at 37°C
- Bright field microscope
- Fume hood
- Processing trays, e.g. 100 × 20 mm Petri dishes

Materials
- Poly-L-Lysine, silane or agarose coated slides
- Low-melting point aqueous agarose
- Tips for Eppendorf pipetters
- Eppendorf tubes 1.5 ml
- 22 × 50 or 24 × 50 mm coverslips

Reagents

Solution for DNA denaturation:	0.1 N HCl; either purchased ready-to-use or prepared by adding the appropriate volume of more concentrated HCl to distilled or reverse osmosis-purified water.
Agarose:	A solution of low melting point agarose (e.g. ThermoFisher Scientific UltraPure™ Low Melting Point Agarose, catalogue reference 16520050) in distilled or reverse osmosis-purified water to a final concentration of 2%.
Lysing solution A:	Solution containing 0.5 M Tris buffer (e.g. Tris Buffer 1.0 M, pH 8.0, molecular biology grade – CAS 77–86-1 from Merck, Germany), 0.02 M DTT (1,4-dithiothreitol), and 50 mM EDTA, in distilled or reverse osmosis-purified water, pH 7.5.
Lysing solution B:	Solution containing 0.5 M Tris buffer, 2 M NaCl, 0.02 M DTT, and 2% SDS (sodium dodecyl sulphate), in distilled or reverse osmosis-purified water, pH 7.5.
Washing solution A:	Tris-borate-EDTA buffer 0.09 M, pH 7.5
Washing solution B:	PBS: Phosphate Buffered Saline
Fixing/dehydrating solutions:	Series of 50%, 70%, 95% and 100% (v/v) ethanol
Staining solution:	Wright Stain solution 5% in PBS (www.sigmaaldrich.com/industries/tissue-diagnostics/wright-stain.html)
Mountant:	e.g. Permount™ (Fisher Chemical™ SP15-100)

Note: Commercial kits are available for the sperm chromatin dispersion test, e.g. Halosperm G2 kit (Halotech DNA, Madrid, Spain; www.halotechdna.com).

Procedure

1. Sperm samples must be adjusted to a final concentration of 5–10×10^6 spermatozoa per ml using any standard sperm-washing medium.
2. Place a 100 μl aliquot of the low melting point agarose in a water bath to warm to 37°C.
3. Mix the agarose at 37°C with 30 μl of the sperm sample and mix using the micropipette to ensure a homogeneous distribution of the sample. Maintain at 37°C in the water bath.
4. Using a clean micropipette tip take 10 μl of the agarose-spermatozoa mixture and place it on the coated slide. This drop must be covered with a coverslip (22 × 50 or 24 × 50 mm) and left to solidify at +4°C for 10 min.
5. Once a microgel has been formed, remove the coverslip to expose the spermatozoa to the different reagents.

Note: Procedure steps #6 to #13 must be performed in a fume hood.

6. Place the slide in a tray with the acid denaturation solution at ambient temperature for 9 min.
7. Block DNA denaturation by washing the slide for 10 min in Tris-borate-EDTA buffer.
8. Transfer the slide to a new tray containing Lysing Solution A and maintain at ambient temperature for 20 min.
9. Transfer the slide to a new tray containing Lysing Solution B and maintain at ambient temperature for 10 min.
10. Transfer the slide to a new tray containing Washing Solution A and maintain at ambient temperature for 5 min.
11. Transfer the slide to a new tray containing Washing Solution B and maintain at ambient temperature for 5 min. The slide is now ready for dehydration/fixation.
12. For dehydration/fixation place the slide in each alcohol concentration (50%, 70%, 95% and 100%) for 2 × 20 min each starting from 50% alcohol concentration.
13. The slides are air dried at ambient temperature.
14. For visualization under brightfield microscopy, stain the slides using Wright Giemsa.
15. Wash the slides with distilled water for 5 min.
16. *Immediate reading:* Although slides can be analysed directly under the microscope using a 40× objective, to achieve better focus the stained slide can be covered with a 24 × 50 mm coverslip directly mounted using water. Using a 100× oil immersion objective on unmounted slides is not recommended due to the risk of contaminating the objective.
17. *Permanent mounted preparations:* Alternatively, leave the slide to air dry and mount with a permanent mounting medium and 22 × 50 or 24 × 50 mm coverslip. These slides provide the best images because they can be examined under a bright field microscope using properly adjusted Köhler illumination and a 100× oil immersion objective.
18. Evaluate at least 300 spermatozoa per patient according to the following criteria:
    Although spermatozoa processing using the SCD test produce a continuous pattern of chromatin dispersion, where a halo of dispersed chromatin surrounding a dense stained core is seen, for scoring systematization four dispersion patterns have been established:
    Large halo: The size of the halo is larger than the diameter of the core
    Medium halo: The size of the halo is equivalent to or slightly larger than the diameter of the core
    Small halo: The size of the halo is smaller than the diameter of the core
    No halo: No halo around the core

Spermatozoa with fragmented DNA present a large or medium halo of dispersed chromatin, the rest of the nuclei must be considered as comprising damaged DNA. The percentage of cells with fragmented DNA with respect to the total number of cells counted represents the percentage of affected spermatozoa.

Calculations and Results

The proportion of spermatozoa containing fragmented DNA is represented by the spermatozoa showing small or no halos. Express this group as a percentage of all the spermatozoa counted.

Reference Limits

Normal range: <15% of spermatozoa with DNA fragmentation
Medium range: 15–30% of spermatozoa with DNA fragmentation
Abnormal values: ≥30% of spermatozoa with DNA fragmentation

Quality Control

For internal quality control, cryopreserved samples previously scored using the same methodology can be processed in parallel.

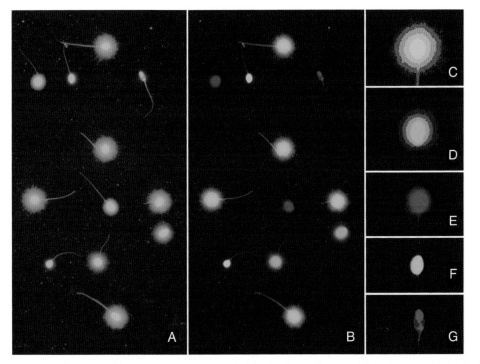

Figure 5.4 Illustration of human spermatozoa processed by the Sperm Chromatin Dispersion test and visualized under fluorescence microscopy: (A) after staining with SYBR Green and captured with a high resolution Nikon DS-Ri2 CCD camera; (B) pseudocoloured image to highlight halos of different sizes; (C–G) green = large halo of dispersed chromatin (no fragmented sperm DNA); blue = medium halo of dispersed chromatin (no fragmented sperm DNA); red = small halo of dispersed chromatin (fragmented sperm DNA); yellow = absence of halo (fragmented sperm DNA); pink = degraded spermatozoon highly fragmented sperm DNA). Image courtesy of Dr Jaime Gosálvez, Halotech DNA, Madrid, Spain; www.halotechdna.com

References

1. Schlegel PN, Sigman M, Collura B, et al. Diagnosis and treatment of infertility in men: AUA/ASRM guideline part I. *Fertil Steril* 2021; **115**: 54–61.

2. Aitken RJ, Bakos HW. Should we be measuring DNA damage in human spermatozoa? New light on an old question. *Hum Reprod* 2021; **36**: 1175–85.

3. Esteves SC, Zini A, Coward RM, et al. Sperm DNA fragmentation testing: summary evidence and clinical practice recommendations. *Andrologia* 2020; **53**: e13874.

4. Evenson D. DNA Damage: sperm chromatin structure assay. Sperm chromatin structure assay test on its fortieth anniversary. In: Agarwal A, Henkel R, Majzoub A, eds. *Manual of Sperm Function Testing in Human Assisted Reproduction.* Cambridge: Cambridge University Press, 2021, 192–201.

5. Rubes J, Selevan SG, Sram RJ, et al. GSTM1 genotype influences the susceptibility of men to sperm DNA damage associated with exposure to air pollution. *Mutat Res* 2007; **625**: 20–8.

6. Steele EK, McClure N, Maxwell RJ, Lewis SE. A comparison of DNA damage in testicular and proximal epididymal spermatozoa in obstructive azoospermia. *Mol Hum Reprod* 1999; **5**: 831–5.

7. Lewis SEM, O'Connell M, Stevenson M, et al. An algorithm to predict pregnancy in assisted conception. *Mol Hum Reprod* 2004; **19**: 1385–90.

8. Greco E, Scarselli F, Iacobelli M, et al. Efficient treatment of infertility due to sperm DNA damage by ICSI with testicular spermatozoa. *Hum Reprod* 2005; **20**: 226–30.

9. Ollero M, Gil-Guzman E, Lopez MC, et al. Characterization of subsets of human spermatozoa at different stages of maturation: implications in the diagnosis and treatment of male infertility. *Hum Reprod* 2001; **16**: 1912–21.

10. Suganuma R, Yanagimachi R, Meistricht M. Decline in fertility of mouse sperm with abnormal chromatin during epididymal passage as revealed by ICSI. *Hum Reprod* 2005; **20**: 3101–8.

11. Cui J, Holmes EH, Greene TG, Liu PK. Oxidative DNA damage precedes DNA fragmentation after experimental stroke in rat brain. *FASEB J* 2000; **14**: 955–67.

12. Sergerie M, Laforest G, Bujan L, et al. Sperm DNA fragmentation: threshold value in male fertility. *Hum Reprod* 2005; **20**: 3446–51.

13. Evenson DP, Jost LK, Marshall D, et al. Utility of the sperm chromatin structure assay as a diagnostic and prognostic tool in the human fertility clinic. *Hum Reprod* 1999; **14**: 1039–49.

14. Fernández JL, Muriel L, Rivero MT, et al. The sperm chromatin dispersion test: a simple method for the determination of sperm DNA fragmentation. *J Androl* 2003 **24**: 59–66.

15. Fernández JL, Muriel L, Goyanes V, et al. Simple determination of human sperm DNA fragmentation with an improved sperm chromatin dispersion test. *Fertil Steril* 2005; **84**: 833–42.

16. Enciso M, Sarasa J, Agarwal A, et al. A two-tailed Comet assay for assessing DNA damage in spermatozoa. *Reprod Biomed Online* 2009; **18**: 609–16.

17. Fernandez JL, Vazquez-Gundin F, Delgado A, et al. DNA breakage detection-FISH (DBD-FISH) in human spermatozoa: technical variants evidence different structural features. *Mutat Res* 2000; **453**: 77–82.

18. Manicardi GC, Bianchi PG, Pantano S, et al. Presence of endogenous nicks in DNA of ejaculated human spermatozoa and its relationship to chromomycin A3 accessibility. *Biol Reprod* 1995; **52**: 864–67.

19. Singh NP, MacCoy MT, Tice RR, Schneider EL. A simple technique for quantification of low levels of DNA damage in individual cells. *Exp Cell Res* 1998; **175**: 184–91.

20. Singh N., Danner D, Tice R, et al. Abundant alkali-sensitive sites in DNA of human and mouse sperm. *Exp Cell Res* 1989; **184**: 461–70.

21. Gorczyca W, Gong J, Darzynkiewicz Z. Detection of DNA strand breaks in individual apoptotic cells by the in situ terminal deoxynucleotidyl transferase and nick translation assays. *Cancer Res* 1993; **53**: 945–51.

22. Duran EH, Morshedi M, Taylor S, Oehninger S. Sperm DNA quality predicts intrauterine insemination outcome: a prospective cohort study. *Hum Reprod* 2002; **17**: 3122–8.

23. Alvarez JG. Efficient treatment of infertility due to sperm DNA damage by ICSI with testicular spermatozoa. *Hum Reprod* 2005; **20**: 2031–2.

24. Borini A, Tarozzi N, Bizzaro D, et al. Sperm DNA fragmentation: paternal effect on early post-implantation embryo development in ART. *Hum Reprod* 2006; **21**: 2876–81.

25. Muriel L, Meseguer M, Fernandez JL, et al. Value of the sperm chromatin dispersion test in predicting pregnancy outcome in intrauterine insemination: a blind prospective study. *Hum Reprod* 2006; **21**: 738–44.

26. Negoescu A, Guillermet C, Lorimier P, et al. Importance of DNA fragmentation in apoptosis with regard to TUNEL specificity. *Biomed Pharmacother* 1998; **52**: 252–8.

27. Evenson DP, Djira G, Kasperson K, Christianson J. Relationships between the age of 25,445 men attending infertility clinics and sperm chromatin structure assay (SCSA®) defined sperm DNA and chromatin integrity. *Fertil Steril* 2020; **114**: 311–20.

28. Jerre E, Bungum M, Evenson D, Giwercman A. Sperm chromatin structure assay high DNA stainability sperm as a marker of early miscarriage after intracytoplasmic sperm injection. *Fertil Steril* 2019; **112**: 46–53.

29. Wyrobek AJ, Eskenazi B, Young S, et al. Advancing age has differential effects on DNA damage, chromatin integrity, gene mutations, and aneuploidies in sperm. *Proc Natl Acad Sci* 2006; **103**: 9601–6.

30. Alvarez JG, Ollero M, Larson-Cook KL, Evenson DP. Selecting cryopreserved semen for assisted reproductive techniques based on the level of sperm nuclear DNA fragmentation resulted in pregnancy. *Fertil Steril* 2004; **81**: 712–13.

31. Werthman P, Wixon R, Kasperson K, Evenson DP. Significant decrease in sperm deoxyribonucleic acid fragmentation after varicocelectomy. *Fertil Steril* 2007; **90**: 1800–4.

32. Roque M, Esteves SC. Effect of varicocele repair on sperm DNA fragmentation: a review. *Int Urol Nephrol* 2018; **50**: 583–603.

33. Casanovas A, Ribas-Maynou J, Lara-Cerrillo S, et al. Double-stranded sperm DNA damage is a cause of delay in embryo development and can impair implantation rates. *Fertil Steril* 2019; **111**: 699–707.

34. Simon L, Aston KI, Emery BR, et al. Sperm DNA damage output parameters measured by the alkaline Comet assay and their importance. *Andrologia* 2017; **49**. https://doi.org/10.1111/and.12608

35. Simon L, Proutski I, Stevenson M, et al. Sperm DNA damage has a negative association with live-birth rates after IVF. *Reprod Biomed Online* 2013; **26**: 68–78.

36. Sakkas D, Alvarez JG. Sperm DNA fragmentation: mechanisms of origin, impact on reproductive outcome, and analysis. *Fertil Steril* 2010; **93**: 1027–36.

Computer-Aided Sperm Analysis

Introduction

Seventy years ago, Macleod and Gold stated that *'The quality of sperm motility is a prime factor to be considered in semen analysis. Achievement of intra- and inter-observer standardization is essential in any method used to assess sperm motility, and observers must be properly trained.'* [1]. While trained observers can reliably categorize sperm progression as rapid, slow and non-progressive motility by eye [2] as described in Chapters 3 and 12, patterns of sperm movement cannot; hence the need for computer-aided sperm analysis (CASA).

Despite greatly improved technology since its first introduction in 1985, CASA is still not widely used in routine diagnostic andrology laboratories. This has been attributed to unrealistic expectations of the technology, and early attempts to sell CASA systems as automated semen analysers [3]. Detailed discussions of the history of CASA, and the development of CASA technology, are beyond the scope of this chapter, and interested readers are referred to relevant review articles [2–10], reports from expert consensus workshops [11–13], as well as more recent updates on the status of CASA technology which have also been published [14,15]. Much of the responsibility for the persistent misuse of CASA technology must lie with its users who, rather than promoting the measurement of traditional semen characteristics known to have only limited clinical predictive value, should have applied the advanced capabilities of CASA technology to assess sperm characteristics with greater biological significance, notably ones based on sperm movement characteristics ('Kinematics', see below).

It is now well-established that it is dynamic sub-populations of motile spermatozoa with appropriate movement characteristics that determine whether a man's spermatozoa can penetrate his partner's cervical mucus, or penetrate the cumulus-oocyte complex and fertilize the oocyte [2,13–15]. Standardized protocols that apply CASA technology to investigate such sperm functional potential must be promoted (see Chapter 7).

Of key importance is that any test in the clinical laboratory which is automated must take into account the limitations inherent to automated laboratory processes [16]. Importantly, it must be noted that automation can involve a loss of technical knowledge and manual skills which have been acquired through decades of experience with conventional methods [17]. Therefore, while it is undeniable that CASA can make life much easier, it turns out that some specific, practical skills might well be lost over time. Overall, automation tends to limit the experience of laboratory technicians and technologists on a daily basis, thus potentially leading to decreased skills and expertise in analytical procedures, including, among other issues, potentially leading to quality controls becoming unnecessary, or to reducing the ability to apply pressure on companies for innovation [16,17]. Introducing a CASA instrument into an andrology laboratory does not mean that the quality of sperm analysis increases immediately. To that end, it is necessary to ensure that its operation and use is optimal, as with any other laboratory procedure. Training the users of CASA is fundamental for this.

Because the technical limitations of CASA technology can dramatically affect the correct use of CASA instruments, even to the extent of rendering results completely meaningless, it is essential that users understand both the technology and its limitations, and adhere to the consensus recommendations for its correct application [13,15]. These dictates apply not only to traditional CASA instruments but also to point-of-care and mobile-phone-based analysis systems; these emergent technologies are discussed in a dedicated section towards the end of this chapter.

Table 6.1 Non-exhaustive list of current CASA systems or devices and their manufacturers

Manufacturer	System/device	Location
CASA platforms		
Hamilton Thorne Inc	CEROS, IVOS (legacy software) CEROS-II, IVOS-II (2nd generation software)	Beverly, MA, USA www.hamiltonthorne.com
Microptic	Sperm Class Analyzer (SCA) SCAScope	Barcelona, Spain www.micropticsl.com and www.scascope.com
MMCSoft	MMC Sperm	Saint Petersburg, Russia www.mmcatalog.com/en/sperm/mmcsperm.html
Proiser R+D	ISAS v1, ISAS Lab, ISAS PSus	Paterna, Spain www.proiser.com
Compact/point-of-care devices		
BonRayBio	LensHooke™ X1 Pro	Taiwan www.bonraybio.com
MES (Medical Electronics Systems)	Sperm Quality Analyzer, current models are the SQA-Vision and the SQA-V Gold	Los Angeles, CA, USA www.mes-global.com

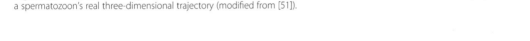

Curvilinear path	———	"Risers"	··················
Average path	- - - - - - -	• largest riser x 2	= ALHmax,
Straight line path	— — — -	• mean of all risers	= ALHmean

Figure 6.1 Illustration showing how the currently used kinematic measures are derived from the two-dimensional projection of a spermatozoon's real three-dimensional trajectory (modified from [51]).

A list of current major commercial CASA systems and details of their manufacturers are provided in Table 6.1

Kinematic Measures of Human Sperm Motility

Although it is the sperm tail which creates motility, modern CASA systems still cannot analyse flagellar beating, and hence we must continue to analyse motility by tracking the sperm head. Current sperm kinematic measures are based on studies using 50 fps microcinematography (see Figure 6.1) [18]. It must be remembered that all current standard kinematic measures are derived from the analysis of two-dimensional projections of the real world three-dimensional swimming pattern of spermatozoa. That spermatozoa roll as they swim was first discussed by Phillips in the early 1970s [19] and flagellar beat asymmetry described as the basis for this pattern of movement since the 1980s [20–24]. A fundamental requirement for flagellar beat asymmetry is due to the low Reynolds number of the system whereby spermatozoa swim in aqueous environments [25]. Direct three-dimensional analysis of swimming spermatozoa has also been reported in recent years [26–27].

While most modern CASA instruments employ 60 images/s, which has generally been considered adequate for spermatozoa in seminal plasma [28], the ideal image sampling frequency has been estimated

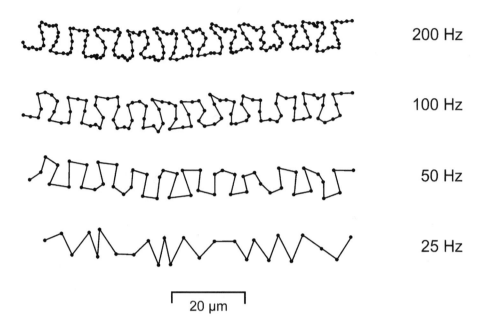

200 Hz

100 Hz

50 Hz

25 Hz

20 µm

Figure 6.2 Illustration of the effect of image sampling frequency (frame rate) on the perceived curvilinear velocity (VCL) of a spermatozoon (modified from [28]).

as closer to 130 Hz [29]. For analysing capacitating populations of human spermatozoa, although 60 images/s has been widely accepted as a technological compromise, a higher image sampling frequency of at least 120 Hz would provide more accurate track reconstruction.

Analyses of sperm movement derived from tracking the head can provide a great deal of useful information on sperm movement in semen and washed sperm populations [6,8,13,30], although it was from observations on flagellar beating that descriptions of hyperactivated motility were based [6,31].

Curvilinear velocity (VCL), sometimes referred to as 'track speed', is calculated from the sum of the straight lines joining the sequential positions of the sperm head along the spermatozoon's track. VCL is therefore the two-dimensional projection of the true three-dimensional helical path of the spermatozoon as revealed by the time resolution of the imaging method used – making it highly sensitive to the frame rate (see Figure 6.2) [28]. VCL values are reported in µm/s to one decimal place.

Average path velocity (VAP) is the velocity along the 'average' path of the spermatozoon. However, because the average path is derived by CASA machines using a variety of algorithms [2,4,6,13,15,32], the precise method used for its derivation must always be stated. For example, 5-point smoothing is *not* adequate for progressive human spermatozoa when tracked at 50 or 60 images/s, where the frame rates typically require more like 11-point smoothing or, better, adaptive smoothing algorithms. VAP values are reported in µm/s to one decimal place.

Straight-line velocity (VSL) is the linear or 'progression' velocity of the spermatozoon and is calculated from the straight-line distance between the start and end of the observed track. VSL values are reported in µm/s to one decimal place.

Three *progression ratios*, all expressed as integer percentages, can be calculated from the three velocity measurements described above:

Linearity	LIN	VSL/VCL × 100
Straightness	STR	VSL/VAP × 100
Wobble	WOB	VAP/VCL × 100

Amplitude of lateral head displacement (ALH) is calculated from the amplitudes of the lateral deviations of the sperm head about the cell's axis of progression (average path). Different CASA programmes use either an average value (ALHmean) calculated from the individual measurements made over the length of the track, or the maximum value (ALHmax) of all the measurements. Historically the ALH concept was based on track width measurements obtained from photomicrographic analyses of sperm movement and hence, by international agreement [15,32], ALH measurements are to be expressed as the width across the whole track [18], i.e. twice the average or maximum individual measurement; and are expressed in μm to one decimal place.

Beat/cross frequency(BCF) is the number of times that the curvilinear track crosses the average path per unit time. It is expressed in Hz, to one decimal place. In reality, BCF is a derivation of the true flagellar beat frequency and the frequency of rotation (ROF) of the sperm head (the number of times the sperm head rotates through 360° per unit time). A human spermatozoon swimming in seminal plasma will usually rotate through 180° at the apex of each lateral deviation of the head about the axis of progression. Unfortunately, ROF, and hence BCF, cannot be analysed reliably by current commercial CASA systems due to imaging frequency limitations that result in aliasing errors (see [6] for further explanation); reported values greater than half the image sampling frequency (sometimes called the frame rate) must be considered suspect.

Fractal dimension (D or 'FDM') is the 'quantitative assessment of the "space-filling" properties of curves on a plane' [33]: while a straight line has one dimension and a plane has two dimensions, a curved line has a dimension that lies between 1.0 and 2.0 (x and y coordinates). The simplest sperm tracks have D values close to 1.0, more complex tracks have values approaching 2.0, and recursive trajectories can have D values between 2.0 and 3.0, with the 'layering' of the trajectory being seen as analogous to the involvement of the third dimension (z coordinate). D is independent of scale, although still influenced by the image sampling frequency [34–36]. D needs to be derived from tracks of at least 0.5 s at 60 Hz (i.e. 31 track points) [37], and while D >1.30 can describe human sperm hyperactivated motility, it is unlikely to identify hyperactivated tracks consistently if used in isolation [38]. See 'Computer-Aided Sperm Analysis of Sperm Hyperactivation', below.

Factors that Limit Computer-Aided Sperm Analysis's Functionality for Human Semen Analysis

While CASA technology is widely used with excellent results in animal production laboratories and on wildlife species, the same is not yet true for human clinical laboratories [14]. Laboratories that use it for this purpose have presumably accepted that its results are more robust than what might be obtained from inadequately trained semen analysis technicians, and/or the lower determination cost precludes the use of more accurate assessments. CASA works extremely well on washed human sperm populations, which typically have very high motility and minimal contamination with other cells and debris, but the limitations affecting CASA's ability to provide accurate results for human sperm concentration and percentages of motile or progressively motile spermatozoa in semen, based on the reviews already cited in this chapter, fall into three major categories: biological, technological and technical.

It must be noted that the discussion here focuses on human spermatozoa, various aspects of cell identification and tracking, and factors that influence their accuracy, which are different for other species' spermatozoa.

Biological Issues

Human semen is probably the hardest type of specimen to have CASA systems analyse. Table 6.2 summarizes these issues and compares them to the semen of most other animal species.

Technological Limitations

These centre on issues relating to digital image analysis and the fundamental differences between how human operators and CASA instruments define and classify motility.

Table 6.2 A comparison of biological and technical issues in the analysis of human semen and semen from domesticated mammals using computer-aided sperm analysis (From ref. [32])

Criterion	Domesticated mammals	Humans
General fertility	Selected for high fertility over many generations	A low fecundity species (maximum reported 28%)
Semen cleanliness (presence of other cells, debris, etc.)	Generally 'clean'	Typically very 'dirty' ejaculates (high background noise)
Semen viscosity	Relatively low in most species	Generally high, with micro-heterogeneity
Possibility for dilution prior to analysis	Ejaculates are typically highly diluted with an 'extender' before analysis (many domesticated and wildlife species have $>1000 \times 10^6$ sperm/ml)	Generally $<200 \times 10^6$/ml, often very low ($<25 \times 10^6$/ml); dilution requires homologous seminal plasma to preserve motility kinematics
Proportion of motile spermatozoa	Typically well over 60%, often higher	Typically lower, often $<50\%$; many dead spermatozoa with aggregation
Sperm morphology	Highly consistent in very many species (although in some groups there can be many types of abnormalities, e.g. carnivores)	Highly pleiomorphic

Table 6.3 Example definitions for the classification of human sperm motility using traditional (manual/visual) and computer-aided sperm analysis technologies

Motility categories	Definitions	
	Manual/visual assessment	CASA approaches
Immotile	No tail beating seen	No movement of the sperm head. Actually based on the sperm head changing position by less than a proportion (e.g. half) of its size (usually based on length, sometimes on width)
Motile	Tail beating seen	Movement of the sperm head
Non-progressive motility	Tail beating seen but no net space gain (movement <5 μm/s)	The sperm head changes position by at least a proportion (e.g. half) of its size (usually based on length, sometimes on width), and VAP (sometimes VSL) of <5 μm/s
Progressive motility	Space gain (equivalent to VSL) of ≥ 5 μm/s but <25 μm/s	VAP (sometimes VSL) of ≥ 5 μm/s but <25 μm/s
Rapid progressive motility	Space gain (equivalent to VSL) of ≥ 25 μm/s	VAP (sometimes VSL) of ≥ 25 μm/s

Human observers base their assessments on flagellar beating and spatial displacement of the cell (Table 6.3), but current commercial CASA instruments cannot analyse flagellar beating directly and must rely on tracking the movement of the sperm head. In extreme situations, Brownian motion of immotile objects of similar size and appearance to sperm heads can be mistaken for sperm motility, and even establishing a robust definition for non-progressive motility (NPM) can be difficult when movement of the flagellum is not used. Consequently, the reported NPM sub-population differs when comparing CASA against motility assessments performed by a trained technician. While this issue will affect software validation, NPM spermatozoa cannot penetrate the cervical mucus *in vivo*, and hence have no chance of contributing to a conception – they can be considered as 'biological junk' [6,39]. CASA software validations should therefore focus on the progressively motile spermatozoa.

Many image-analysis problems stem from errors in discriminating between spermatozoa and non-sperm objects, and between immotile and motile objects. While more modern software can reduce this problem (e.g. CASA-II software on the Hamilton Thorne *IVOS-II* and *CEROS-II* platforms, the

Microptic *SCAScope*, and Proiser *ISAS Lab* and *ISAS PSus* systems with the introduction of tail recognition algorithms), core problems remain in many systems.

- When even as few as two spermatozoa are clumped together, or with debris, the resulting contiguous digitized object can be too large to be classified as a sperm head and is therefore rejected from the analysis. Consequently, the overall sperm concentration is reduced and, since such spermatozoa are typically non-progressive or immotile, the proportion of progressive cells is increased. Unfortunately, such 'micro-aggregates' are very common in human semen samples.

- When negative phase contrast optics or dark ground illumination are used, the incorrect identification of non-sperm objects (e.g. large pieces of debris) as 'spurious' spermatozoa can be a significant source of error, increasing the apparent total number of spermatozoa within the field of view [e.g. 40], see Figure 6.3.

- There is considerable debate regarding the choice of optics for use with CASA because tracking motile spermatozoa is greatly facilitated using negative phase contrast/dark ground illumination, and it works well for washed human sperm preparations as well as other species' seminal spermatozoa for determining concentration as well; it is just the 'dirty' nature of human semen that causes the problems when trying to use CASA for human semen analysis. Positive phase contrast optics are only useful in certain species, which includes human spermatozoa [41]. Hence most CASA systems use negative phase contrast/dark ground optics for their human semen analysis software, e.g. those listed above and also the MMC Sperm system.

- Immotile spermatozoa or similarly sized debris can be 'stirred' by nearby motile spermatozoa and erroneously classified as motile spermatozoa. This increases the apparent motility, as well as the total number of spermatozoa in the case of agitated debris or non-sperm cells.

- Tracking motile spermatozoa through collisions (real or even 'perceived' collisions as spermatozoa swim close by each other within the temporal-spatial discrimination of the instrument) can cause track fragmentation and so increase the perceived concentration and proportions of motile and progressively motile spermatozoa. Even with smart collision-correcting algorithms there can still be disturbances in the cells' trajectories, and hence their kinematics.

While many CASA systems include functions for the operator to edit the objects identified within each analysis field to correct for missed or spurious spermatozoa, it is very time consuming and consequently is rarely done in routine practice – so inaccurate results are generated. It would seem necessary that a CASA system truly fit-for-purpose should not require human input into such a basic process step.

Because of these issues, the CASA-determined sperm concentration in human semen samples is often incorrect – and hence the proportions of motile spermatozoa will also be incorrect. With clean semen samples (often a rarity in clinical andrology labs) this issue is greatly reduced, and non-existent when analysing washed sperm populations.

Technical Issues

- The key issue here is the impossibility of mixing such a viscous fluid as human semen to achieve completely random distribution of the cells throughout the sample; there is always a degree of 'micro-heterogeneity'.

- A fixed depth preparation must be made for analysis in the instrument, and it really cannot exceed 20 μm for reliable tracking of the spermatozoa under a 10× objective. While many commercial slides/chambers exist for making these preparations, all those with a fixed cover glass require loading by capillary action and are therefore subject to the Segré-Silberberg effect that influences the perceived sperm concentration as a result of laminar flow artefacts, resulting in a viscosity-dependent underestimation of up to 30% at aqueous viscosity [42,43]. Devices such as the *Makler chamber* (10 μm), *2X-CEL* and *Cell-VU* slides (both 20 μm), and both 10 μm and 20 μm *Spermtrack* chambers (Proiser), which use a separate cover glass over drops of sperm suspension ('drop-loading') are not subject to this error.

- The inherent sampling variability when taking aliquots of just 2–5 μl to load Makler chambers or fixed-depth slides is substantial, and confounds replicate analyses [5,13,15].

135

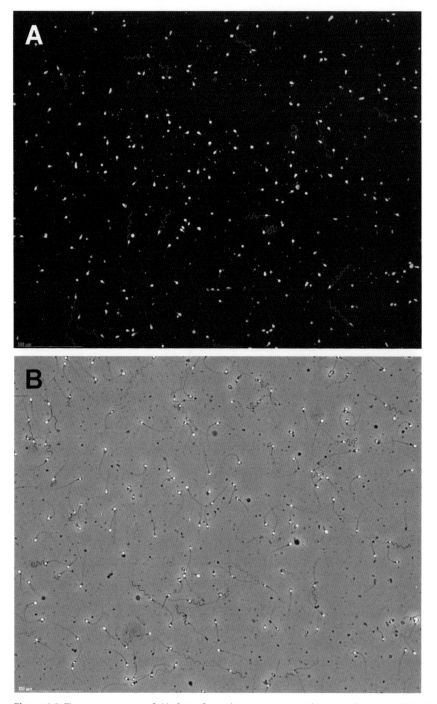

Figure 6.3 The same microscope field of view from a human semen sample seen under positive (A) and negative (B) phase contrast. Motile spermatozoa are obviously not located in the same position in each image due to their movement between captures. (Images courtesy of Professor Gerhard van der Horst, taken from the Sperm Class Analyzer v6.)

Note: If a CASA instrument evaluation compared un-corrected sperm concentration values determined using capillary-loaded slides against haemocytometry-derived reference values and found good equivalence, then it would, in effect, be establishing that the CASA instrument actually had a variable over-estimation, and hence the study outcome was
fortuitous.

For example, a meticulous study comparing the *Makler chamber*, *Leja* slide and Improved Neubauer haemocytometer for determining sperm concentration showed that while the Makler chamber was highly inaccurate (typically giving significantly high values), the *Leja* slide achieved sufficient comparability to the haemocytometer for it to be considered for clinical use [44]. But this equivalence was only achieved by timing how long it took for the chamber to load by capillary action and then applying a correction factor for the Segré-Silberberg effect [45], and also by pre-diluting the semen: neither of which steps are taken when these chambers are used in routine clinical lab practice.

- Specimen drift is also a problem and analyses must not be commenced until all visible flow has ceased, although incorporating a 'drift filter' can counter this artefact [14].

Expert Recommendations on the Use of Computer-Aided Sperm Analysis

The following recommendations on the practical application of CASA technology are closely based on the expert consensus published by the ESHRE Special Interest Group in Andrology [13]. The great majority of these recommendations, concerns and limitations originally made in 1997 remain valid today, especially since many older CASA systems remain in use [9]. While most recent CASA systems employ significantly improved technology and/or software [46,47] core aspects of the routine use of CASA must still be recognized. Relevant updates are shown in italics.

General Recommendations for All Mammalian Species

- Standardization and quality control (both internal and external) are paramount fundamental requirements for CASA, just as they are for any other diagnostic andrology laboratory procedure.
- As for all biological measurement systems, it is the responsibility of users to ensure that an appropriate number of cells is sampled in order to achieve the statistical requirements for a proper interpretation of the obtained results with CASA, including sensitivity and specificity.
- It is mandatory that technicians are trained to understand the theory behind CASA, as well as the influence that the initial settings can have on the data produced. *Even the latest CASA technology is not able to operate reliably at the simple push of a button.*
- Each laboratory using CASA must have quality control (QC) procedures.
- In any manuscript or report, methods *[must]* should be presented in sufficient detail to establish that accepted relevant CASA guidelines were followed. These include image acquisition rate, track sampling time, smoothing algorithm(s) employed, number of cells sampled, type of chamber including its depth, as well as instrument model and software version numbers, and microscope optics and magnification.
- Chamber depth must be sufficient for unconstrained sperm motion. This will vary depending on the species. Chamber depth must match optics to achieve an appropriate depth of focus.
- In all CASA analyses, the user must verify that all motile spermatozoa in the field of view are being tracked.

Basic Instrumentation

- When used for kinematic analysis of non-capacitated spermatozoa in seminal plasma, the magnification of the CASA instrument should be such that the majority of spermatozoa are tracked for 0.5 s before leaving the field of view. Hence, for human spermatozoa, the minimum field of view should be no less than 200 μm by 200 μm, allowing optimal tracking of spermatozoa with VSL values up to 100 μm/s.

- For human spermatozoa, an objective with maximum 10× magnification and suitable numerical aperture must be used so as to provide an adequate depth of focus.
- Reliable analysis of human sperm motility ideally requires a minimum acquisition frequency of 50 Hz. *Current recommendations are to use at least 60 Hz, with 120 Hz providing better analysis of washed spermatozoa which swim faster* [14].
- A minimum sampling time of 0.5 s is needed to acquire reliable kinematic values for a track (see [12] for further details).

Determination of Sperm Concentration

- This must not be a primary reason for acquiring a CASA instrument.
- A user wishing to use a CASA instrument to determine sperm concentration must establish that the intended measurement procedure provides accurate results compared to established reference methods (e.g. haemocytometry).
  Note: This is further compounded by the specific error associated with the capillary-loading of shallow chambers, as are used by many laboratories using CASA [42,43], although it might be possible to apply a correction factor in order to achieve the correct result [45].
- *Essentially these points remain valid today. However, if a modern CASA instrument is to be considered for this purpose, it must have been properly validated as being fit-for-purpose [15,32]. A suggested procedure for this is provided later in this chapter.*

Determination of the Proportion of Motile Spermatozoa

- This should not be considered a primary reason for acquiring a CASA instrument.
- If used in the routine analysis of seminal spermatozoa, CASA should be used to determine the concentration of progressively motile spermatozoa. CASA can determine this value accurately if care is taken with specimen preparation, instrument use and appropriate user-defined criteria. Current CASA instruments should not be used for the determination of the proportion of motile spermatozoa, since they cannot be relied upon to distinguish between debris and dead spermatozoa while tracking live spermatozoa at the same time.
- *Essentially these points remain valid today. However, if a modern CASA instrument is to be considered for this purpose, it must have been properly validated as being fit-for-purpose [15,32]. A suggested procedure for this is provided later in this chapter.*

Determination of Sperm Movement of Ejaculated Spermatozoa

- Semen samples with sperm concentrations higher than those recommended by the CASA instrument manufacturer must be diluted using cell-free autologous seminal plasma.
  Note: Using culture medium will change the semen viscosity and hence alter the sperm kinematics.
- All CASA analyses should be performed at body temperature (37°C for human spermatozoa). Velocity is extremely temperature labile, increasing by 60–100% when measured at 37°C *c.f.* 25°C [48].
- A minimum chamber depth of 10 μm must be used, although depths >20 μm are unlikely to be of any benefit.
- At least 200 motile spermatozoa should be analysed per sample.
- *Ideally replicate analyses should be performed and their results combined if concordant.*
- Population-averaged kinematics are considered to be of limited value because values are often not normally distributed, making the mean an inappropriate estimate of the sample. Consequently:
  - Median and range or centile values are statistically more meaningful than mean values.

- Multiparametric kinematic definitions, which allow the classification of individual spermatozoa into specific sub-populations that are correlated with relevant functional endpoints (e.g. 'good mucus penetrating' spermatozoa), should be made.
- For critical analysis of data, it is recommended that individual track values be saved in a database so that their distribution may be examined in order to select the most appropriate statistic for either describing the sample or comparing it with others (e.g. fertile vs infertile men or treated/exposed vs control/unexposed animals.

Computer-Aided Sperm Analysis of Sperm Hyperactivation

- Spermatozoa for hyperactivation studies should not be prepared from liquefied semen using techniques that have been demonstrated to have potentially deleterious effects on sperm function, e.g. initial centrifugation to separate spermatozoa from seminal plasma.
- A culture medium capable of supporting capacitation *in vitro* should be employed. Hence at least 25 mM HCO_3^- and millimolar quantities of Ca^{2+} and glucose, with sufficient albumin to minimize the sticking-to-glass phenomenon, ideally at least 10 mg/ml.
  This is now considered a 'must' requirement.
- All hyperactivation analyses must be performed at body temperature (i.e. 37°C for human spermatozoa).
- Preparations of sufficient depth to not constrain hyperactivated movement must be used. For human spermatozoa, a minimum chamber depth of 30 μm is essential (50 μm is probably ideal but can only be employed if the optical system used is capable of resolving this depth of focus).
  Since 30 μm and 50 μm chambers are not easily available commercially, 20 μm chambers can be used with human spermatozoa, but recognizing that they will constrain the movement of hyperactivating cells to reduce the appearance of the 'whiplash' or 'thrashing' pattern, while not affecting the overall prevalence of hyperactivation. Chambers that are not loaded by capillary action are strongly recommended.
- Definitions for hyperactivated motility must take into account the image acquisition frequency and should use kinematic criteria which have been validated for that CASA instrument.
  This is vital. See the later discussions on the impact of system-specific algorithms for average path calculation, ALH determination, and hence hyperactivated status. A definition based on the fractal dimension should be used instead [14].

Morphology Assessment by Computer-Aided Sperm Analysis

- The current generation of CASA instruments are not capable of analysing human sperm morphology in a manner adequate for routine clinical applications. In particular, the inability to include assessment of the midpiece and tail regions is considered to be a major weakness. Consequently, the use of CASA instruments for the clinical assessment of human sperm morphology is not supported at this time.
  Some modern CASA systems are able to provide some analysis of the neck/midpiece region, see the following section on sperm morphology assessment using CASA.

Clinical Application of Computer-Aided Sperm Analysis

- In the context of male fertility diagnosis, CASA should not be used without first undertaking a proper clinical assessment of the patient (including a clinical history and physical examination).
- For the present, CASA should not be undertaken in a clinical setting without first having constructed a basic semen profile according to recognized guidelines.
- Clinicians should understand that correct sample handling prior to analysis is critical for obtaining useful information. This is true for all semen assessments, not just CASA. Hence the length of abstinence (ideally in hours) and the ejaculation-to-analysis delay must be known accurately.

- Studies are required, using the current generation of CASA systems, to define:
  - The limits of normal semen quality in fertile men.
  - The relationships between CASA variables and the time to pregnancy.
  - The relationships between CASA variables (especially hyperactivation) and IVF outcome.
- *There has been little real progress in this area because significant clinical studies are still lacking.*

Applications of Computer-Aided Sperm Analysis in Reproductive Toxicology

- For toxicological studies on epididymal or vasa deferentia spermatozoa, accepting that samples must be diluted, the user must demonstrate that:
  - The process of dilution does not damage the spermatozoa.
  - The medium used supports consistently normal motility over the period of analysis.
  - The sperm concentration has been adjusted and controlled to minimize artefacts induced by crowding.
- Magnification should be adjusted according to sperm size and velocity (e.g. 4× is appropriate for rat spermatozoa which are considerably larger and faster than human spermatozoa) and chamber depth should allow unimpeded motion (e.g. >40 µm for rat spermatozoa).
- Users must verify that instrument settings have been optimized to detect all motile spermatozoa.
- Users must verify that the temperature at which images are captured is the body temperature for that species.
- With rodent sperm preparations, CASA can be used to determine both % motile and % progressively motile. User-defined thresholds for progressiveness should be justified based upon distributions of these endpoints in control samples.
- A permanent video record of samples is recommended so that data can be verified at any time and re-analysed as necessary when improvements in software become available. Fields should be recorded in a predetermined order so that the user does not bias the results by selecting or rejecting fields on the basis of their appearance.
- New users should compare their sample preparation methods and velocity data with those in the literature to achieve minimum standards in line with current practice.

Issues of Non-Comparability of Kinematics between Computer-Aided Sperm Analysis Systems

Image capture frequency dramatically affects the observed sperm track (Figure 6.2), with lower sampling rates giving simpler tracks that have reduced curvilinear velocity (VCL) and modified ALH values, affecting the proportion of tracks that meet any pre-defined criteria [8,28]. The reason that VCL is affected is relatively straightforward – fewer points along the track mean fewer deviations from a straight-line track – but why ALH is affected is more complex, since it depends on the robustness of the derived average path from which it is calculated [5,8,15,28].

Applying a fixed-point smoothing algorithm to all tracks in a population will result in many tracks being under- or over-smoothed, so clearly different sperm tracks require different degrees of smoothing to derive an optimum average path, and a CASA system that employs 'adaptive smoothing' algorithms to optimize the smoothing of each track will achieve more robust derivation of ALH values [8,15,32]. As an added unnecessary complication, some CASA systems do not conform to the consensus definition for ALH, and only present the scale-corrected riser value (i.e. a classical wave amplitude value) rather than the full track width (i.e. 2× riser values). A final issue is that some CASA systems report track-averaged values (ALHmean) while others report the maximum value for the track (ALHmax). Together these issues mean that:

- Conducting meaningful comparisons between published studies using different CASA instruments is essentially impossible; even knowing the differences in their algorithms will not permit adjustment of values since specific corrections cannot be applied to each track in retrospect.

- A threshold definition, e.g. for hyperactivation, validated for one CASA software will not be valid for a different system, *post hoc* corrections will not be possible, and *de novo* validation of a system-specific definition will be needed.

- Relationships between sperm kinematics and clinical endpoints such as threshold or cut-off values determined using one instrument will not be the same when another system is used – and might not even exist.

Computer-Aided Sperm Analysis and Human Semen Analysis

There is still considerable debate as to the clinical usefulness of the traditional descriptive semen analysis, which is held to exhibit very little prognostic value and limited diagnostic value since there is no 'disease' of 'infertility' [49]. While it is clearly impossible to try and resolve such arguments here, it can be concluded that only with the widespread use of robust, accurate methods could we expect to be able to establish real clinical utility for semen analysis, and that such utility would be greatly enhanced by including aspects of sperm functional ability [49] (also see Chapter 7).

There are two fundamental approaches to understanding the clinical utility of semen analysis:

- As a means of assessing the man's reproductive health.

- Whether the man's ejaculate contains sufficient potentially functional spermatozoa to effectively colonize his partner's reproductive tract and reach the site of fertilization in the Fallopian tube.

In the latter regard, that sperm population is contained within the rapid progressive motility (WHO4/6 grade *a*) fraction [50], and can be described kinematically as having 'good mucus penetrating' characteristics [6,15,51,52]. Experts considered this capability of CASA software to be fundamentally important more than two decades ago [13], representing the best approach to defining clinically useful measures with both discriminative and prognostic value in regard to *in-vivo* fertility endpoints [13,15,32,51,52].

This approach will provide more biologically important information than the traditional descriptive semen analysis for guiding the management of, and identifying appropriate ART treatment options for, infertile couples [53,54].

Because the precise operation of CASA instruments varies widely between makes and models, it is not practical to provide detailed SOPs here, although an example can be found elsewhere [52].

Sperm Concentration

In 1998, the ESHRE Special Interest Group in Andrology concluded that this must not be a primary reason for acquiring a CASA instrument because the then current technology did not provide accurate, reproducible values for sperm concentration unless an imaging method capable of differentiating spermatozoa from other cells and debris by a specific staining method (e.g. fluorescent staining of DNA for quantitation of nuclear size) was used [13,55].

Newer CASA instruments that use regular positive phase contrast rather than negative phase contrast/dark ground illumination do perform better in determining sperm concentration in human semen since these images are much less affected by debris that looks like sperm heads [14], but no such CASA instrument has yet been definitively validated against reference methodology. Consequently, anyone using a CASA instrument for this purpose must establish that their protocol provides accurate results compared to established reference methodology such as haemocytometry.

Notes: 1) Any dilutions must be made using positive displacement-type pipetters and not air displacement pipetters with disposable plastic tips which have a large air dead space inside the handle and the shaft of the device.

2) Thorough mixing is essential, but 'needling' and vortexing must be avoided.

Sperm Motility Percentages

Again, the ESHRE Special Interest Group in Andrology concluded that this aspect of semen analysis should not be considered a primary reason for acquiring a CASA instrument [13]. Unless a CASA instrument can be relied upon to distinguish between debris and dead spermatozoa in semen while tracking live spermatozoa simultaneously, it should not be used to determine the *proportion* of motile spermatozoa. However, CASA technology can be used to determine the *concentration* of progressively motile spermatozoa in routine semen analysis, since this value can be determined accurately if care is taken with specimen preparation, instrument use and appropriate user-defined criteria.

Sperm Morphology

The current generation of CASA instruments remain unable to analyse human sperm morphology, including assessment of the midpiece and tail regions as required by current WHO guidelines [56,57], and for the determination of the Teratozoospermia Index (see Chapter 3). While CASA systems have been able to provide reliable morphometric analysis of human sperm heads since the 1990s, it seems that few routine laboratories employ this technology [7,14], primarily because it provides little or no benefit in time compared to trained technicians. Consequently, the ESHRE Special Interest Group in Andrology does not currently support the use of CASA instruments for the clinical assessment of human sperm morphology [13].

Robust sperm morphology assessment requires the analysis of all regions of the cell – head, neck, midpiece and tail – often based on polychromatic staining techniques. In addition, a sound under-standing of the relationships between sperm structure and function at the sub-cellular, cellular and organism (sperm approximation and fertilization) levels [58–62], is key. See also Chapter 3.

Compared to assessments of sperm concentration and motility, where good resolution and high frame rate are key but colour is not necessary, robust sperm morphology assessment requires the use of high resolution colour cameras to take advantage of polychromatic staining methods, combined with sophisticated morphometric and textural analytical techniques. Without colour image analysis capabil-ities, it seems unlikely that CASA machines will be able to achieve fully the sophistication of analysis inherent to human visual perception. Specimen preparation is extremely important for morphological/morphometric analysis, especially the making and staining of preparations [63–66].

Although an automated system capable of performing multiparametric morphological assessments of human spermatozoa was developed in the early 1980s [67], it was never commercialized, and its capabilities were not adopted or emulated by any of the CASA manufacturers. This remains an area of active research [68], although the new Microptic *SCAScope* and Proiser *ISAS* systems are coming closer.

Many CASA systems are able to provide reliable morphometric analysis of human sperm heads [69–74], but early CASA morphology packages analysed only the sperm head and required both manual corrections and entry of human observations regarding the other regions of each spermatozoon [e.g. 74], making the process of analyzing a morphology slide too laborious, greatly hindering acceptance of the technology. More recent systems are more robust [e.g. 40], several can measure midpiece length [e.g. 75], and some can analyse all regions of the cell and even derive a value for TZI [14]. While full validations against reference experts remain to be published, this is a very promising evolution of the technology.

A brief overview of the possible future application of artificial intelligence (AI)-enhanced software for automated sperm morphology assessment is included under 'Future Computer-Aided Sperm Analysis Technology', below.

Sperm Vitality

In routine semen analysis, sperm vitality assessments are performed when the sperm motility is low (typically <40%), to establish whether the immotile spermatozoa are alive or dead, using a combination of eosin as the vital stain and nigrosin as a purple background stain to facilitate observation of the unstained live cells (see Chapter 3). Fluorescence-based methods are also available (e.g. Hoeschst 33258 [76]), but few clinical andrology labs have a fluorescence microscope.

Several late generation CASA systems are able to analyse eosin-nigrosin preparations: Microptic *SCA* systems [14], *MMC Sperm*, and Proiser *ISAS* systems. Some CASA systems have fluorescence imaging options that permit evaluation of sperm vitality, e.g. the Hamilton Thorne *VIADENT* system.

Computer-Aided Sperm Analysis and the Assessment of Sperm Functional Potential

Although CASA analysis results have been correlated with *in-vivo* fertility [e.g. 77,78], it is generally understood that using CASA to define specific sub-populations of potentially functional spermatozoa, rather than considering population-averaged kinematic measures, will provide more meaningful results for patient diagnosis and management [6,13–15].

Sperm-Mucus Penetration

Sperm kinematics are key for successful sperm cervical mucus interaction, and a small number of men have been identified whose motile spermatozoa are completely unable to penetrate into or migrate through cervical mucus, a defect caused by extremely small ALH ('sliding spermatozoa') [79–82]. Good progression (e.g. VSL or VAP ≥25 µm/s) with large ALH (e.g. ALHmean >2.5 µm) are important discriminators in predicting the outcome of *in-vitro* sperm-mucus interaction tests. See Figure 6.4.

This understanding was used to describe a subpopulation of human spermatozoa that are better able to penetrate cervical mucus and quantify it during a more functional semen analysis [6,15,51,52]. The following Boolean criteria have been proposed for identifying spermatozoa with 'good mucus penetrating ability':

$$\text{VAP} \geq 25 \ \mu\text{m/s} \quad \text{AND} \quad \text{STR} \geq 80\% \quad \text{AND ALH} \geq 2.5 \ \mu\text{m} \quad \text{AND} \quad \text{ALH} < 7.0 \ \mu\text{m}$$

The fourth term serves to exclude spermatozoa whose motility has been compromised by ROS-induced damage, which can cause a quasi-hyperactivation pattern of movement.

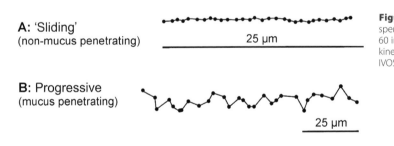

A: 'Sliding'
(non-mucus penetrating)

25 µm

B: Progressive
(mucus penetrating)

25 µm

Figure 6.4 Illustration of human sperm tracks seen in semen, plotted at 60 images/s for 0.5 s (31 points); kinematics were analysed using an IVOS-II system (modified from [32]).

Kinematics		Sliding	Progressive
VCL	(µm/s)	25.4	131.3
VSL	(µm/s)	23.3	96.3
VAP	(µm/s)	23.6	101.2
LIN	(%)	92	73
STR	(%)	99	95
WOB	(%)	93	77
ALHmean	(µm)	n/a	n/a
ALHmax	(µm)	0.89	4.8
D		1.03	1.10

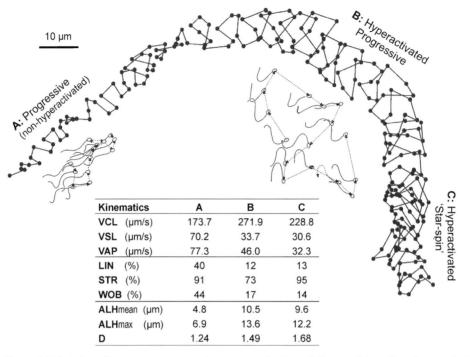

Kinematics	A	B	C
VCL (µm/s)	173.7	271.9	228.8
VSL (µm/s)	70.2	33.7	30.6
VAP (µm/s)	77.3	46.0	32.3
LIN (%)	40	12	13
STR (%)	91	73	95
WOB (%)	44	17	14
ALHmean (µm)	4.8	10.5	9.6
ALHmax (µm)	6.9	13.6	12.2
D	1.24	1.49	1.68

Figure 6.5 Illustration of human sperm movement as seen in washed/capacitating populations. The cell was tracked manually at 60 images/s for 3.77 s (227 points) and shows the three common phases of movement between which such spermatozoa switch spontaneously. Illustrative sperm-tail beating patterns are shown for the non-hyperactivated and hyperactivated progressive regions of the track. Note the much larger amplitude proximal waves in the hyperactivated phase. Kinematic values were analysed using Excel. (Modified from ref. [32])

Analysis of Sperm Hyperactivation

Hyperactivated motility is a high-energy pattern of movement characterized by the development of high amplitude flagellar waves, but with little net space gain (Figure 6.5). It occurs in all Eutherian spermatozoa studied, is a concomitant of capacitation *in vitro*, and has been observed in free-swimming spermatozoa in the oviduct *in situ*.

The physiological importance of hyperactivation is generally accepted, and while low levels of hyperactivation have been associated with reduced fertilizing ability *in vivo* and *in vitro* [6,8,83] the full clinical significance of its assessment is still under investigation (see Chapter 5). For populations of capacitating human spermatozoa, hyperactivated motility includes cells showing both the 'transition' and 'thrashing' patterns. Both patterns are characterized by the development of very large amplitude proximal flagellar waves with very rapid propagation, but the latter pattern (also described as 'whiplash', 'star-spin' and 'dance') shows a delay in propagation causing the sperm head to be turned back into a reflexed position upon the axis of the cell so that when the wave is propagated, the cell appears to thrash about wildly.

The identification of hyperactivated motility using sperm-head-derived tracks is sub-optimal [6], but routine flagellar analysis remains impractical [15,31]. Validated criteria for identifying hyperactivated human spermatozoa have been established and validated for both the first and second generations of CASA software on the Hamilton Thorne *IVOS* and *CEROS*, and *IVOS-II* and *CEROS-II* systems, respectively, operating at 60 Hz frame rates [51,52]:

$$\text{CASA} - \text{I} \qquad \text{VCL} \ge 150 \ \mu m/s \ \text{AND LIN} \ \le 50\% \ \text{AND ALH} \ge 7.0 \ \mu m$$

$$\text{CASA} - \text{II} \qquad \text{VCL} \ge 150 \ \mu m/s \ \text{AND D} \ge 1.20$$

As discussed already in this chapter, the use of these – or other – 'sort' criteria with other CASA systems must be independently validated using flagellar analysis studies.

Sperm DNA Fragmentation

The most common type of sperm DNA fragmentation analysis performed in diagnostic andrology labs is based on sperm chromatin dispersion, with the *Halosperm G2* Kit being the primary commercial product (HalotechDNA, Madrid, Spain; www.halotechdna.com), see Chapter 5. Several CASA systems are able to read these slides, removing observer subjectivity in estimating halo size and enabling the test result to be based on a larger number of cells [14,40,84].

Other Tests of Sperm Fertilizing Ability

Although numerous tests of sperm fertilizing ability were described over the past 50 years, almost all are now considered either too complex for a routine diagnostic andrology lab or have failed to achieve widespread acceptance [2,12], see Chapter 7. Beyond assessing sperm hyperactivation, the only other sperm function test that remains of serious current interest is evaluating the acrosome reaction in response to an ionophore challenge (the 'ARIC' test). Acrosome status is determined using fluorescence-labelled lectins, most often peanut agglutinin (PNA) that binds to the outer acrosomal membrane, ideally in conjunction with a fluorescent vital stain [76,85]. Microptic sells a *FluoAcro* kit based on this methodology and the *SCA* platform has a software package to analyse the results.

Conclusions

Computer-aided sperm analysis has enormous potential as a research tool, in reproductive toxicology, in animal production, and for human clinical analyses. There is no doubt that future CASA systems will incorporate more functional tests of sperm quality that will better enable quantifying relative fertility, rather than merely measuring the traditional descriptive semen parameters.

As human clinical andrology laboratories become ever more regulated and more broadly subject to accreditation, the methodologies they employ will need to be rigorously tested and conform to the differing needs of andrology laboratories, domesticated animal production laboratories, and reproductive toxicology testing and research laboratories.

Of particular importance in the human clinical semen analysis field, we should stop trying to use CASA for applications that are inherently problematic for the underlying technology – at least until the technology has been improved and definitively validated. In the absence of such instrumentation, human clinical andrology laboratories need to focus on what CASA can do *accurately*, which in terms of human sperm analysis at this time comprises:

Semen analysis: the concentration of that sub-population of spermatozoa that has the right kinematics to penetrate cervical mucus, sperm vitality assessment;

Washed sperm preparation analysis: sperm concentration and motility class percentages;

Sperm fertilizing ability: evaluation of sperm hyperactivation (perhaps acrosomal status); and

Sperm DNA assessment: DNA fragmentation analysis.

Quality Control for Computer-Aided Sperm Analysis

Quality control (QC) is extremely important in all measurement systems employed in medical laboratories, and each laboratory using CASA must have appropriate QC procedures in place.

It has been suggested that QC for sperm motility analysis should use appropriate video recordings in conjunction with the 'playback' feature of the CASA instrument to ensure that all the motile spermatozoa are being identified using each set of system parameters. However, this approach is not logical, as it fails to control for the most important aspects of instrument operation that can affect reliable tracking and analysis of spermatozoa (since the correct derivation of kinematic values from a track by the software should not be in doubt). Moreover, it is likely that different setup parameters will need to be used for video recordings compared to 'live' specimens – and that system setup parameters have not been changed can easily be verified by inspecting the setup screen (indeed, most systems allow supervisors to prevent technical operators from changing these parameters). It is, therefore, more important to follow a daily QC procedure similar to the following:

1. Basic system operation and magnification calibration can be verified by analysing known-concentration preparations of microscopic beads as surrogates for sperm heads (e.g. *Accubeads*®; Hamilton Thorne). The concentration of beads obtained from the CASA instrument must be within the stated reference range.

2. Verify that the CASA instrument's imaging system (illumination intensity and focus) and setup parameters are properly matched. This will ensure that:

   - Spermatozoa will be correctly identified.
   - Debris particles will not contribute undue numbers of spurious spermatozoa.
   - Moving spermatozoa will be tracked reliably.

To do this, analyse a field from a *live* specimen and then use the 'playback' function to make sure that:

   a) The great majority of the spermatozoa in the field have been identified correctly (e.g. at least 90% of visually identifiable sperm tracks or immotile heads have been tagged by the system).
   b) Debris has not been excessively identified as spurious sperm heads (e.g. <10% of the number of sperm identified should be suspect).
   c) All the moving cells have been tracked, and that the tracks appear intact (i.e. not fragmented into shorter lengths). A track that was truncated due to colliding with another cell or piece of debris is not considered a tracking problem.

Then check 10 to 20 individual tracks (e.g. using the 'Edit Tracks – Zoom' function for Hamilton Thorne systems) and verify that only occasional track points have been lost (e.g. no more than two missed points, either individually or in sequence), and that adjacent short tracks are not fragments of a single longer track. The latter aspect can be identified from the image numbers for the track points that make up each track; a complete intact track will contain points from the first image through to the end of the sequence, e.g. 31 points.

Document that the CASA instrument has passed the QC check and is now OK to use. In the case of any non-compliant elements, document their resolution and then that the instrument passed the QC check.

Note: This procedure must be repeated for each variation of illumination and optics used.

Validating a Computer-Aided Sperm Analysis System for Human Semen Analysis

During the late 1980s and the 1990s ('the early CASA era') most attempts to validate CASA technology for human semen analysis applications suffered from fundamental technical issues that undermined the data quality, and hence the possible clinical value of the CASA results [6–8,11–13]. That few clinical andrology labs used robust semen analysis methods, or had thoroughly trained competent staff working within a quality-managed environment [86], resulted in very poor comparability between CASA and routine semen analysis results, especially when appropriate statistical methodology such as 'discrepancy analysis' Bland and Altman plots were used instead of simple linear regression with no consideration of slope or intercept. Unsurprisingly, comparing poor-quality data against diagnostic or prognostic end-points had limited success, frustrating both CASA users and CASA vendors.

Reference methods for sperm concentration are flow cytometry and haemocytometry by competent operators [86]. While positive phase contrast-based CASA can come close to such results, no system has yet been definitively validated against reference methodology. CASA results are certainly more reproducible, but this is obviously insufficient without evidence of accuracy [15,86]. Various papers report perceived agreement between CASA and routine semen analysis, but the range of discrepancies between results remains significant [10,44,87–89]. Many studies do not reveal the magnitude of such differences [e.g. 44], while others consider substantial differences in results as 'acceptable' [87]. That CASA operators must be well-trained is a common theme.

Expectations of Accuracy and Precision

Standards for medical laboratories are well-established and clearly defined in ISO 15189:2012 [90]. As for any medical laboratory test, the results of a semen analysis must be accurate to have any real world value [15,49,57,91]. Any quantitative result must be within an acceptable range of the 'right answer', i.e. its Measurement Uncertainty (MU) must be known relative to established reference standards or methods [92,93].

Expert opinion requires that results for semen analysis characteristics obtained using CASA in a clinical andrology laboratory setting need to be within ±10% of reference values for an expert andrology laboratory, although ±20% might be adequate for a general diagnostic laboratory [15,49]. However, the assumption here is that all clinical andrology laboratories conform to current accepted 'Gold Standard' semen analysis methodology, with all laboratory staff having been properly trained in all the protocols and quality control systems [86], although poor conformity to international guidelines is well known [94,95]. The recent publication of the ISO 23162 technical standard for basic semen analysis provides true reference methodology against which CASA needs to be validated [96].

Comparisons between systems cannot be based on average values or on correlations/linear regression between paired values. Both techniques conceal the real differences that exist between specific replicate determinations. Instead, Bland and Altman 'limits of agreement' or 'discrepancy' plots must be used [2,86,97], which plot the actual differences between the paired values, and can hence be used to establish whether each 'new method' (or 'trainee') value is within ±10% of the reference method or value. Reports using other statistical approaches, many of which typically conceal the true extent of the existing discrepancy, must be viewed with caution (see Chapter 12).

Recommended Strategy for Validating a Computer-Aided Sperm Analysis System for Semen Analysis

A framework to validate a CASA system for human semen analysis, based on the fundamental principles discussed in this chapter and in Chapter 12, requires that:

- The study must be performed in an expert andrology laboratory whose staff are all trained (with evidence of competency) in, and employ, reference methodology. The laboratory must function within a proper quality-managed operational environment.
- Sufficient clinical specimens for a robust statistical comparison must be analysed in parallel using reference methodology and by the CASA system. Ideally several hundred ejaculates need to be analysed, covering the spectrum of ejaculate quality that exists in the population, but 120 should be considered a minimum.
- Each semen characteristic assessment must be performed in at least duplicate, with verification of adequate reproducibility of the replicates before calculating the final result.
- If CASA analyses included human intervention to correct the detection and recognition of spermatozoa within the image analysis process, this must be stated, and such intervention must then become a required step in the subsequent routine clinical use of the instrument.
- Expression of results to an appropriate degree of precision based on the methodology, i.e. no 'false precision'.
- Data must be subjected to appropriate statistical analysis.
- The CASA-derived result must have an established MU or error and needs to fall within ±10% of the reference method's result.

- Reports need to be published at least on the vendor's website, but ideally in a respected peer-reviewed journal (e.g. impact factor of at least 2.0) using an open access model.

Obviously, results can only be reported if an actual measurement was made. For example, if a device reports a '% normal morphology, result based entirely on an algorithm that derives the value indirectly from associated sperm concentration and motility data, it cannot be validated as there are no actual values to compare with reference results.

Without proper validation, no claims of suitability for purpose (e.g. 'automated semen analyser') should be made. Hopefully, the evolving modern regulatory environment will lead to improvements in the performance of CASA systems – but this will very likely depend on manufacturers undertaking robust validation studies or, perhaps better, supporting their performance in recognized expert laboratories that conform fully to reference methodology, quality management and ensure staff competency.

Future Computer-Aided Sperm Analysis Technology

New Technology

Three new imaging and software approaches have recently been reported for research applications.

- An open-source CASA software called *OpenCASA* has been developed and released in a version control system at Github (https://github.com/calquezar/OpenCASA), which, as well as analysing the classic parameters of semen, also reports sperm chemotactic behaviour and recognizes five sperm subpopulations according to their fluorescence patterns associated with the plasma membrane and acrosomal status [98,99].
- Analysis of the natural three-dimensional pattern of sperm movement using a 'holographic' CASA system (Proiser *ISAS 3D-Track*) [41].
- The *FAST* (Flagellar Analysis and Sperm Tracking) software tool enables high-throughput, repeatable, accurate and verifiable analysis of sperm flagellar waveform tracking [100].

Application of Artificial Intelligence Techniques

The rapid development of AI technology for use in reproductive medicine opens new possibilities, but there is also a risk of pitfalls [101,102]. AI is being widely mentioned in regard to semen analysis (although not always with full understanding of what it involves), with expectations of performing semen analysis more reliably than manual assessments and at a low cost compared to present CASA systems.

Some of the AI algorithms are working especially well for image analysis and can be used to carry out the classification of spermatozoa. Supervised machine learning (ML) algorithms have been shown to perform well in distinguishing normal and abnormal spermatozoa [103]. However, these approaches depend on manually annotated training data, thereby being time-consuming and possibly introducing human bias. Deep learning (DL) algorithms represent an advancement in ML, and the state of the art for image analysis is convolutional neural networks (CNNs) inspired by the principles of processing data in the visual cortex of the brain. CNNs learn image features by memorizing and applying different kernels to the images. The resulting features are able to describe patterns in the data that are often not visible to humans and can be used as input to other ML algorithms.

Several research groups are working on applying ML/DL techniques, in particular using CNN-based methods, to analyse digital videos and images to identify and classify human sperm motility and morphology types [104]. While early results are promising, such CNN-based technology has not yet seen mainstream commercial application, although the BonRayBio *LensHooke™ X1 Pro* device has been described as using a novel AI optical microscopic technology [87].

Segmentation is often used in developing DL models for sperm morphology assessment, by which the spermatozoon is divided into segments, each comprising sets of pixels. For example, when employing algorithms to assess the shape of the head, pixel-accurate segmentation masks are necessary. An accurate annotated image dataset, either frame-wise or with segmentations representing parts of the spermatozoon, is a prerequisite for developing and evaluating supervised methods (learning of labelled data).

Annotating large image datasets could be a challenge, and can also be dependent on which part of the spermatozoon should be segmented and how detailed this segmentation has to be. In general, more detailed annotations lead to a more detailed analysis, but at the same time the annotation will need more time. Automatic segmentation of stained spermatozoa has been developed using various unsupervised learning approaches, depending on the part of the spermatozoon that should be examined [105]. However, even if unsupervised methods do not necessarily need annotated training data, such data will still be required for evaluation of the performance.

The AI approach could be to classify the whole or parts of the spermatozoon as normal or abnormal. Data sets of both stained and unstained spermatozoa have been used. Recently, two DL algorithms (deep transfer learning and deep multi-task transfer learning) were applied to classify the head of the spermatozoon as well as the vacuole and acrosome as normal or abnormal [106]. Both algorithms achieved an accuracy of more than 80% for the head and acrosome label and over 90% for the vacuole. The dataset in this study was unstained, noisy, and of low resolution (64×64 pixels each), in contrast to the stained dataset of high resolution used in several other studies. The classification of images in real-time, i.e. unstained, is a prerequisite for developing algorithms suitable for selecting the spermatozoon for ICSI. However, the sample size used in the above-mentioned study was limited and cannot be generalized to other data.

A smartphone-based system has recently been introduced, consisting of an automatic segmentation step and a classification step of normal/abnormal spermatozoa [107]. This system outperformed the conventional ML methods included in the study for comparison and achieved an accuracy of 87%.

To develop the most reliable and accurate AI models for sperm morphology assessments requires studies that compare performance using the same datasets based on the same technology and protocols. An important factor is also to test models across different datasets, since otherwise generalizability is not given. In addition, the evaluation of the results should include a set of metrics and not just accuracy. This is important since some problems such as overfitting or bias from underrepresented classes cannot be seen from one metric only. Unbiased and representative datasets must be used for training the models. For AI-guided selection of spermatozoa for ICSI, clinical studies based on standardized methods must be performed to elucidate the robustness and predictive value of the algorithms.

Point-of-Care Computer-Aided Sperm Analysis Devices

As in so many branches of laboratory medicine, there is a trend for automation to create point-of-care testing devices.

Various iterations of the *Sperm Quality Analyzer* ('*SQA*') have been commercialized over the past three decades, with current models being the *SQA-Vision* and the *SQA-V Gold*. While studies have been published in support of these instruments, the perceived acceptability of their results, and the robustness of their comparisons with manual/visual semen analysis methods (not always true reference methodology) [e.g. 40], are typically less rigorous than the approach now recommended; most have only been conference presentations, not published in peer-reviewed journals.

The latest point-of-care type device is the *LensHooke™ X1 Pro*. However, the evaluation study was willing to accept wider ranges of difference between results obtained using the device and by routine methodology, including +20% and +12% systematic differences in the motile and progressively motile sperm concentrations [87]. Unfortunately, the routine sperm concentration results were obtained using a Makler chamber rather than reference methodology.

Mobile Phone Computer-Aided Sperm Analysis

Several mobile-phone-based sperm analysis systems have been reported in the literature [e.g. 107–110], but none have been subjected to rigorous validation against reference methodology. These systems are intended for home use (see Appendix 3) rather than in diagnostic laboratories.

References

1. MacLeod J, Gold RZ. The male factor in fertility and infertility. III. An analysis of motile activity in the spermatozoa of 1000 fertile men and 1000 men in infertile marriage. *Fertil Steril* 1951; **2**: 187–204.

2. Mortimer D. *Practical Laboratory Andrology.* New York: Oxford University Press, 1994.

3. Davis RO, Katz DF. Computer-aided sperm analysis: technology at a crossroads. *Fertil Steril* 1993; **59**: 953–5.

4. Boyers SP, Davis RO, Katz DF. Automated semen analysis. *Curr Probl Obstet Gynecol Fertil* 1989; **XII**: 167–200.

5. Mortimer D. Objective analysis of sperm motility and kinematics. In: Keel BA, Webster BW, eds. *Handbook of the Laboratory Diagnosis and Treatment of Infertility.* Boca Raton: CRC Press, 1990.

6. Mortimer ST. A critical review of the physiological importance and analysis of sperm movement in mammals. *Hum Reprod Update* 1997; **3**: 403–39.

7. Mortimer D, Mortimer ST. Value and reliability of CASA systems. In: Ombelet W, Bosmans E, Vandeput H, et al., eds. *Modern ART in the 2000s.* Carnforth: Parthenon Publishing, 1998.

8. Mortimer ST. CASA – practical aspects. *J Androl* 2000; **21**: 515–24.

9. Amann RP, Waberski D. Computer-assisted sperm analysis (CASA): capabilities and potential developments. *Theriogenology* 2014; **81**: 5–17.

10. Tomlinson MJ, Naeem A. CASA in the medical laboratory: CASA in diagnostic andrology and assisted conception. *Reprod Fertil Dev* 2018; **30**: 850–9.

11. Mortimer D, Aitken RJ, Mortimer ST, Pacey AA. Workshop report: Clinical CASA – The quest for consensus. *Reprod Fertil Dev* 1995; **7**: 951–9.

12. ESHRE Andrology Special Interest Group. Consensus workshop on advanced diagnostic andrology techniques. *Hum Reprod* 1996; **11**: 1463–79.

13. ESHRE Andrology Special Interest Group. Guidelines on the application of CASA technology in the analysis of spermatozoa. *Hum Reprod* 1998; **13**: 142–5.

14. Mortimer ST, van der Horst G, Mortimer D. The future of computer-aided sperm analysis. *Asian J Androl* 2015; **17**: 545–53.

15. Mortimer D, Mortimer ST. Routine application of CASA in human clinical andrology and ART laboratories. In: Björndahl L, Flanagan J, Holmberg R, Kvist U, eds. *XIIIth International Symposium on Spermatology.* Switzerland: Springer Nature, 2021, 183–97.

16. Lippi G, Da Rin G. Advantages and limitations of total laboratory automation: a personal overview. *Clin Chem Lab Med* 2019; **57**: 802–11.

17. Thomson RB Jr, McElvania E. Total laboratory automation: what is gained, what is lost, and who can afford it? *Clin Lab Med* 2019 **39**: 371–89.

18. Serres C, Feneux D, Jouannet P, David G. Influence of the flagellar wave development and propagation on the human sperm movement in seminal plasma. *Gamete Res* 1984; **9**: 183–95.

19. Phillips DM. Comparative analysis of mammalian sperm motility. *J Cell Biol* 1972; **53**: 561–73.

20. Woolley DM. Interpretation of the pattern of sperm tail movements. In: Fawcett DW, Bedford JM, eds. *The Spermatozoon. Maturation, Motility, Surface Properties and Comparative Aspects.* Baltimore: Urban & Schwarzenberg, 1979.

21. Woolley DM. A method for determining the three-dimensional form of active flagella, using two-colour darkground illumination. *J Microsc* 1981; **121**: 241–4.

22. Phillips DM. The direction of rolling in mammalian spermatozoa. In: Andre J, ed. *The Sperm Cell. Fertilizing Power, Surface Properties, Motility, Nucleus and Acrosome, Evolutionary Aspects.* The Hague: Martinus Nijhoff, 1983.

23. Serres C, Escalier D, David G. Ultrastructural morphometry of the human sperm flagellum with a stereological analysis of the lengths of the dense fibres. *Biol Cell* 1983; **49**: 153–62.

24. Denehy MA. Herbison-Evans D, Denehy BV. Rotational and oscillatory components of the tailwave in ram spermatozoa. *Biol Reprod* 1975; **13**: 289–97.

25. Purcell EM. Life at low Reynolds number. *Am J Phys* 1977; **45**: s3–11.

26. Corkidi G, Taboada B, Wood CD, et al. Tracking sperm in three-dimensions. *Biochem Biophys Res Commun* 2008; **373**: 125–9.

27. Su T-W, Choi I, Feng J, et al. Sperm trajectories form chiral ribbons. *Sci Rep* 2013; **3**: 1664. https://doi.org/10.1038/srep01664

28. Mortimer D, Serres C, Mortimer ST, Jouannet P. Influence of image sampling frequency on the perceived movement characteristics of progressively motile human spermatozoa. *Gamete Res* 1988; **20**: 313–27.

29. Castellini C, Dal Bosco A, Ruggeri S, Collodel G. What is the best frame rate for evaluation of sperm

motility in different species by computer-assisted sperm analysis? *Fertil Steril* 2011; **96**: 24–7.

30. Mortimer ST, Mortimer D. Kinematics of human spermatozoa incubated under capacitating conditions. *J Androl* 1990; **11**: 195–203.

31. Mortimer ST, Schoëvaërt D, Swan MA, Mortimer D. Quantitative observations of flagellar motility of capacitating human spermatozoa. *Hum Reprod* 1997; **12**: 1006–12.

32. Mortimer D, Mortimer ST. The future of computer-assisted semen analysis in the evaluation of male infertility. In: Patuszak A, Hotaling, J, Carrell D, eds. *Comprehensive Guide to Modern Andrology*. Cambridge: Cambridge University Press, 2021, (in press).

33. Katz MJ, George EB. Fractals and the analysis of growth paths. *Bull Math Biol* 1985; **47**: 273–86.

34. Mortimer ST, Swan MA. Effect of image sampling frequency on established and smoothing-independent kinematic values of capacitating human spermatozoa. *J Androl* 1999; **14**: 997–1004.

35. Davis RO, Siemers RJ. Derivation and reliability of kinematic measures of sperm motion. *Reprod Fertil Dev* 1995; **7**: 857–69.

36. Mortimer ST, Swan MA. The development of smoothing-independent kinematic measures of capacitating human sperm movement. *Hum Reprod* 1999; **14**: 986–96.

37. Mortimer ST. Minimum sperm trajectory length for reliable determination of the fractal dimension. *Reprod Fertil Dev* 1998; **10**: 465–9.

38. Mortimer ST, Swan MA, Mortimer D. Fractal analysis of capacitating human spermatozoa. *Hum Reprod* 1996; **11**: 1049–54.

39. Mortimer D. Sperm transport in the female genital tract. In: Grudzinskas JG, Yovich JL, eds. *Cambridge Reviews in Human Reproduction, Volume 2: Gametes – The Spermatozoon*. Cambridge: Cambridge University Press, 1995.

40. Schubert B, Badiou M, Force A. Computer-aided sperm analysis, the new key player in routine sperm assessment. *Andrologia* 2019; **51**: e13417.

41. Soler C, Picazo-Bueno JÁ, Micó V, et al. Effect of counting chamber depth on the accuracy of lensless microscopy for the assessment of boar sperm motility. *Reprod Fertil Dev* 2018 **30**: 924–34.

42. Douglas-Hamilton DH, Smith NG, Kuster CE, et al. Particle distribution in low-volume capillary-loaded chambers. *J Androl* 2005; **26**: 107–14.

43. Douglas-Hamilton DH, Smith NG, Kuster CE, et al. Capillary-loaded particle fluid dynamics: effect on estimation of sperm concentration. *J Androl* 2005; **26**: 115–22.

44. Lammers J, Splingart C, Barrière P, Jean M, Fréour T. Double-blind prospective study comparing two automated sperm analyzers versus manual semen assessment. *J Assist Reprod Genet* 2014; 31: 35–43.

45. Rijnders S, Bolscher JG, McDonnell J, Vermeiden JP. Filling time of a lamellar capillary-filling semen analysis chamber is a rapid, precise, and accurate method to assess viscosity of seminal plasma. *J Androl* 2007; **28**: 461–5.

46. van der Horst G, Maree L, du Plessis SS. Current perspectives of CASA applications in diverse mammalian spermatozoa. *Reprod Fertil Dev* 2018; **30**: 875–88.

47. Valverde A, Castro-Morales O, Madrigal-Valverde M, Soler C. Sperm kinematics and morphometric subpopulations analysis with CASA systems: a review. *Int J Trop Biol* 2019; **67**: 1473–87.

48. Milligan MP, Harris SJ, Dennis KJ. The effect of temperature on the velocity of human spermatozoa as measured by time-lapse photography. *Fertil Steril* 1978; **30**: 592–4.

49. Björndahl L. What is normal semen quality? On the use and abuse of reference limits for the interpretation of semen analysis results. *Hum Fertil* 2011; **14**: 179–86.

50. Barratt CLR, Björndahl L, Menkveld R, Mortimer D. The ESHRE Special Interest Group for Andrology Basic Semen Analysis Course: a continued focus on accuracy, quality, efficiency and clinical relevance. *Hum Reprod* 2011; **26**: 3207–12.

51. Mortimer D, Mortimer ST. Laboratory investigation of the infertile male. In: Brinsden PR, ed. *A Textbook of In-Vitro Fertilization and Assisted Reproduction*, 3rd edn. London: Taylor & Francis Medical Books, 2005.

52. Mortimer D, Mortimer ST. Computer-aided sperm analysis (CASA) of sperm motility and hyperactivation. In: Carrell DT, Aston KI, eds. *Spermatogenesis and Spermiogenesis: Methods and Protocols*. New York: Springer (Humana Press), 2013.

53. Mortimer D. (1999) Structured management as a basis for cost-effective infertility care. In: Gagnon C, ed. *The Male Gamete: From Basic Knowledge to Clinical Applications*. Vienna: Cache River Press, 1999.

54. Mortimer D, Mortimer ST. The case against intracytoplasmic sperm injection for all. In: Aitken J, Mortimer D, Kovacs G, eds. *Male and Sperm Factors that Maximize IVF Success*. Cambridge: Cambridge University Press, 2020.

55. Zinaman MJ, Uhler ML, Vertuno E, et al. Evaluation of computer-assisted semen analysis

(CASA) with IDENT stain to determine sperm concentration. *J Androl* 1996; **17**: 288–92.

56. Rowe PJ, Comhaire FH, Hargreave TB, Mahmoud AMA. *WHO Clinical Manual for the Standardized Investigation, Diagnosis and Management of the Infertile Male.* Cambridge: Cambridge University Press, 2000.

57. World Health Organization. *WHO Laboratory Manual for the Examination and Processing of Human Semen*, 5th edn. Geneva: World Health Organization, 2010.

58. Mortimer D, Menkveld R. Sperm morphology assessment – Historical perspectives and current opinions. *J Androl* 2001; **22**: 192–205.

59. Mortimer D. Sperm form and function: beauty is in the eye of the beholder. In: van der Horst G, Franken D, Bornman R, de Jager T, Dyer S, eds. *Proceedings of 9th International Symposium on Spermatology.* Bologna: Monduzzi Editore, 2002, 257–62.

60. Auger J, Jouannet P, Eustache F. Another look at human sperm morphology. *Hum Reprod* 2016; **31**: 10–23.

61. Gatimel N, Moreau J, Parinaud J, Léandri RD. Sperm morphology: assessment, pathophysiology, clinical relevance, and state of the art in 2017. *Andrology* 2017; **5**: 845–62.

62. Mortimer D. The functional anatomy of the human spermatozoon: relating ultrastructure and function. *Mol Hum Reprod* 2018; **24**: 567–92.

63. Davis RO, Gravance CG. Standardization of specimen preparation, staining, and sampling methods improves automated sperm-head morphometry analysis. *Fertil Steril* 1993; **59**: 412–17.

64. Lacquet FA, Kruger TF, Du Toit TC, et al. Slide preparation and staining procedures for reliable results using computerized morphology. *Arch Androl* 1996; **36**: 133–8.

65. van der Horst G, Maree L. SpermBlue®: a new universal stain for human and animal sperm which is also amenable to automated sperm morphology analysis. *Biotechnic Histochem* 2009; **84**: 299–308.

66. Maree L, du Plessis SS, Menkveld RM, van der Horst G. Morphometric dimensions of the human sperm head depend on the staining method used. *Hum Reprod* 2010; **25**: 1369–82

67. Schoevaert D. Automated recognition and morphological analysis of human spermatozoa. In: Robard D, Forti G, eds. *Computers in Endocrinology.* New York: Raven Press, 1984.

68. Yániz JL, Soler C, Santolaria P. Computer-assisted sperm morphometry in mammals: a review. *Anim Reprod Sci* 2015; **156**: 1–12.

69. Davis RO, Thal DM, Bain DE, et al. Accuracy and precision of the CellForm-Human automated sperm morphometry instrument. *Fertil Steril* 1992; **58**: 763–9.

70. Kruger T. Computer-assisted sperm analysis systems: morphometric aspects. *Hum Reprod* 1995; **10 Suppl. 1**: 46–52.

71. Farrell P, Trouern-Trend V, Foote RH, Douglas-Hamilton D. Repeatability of measurements on human, rabbit, and bull sperm by computer-assisted sperm analysis when comparing individual fields and means of 12 fields. *Fertil Steril* 1995; **64**: 208–10.

72. Hofmann GE, Santilli BA, Kindig S, et al. Intraobserver, interobserver variation of sperm critical morphology: comparison of examiner and computer-assisted analysis. *Fertil Steril* 1996; **65**: 1021–5.

73. Kruger TF, Lacquet FA, Sarmiento CAS, et al. A prospective study on the predictive value of normal sperm morphology as evaluated by computer (IVOS). *Fertil Steril* 1996; **66**: 285–91.

74. Coetzee K, Kruger TF, Lombard CJ. Repeatability and variance analysis on multiple computer-assisted (IVOS) sperm morphology readings. *Andrologia* 1999; **31**: 163–8.

75. Soler C, Gaßner P, Nieschlag E, et al. Utilización del Integrated Semen Analysis System (ISAS)® para el análisis morfométrico espermático humano y su significado en las técnicas de reproducción asistida. *Revista Internacional de Andrología* 2005; **3**, 112–19.

76. Mortimer D, Curtis EF, Camenzind AR. Combined use of fluorescent peanut agglutinin lectin and Hoechst 33258 to monitor the acrosomal status and vitality of human spermatozoa. *Hum Reprod* 1990; **5**: 99–103

77. Irvine DS, Macleod IC, Templeton AA, et al. A prospective clinical study of the relationship between the computer-assisted assessment of human semen quality and the achievement of pregnancy *in vivo*. *Hum Reprod* 1994; **9**: 2324–34.

78. Macleod IC, Irvine DS. The predictive value of computer-assisted semen analysis in the context of a donor insemination programme. *Hum Reprod* 1995; **10**: 580–6.

79. Feneux D, Serres C, Jouannet P. Sliding spermatozoa: a dyskinesia responsible for human infertility? *Fertil Steril* 1985; **44**: 508–11.

80. Aitken RJ, Sutton M, Warner P, Richardson DW. Relationship between the movement characteristics of human spermatozoa and their ability to penetrate cervical mucus and zona-free hamster oocytes. *J Reprod Fertil* 1985; **73**: 441–9.

81. Mortimer D, Pandya IJ, Sawers RS. Relationship between human sperm motility characteristics and sperm penetration into human cervical mucus in vitro. *J Reprod Fertil* 1986; **78**: 93–102.

82. Aitken RJ, Warner PE, Reid C. Factors influencing the success of sperm-cervical mucus interaction in patients exhibiting unexplained infertility. *J Androl* 1986; 7: 3–10.

83. Alasmari W, Barratt CLR, Publicover SJ, et al. The clinical significance of calcium signaling pathways mediating human sperm hyperactivation. *Hum Reprod* 2013; **28**: 866–76.

84. Sadeghi S, García-Molina A, Celma F, et al. Morphometric comparison by the ISAS® CASA-DNAf system of two techniques for the evaluation of DNA fragmentation in human spermatozoa. *Asian J Androl* 2016; **18**: 835–9.

85. Mortimer D, Curtis EF, Miller RG. Specific labelling by peanut agglutinin of the outer acrosomal membrane of the human spermatozoon. *J Reprod Fertil* 1987; **81**: 127–35.

86. Björndahl L, Barratt CLR, Mortimer D, Jouannet P. How to count sperm properly: checklist for acceptability of studies based on human semen analysis. *Hum Reprod* 2016; **31**: 227–32.

87. Agarwal A, Henkel R, Huang C-C, Lee M-S. Automation of human semen analysis using a novel artificial intelligence optical microscopic technology. *Andrologia* 2019; **51**: e13440.

88. Dearing CG, Kilburn S, Lindsay KS. Validation of the sperm class analyser CASA system for sperm counting in a busy diagnostic semen analysis laboratory. *Hum Fertil* 2014; **17**: 37–44.

89. Dearing C, Jayasena C, Lindsay K. Can the Sperm Class Analyser (SCA) CASA-Mot system for human sperm motility analysis reduce imprecision and operator subjectivity and improve semen analysis? *Hum Fertil* 2021; **24**: 208–18. https://doi.org/10.1080/14647273 .2019.1610581

90. International Standards Organization. *ISO 15189:2012 Medical laboratories – Requirements for quality and competence.* Geneva: International Standards Organization, 2012.

91. Palacios ER, Clavero A, Gonzalvo MC, et al. Acceptable variability in external quality assessment programmes for basic semen analysis. *Hum Reprod* 2012; **27**: 314–22.

92. Sanders D, Fensome-Rimmer S, Woodward B. Uncertainty of measurement in andrology: UK best practice guideline from the Association of Biomedical Andrologists. *Br J Biomed Sci* 2017; **74**: 157–62.

93. International Standards Organization. *ISO/TS 20914:2019 Medical laboratories – Practical guidance for the estimation of measurement uncertainty.* Geneva: International Standards Organization, 2019.

94. Keel BA, Quinn P, Schmidt CF Jr., et al. Results of the American Association of Bioanalysts national proficiency testing programme in andrology. *Hum Reprod* 2000; **15**: 680–6.

95. Bailey E, Fenning N, Chamberlain S, et al. Validation of sperm counting methods using limits of agreement *J Androl* 2007; **28**: 364–73.

96. International Standards Organization. *ISO 23162:2021 Basic semen examination – Specification and test methods.* Geneva: International Standards Organization, 2021.

97. Bland JM, Altman DG. Statistical methods for assessing agreement between two methods of clinical measurement. *Lancet* 1986; **I**: 307–10.

98. Alquezar-Baeta C, Gimeno-Martos S, Miguel-Jimenez S, et al. OpenCASA: a new open-source and scalable tool for sperm quality analysis. *PLoS Comput Biol* 2019; **15**: e1006691.

99. Yániz J, Alquézar-Baeta C, Yagüe-Martínez J, et al. Expanding the limits of computer-assisted sperm analysis through the development of open software. *Biology (Basel)* 2020; **9**: 207.

100. Gallagher MT, Cupples G, Ooi EH, et al. Rapid sperm capture: high-throughput flagellar waveform analysis. *Hum Reprod* 2019; **34**: 1173–85.

101. Chu KY, Nassau DE, Arora H. Artificial intelligence in reproductive urology. *Curr Urol Rep* 2019; **20**: 52. https://doi.org/10.1007/s11934 -019-0914-4

102. Riegler M, et al. Artificial intelligence in the fertility clinic – status, pitfalls, and possibilities. *Hum Reprod* 2021; **36**: 2429–42. https://doi.org/ 10.1093/humrep/deab168

103. Chang V, Garcia A, Hitschfeld N, et al. Gold-standard for computer-assisted morphological sperm analysis. *Comput Biol Med* 2017; **83**: 143–50.

104. Hicks SA, Andersen JM, Witczak O, et al. Machine learning-based analysis of sperm videos and participant data for male fertility prediction. *Sci Rep* 2019; **9**: 16770. https://doi.org/10.1038/ s41598-019-53217-y

105. Movahed RA, Mohammadi E, Orooji M. Automatic segmentation of sperm's parts in microscopic images of human semen smears

using concatenated learning approaches. *Comput Biol Med* 2019; **109**: 242–53.

106. Abbasi A, Miahi E, Mirroshandel SA. Effect of deep transfer and multi-task learning on sperm abnormality detection. *Comput Biol Med* 2021; **128**: 104121. https://doi:10.1016/j.compbiomed.2020 .104121

107. Ilhan HO, Serbes G, Aydin N, et al. A fully automated hybrid human sperm detection and classification system based on mobile-net and the performance comparison with conventional methods. *Med Biol Engineer Comput* 2020; **58**: 103845.

108. Kobori Y, Pfanner P, Prins GS, Niederberger C. Novel device for male infertility screening with single-ball lens microscope and smartphone. *Fertil Steril* 2016; **106**: 574–8.

109. Wei SY, Chao HH, Huang HP, et al. A collective tracking method for preliminary sperm analysis. *Biomed Eng Online* 2019; **18**: 112.

110. Ilhan HO, Aydin N. Smartphone based sperm counting – An alternative way to the visual assessment technique in sperm concentration analysis. *Multimed Tools Appl* 2020; **79**: 6409–35.

Chapter

7

Sperm Function Tests

Introduction

During the last three decades of the twentieth century, extensive research on a global basis was directed towards developing tests that might be able to identify particular aspects of sperm pathophysiology that resulted in dysfunction, and hence could help diagnose male factor infertility. In June 1995, the ESHRE Special Interest Group in Andrology held a Consensus Workshop on Advanced Diagnostic Andrology Techniques in Hamburg that seemed to mark a point of closure for much of the research in this field [1]. Certainly, the widespread availability of ICSI from the mid-1990s has led to much less interest in trying to diagnose what might be the aetiology of a man's infertility, and very few diagnostic andrology laboratories nowadays offer testing of sperm fertilizing ability.

This chapter summarizes the current status of what are, or were, the mainstream sperm function tests, and provide experimental protocols for anyone who might need to employ them, either for diagnostic or research purposes. Due to their key involvement in sperm dysfunction and reproductive competence, this chapter begins with a section on reactive oxygen species (free radicals). Tests of sperm chromatin/DNA fragmentation are not really measures of sperm function but rather the integrity of the 'payload', and are covered in Chapter 5.

Sperm Hyperactivation

Principle

Hyperactivated motility is a high-energy pattern of sperm movement seen in all Eutherian species. It is characterized by the development of high amplitude flagellar waves, but their propagation along the sperm tail results in little net space gain (see Figure 6.5). It is a visible concomitant of sperm capacitation *in vitro*, and has been observed in free-swimming spermatozoa in the oviduct *in situ*, and is now generally accepted to have a physiological importance for fertilization both *in vivo* and *in vitro*, especially in the penetration of the zona pellucida [2,3].

The clinical value of human sperm hyperactivation assessment is still not fully established, its investigation being confounded by several factors, including that there is both inter- and intra-individual variation in the proportion of human spermatozoa that exhibit hyperactivated motility, and that spermatozoa do not remain in the hyperactivated state continuously or indefinitely [4].

Although hyperactivation is a flagellar phenomenon, the only practical means for assessing its prevalence in a capacitating sperm population requires the use of specialized computer-aided sperm analysis (CASA) techniques (see Chapter 6). Unless all appropriate assay conditions are met (including careful separation of the spermatozoa from seminal plasma, specific physiological requirements for the incubation medium, and an adequate analysis preparation depth so as not to unduly constrain flagellar movement), hyperactivation studies will produce unreliable results [5,6].

Because the expression of spontaneous sperm hyperactivation is highly variable over time, even for sperm sub-populations within a single ejaculate (Figure 7.1), the need for multiple assessment time points has made the establishment of a robust clinical assay for hyperactivation difficult. However, two hyperactivation agonists, progesterone and pentoxifylline, have been employed to create a similar assay to the ARIC test [7,8]. Exposure of prepared motile sperm populations to 1μg/ml progesterone + 3.6 mM pentoxifylline in a capacitating sperm medium for 60 min induces maximal levels of hyperactivation in

155

the majority of men (Figure 7.2). This 'HAmax' assay contributes significantly towards predicting cases with poor and good IVF fertilization rate (0–49% and 50–100% respectively) even when testing is performed weeks, or even months, prior to the actual treatment cycle: discriminant function analysis $R^2 = 0.884$ with 100% sensitivity (22/22 cases) and 100% specificity (7/7 cases).

Specimen

- Liquefied semen collected, ideally, at the laboratory after a three-day period of prior sexual abstinence. A semen examination should be performed on the specimen.

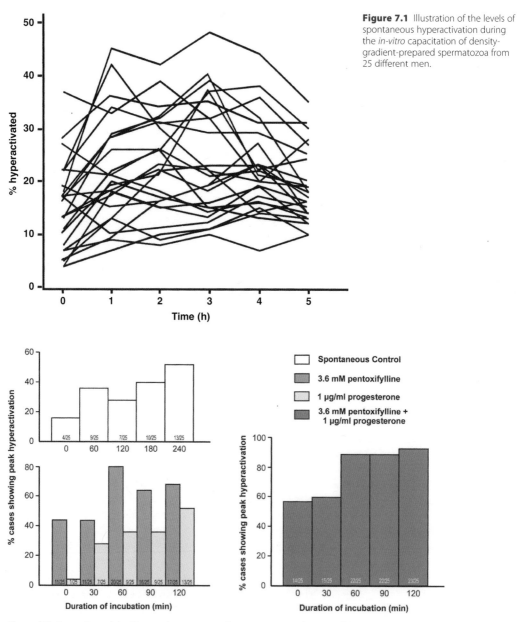

Figure 7.1 Illustration of the levels of spontaneous hyperactivation during the *in-vitro* capacitation of density-gradient-prepared spermatozoa from 25 different men.

Figure 7.2 Proportions of the 25 cases showing sperm hyperactivation within 10% of the peak spontaneous hyperactivation seen for each man level at different time points after either no treatment (control), treatment with 3.6 mM pentoxifylline or 1 μg/ml progesterone, or treatment with both pentoxifylline and progesterone. Based on these results, the optimum test format for the 'HAmax' assay was a 60 min incubation with the combined agonist treatment.

Equipment

See also Appendix 2.

- As for a semen examination
- As for sperm preparation using density gradient centrifugation
- Analytical balance capable of reading to 0.1 mg accuracy
- CO_2 incubator, operating at 6.0% CO_2-in-air if close to sea level. If a CO_2 incubator is not available then gas the tubes with pre-mixed gas containing 6.0% CO_2, cap them tightly and mix by inversion to equilibrate with the gas, and place the tubes in a 37°C incubator with an air atmosphere.
- Hamilton Thorne ('HT') IVOS or CEROS 60 Hz CASA system with the 'Edit Tracks' and 'Sort' function software options installed (see Chapter 6 for further details).

Disposable Materials

- As for semen examination
- As for sperm preparation using density gradient centrifugation
- Fixed-depth chambers for CASA analysis, ideally 50 µm MicroCell HAC chambers (Vitrolife, Göteborg, Sweden), but 20 µm chambers such as the 2X-CEL (Hamilton Thorne Biosciences) can be used for this particular assay if deeper chambers are unavailable.
- Falcon #2003 culture tubes

Reagents

1. *Sperm preparation:* As for sperm preparation using density gradient centrifugation (see Chapter 9).
2. *Sperm medium:* A bicarbonate-based (not HEPES-buffered) culture medium that supports human sperm capacitation (ideally Sydney IVF Sperm Medium, Cook Medical, see www.cookmedical.com/products).
3. *'HAmax' reagent:* This is a 2× concentrated solution of pentoxifylline and progesterone in the same medium as the prepared sperm suspension, which is mixed 1+1 with the prepared sperm suspension. The HAmax reagent contains 7.2 mM pentoxifylline and 2 µg/ml progesterone dissolved in sperm medium with added human serum albumin to give 30 mg HSA/ml and must be prepared for use each day. As supplied, the recommended product contains 10 mg/ml HSA whereas Sydney IVF Fertilization Medium contains only 5 mg/ml.
4. *Stock 1000× progesterone solution:* Dissolve 1.0 mg of progesterone (Sigma P6149) in 1.0 ml of absolute ethanol. Store tightly capped at +4°C for up to six months from date of opening.
5. *Daily use HAmax reagent:*
   a) To 2.0 ml of sterile sperm medium, add 4.0 mg pentoxifylline (Sigma P1784), 4.0 µl of stock progesterone solution and 40 mg of HSA (Sigma A1653).
   b) Mix thoroughly by gentle inversion. Do not shake as this will cause frothing due to the protein content of the medium.
   c) Store loosely capped in a CO_2 incubator at 37°C until required. Discard any unused reagent at the end of the day.

Calibration

The HT CASA instrument must be properly calibrated in terms of its optics and stage temperature (37°C), and the 'Sort' function must be configured to use validated criteria for identifying hyperactivated human spermatozoa using this instrument [see Chapter 6].

With legacy HT CASA software use: VCL ≥150 µm/s AND LIN ≤50% AND ALH ≥7.0 µm

With HT CASA-II software use: VCL ≥150 µm/s AND FDM ≥1.20 (FDM = the fractal dimension, a.k.a. 'D')

There are no other special calibrations required for the performance of this assay.

Quality Control

1. Daily QC is required for the proper operation of the IVOS instrument.
2. A positive control sample (i.e. semen from a control donor who has known HAmax response) should be run for each batch of HAmax reagent.

Procedure

1. Prepare a selected motile population of spermatozoa using a standardized two-layer discontinuous density gradient method (see Chapter 9) in sperm medium at $5-10 \times 10^6$ motile spermatozoa/ml.
2. Label two small Falcon #2003 culture tubes with the patient's name, the Andrology Lab Accession Number and the date, and either 'HA control' or 'HAmax'.
3. Transfer 0.5 ml of the washed sperm preparation into each tube.
4. Add reagents to the tubes:
    a) To the HA control tube add 0.5 ml of sperm medium
    b) To the HAmax tube add 0.5 ml of the HAmax reagent
    c) Mix thoroughly but gently, do not vortex
5. Incubate the tubes loosely capped at 37°C in the CO_2 incubator.
6. After the 60-min incubation, remove the tubes and perform a CASA analysis on each sperm population for the level of hyperactivated motility being expressed.
    Note: Remember to mix each tube thoroughly before taking the aliquots for making the CASA preparations. Do not mix too vigorously because this will cause frothing due to the HSA content of the medium; do not vortex.
7. Once the CASA analyses have been completed, discard the tubes.

Calculations and Results

No calculations are required for this specific procedure. The '% hyperactivation' ('%HA') sort fraction reported by the HT CASA software is the proportion of the motile spermatozoa in the sample that demonstrated movement characteristics indicative of hyperactivated motility.

Report both the spontaneous (control) level of hyperactivation as well as the agonist-induced HAmax value. In those men who show rapid capacitation, the spontaneous value might exceed the HAmax value (which can be reduced in cases of 'burn-out' caused by the powerful agonists employed). The higher value is taken as the maximum likely level of hyperactivation typical of the sperm population assayed.

Interpretation Guidelines and Notes

1. *Normal result:* Control shows >20% spontaneous HA and HAmax >50%. Suitable for any form of treatment.
2. *Good result:* Spontaneous HA and HAmax >20%. Recommended treatment options would be natural intercourse or IUI (with or without ovarian stimulation) or IVF (unless otherwise contra-indicated).
3. *Low result:* Spontaneous HA <20% and/or HAmax <20%. Recommended treatment options would be IUI (with or without ovarian stimulation), but if no pregnancy ensues after three cycles, proceed direct to ICSI.
4. *Abnormal results:* Spontaneous HA <20% and HAmax <10%; or if the results diverge by >20–30%. Recommended treatment option is ICSI.

Note: Treatment option decisions must only be made by a medical infertility specialist with particular expertise in andrology.

Acrosome Reaction Testing

Principle

Because the fertilizing spermatozoon undergoes its acrosome reaction (AR) on the surface of the zona pellucida, in response to binding to the putative sperm receptor, the zona glycoprotein ZP3, studies of the spontaneous AR have little positive predictive value for clinical applications. Because human zonae are so scarce, the true physiological inducer of the AR cannot be used in diagnostic laboratory practice, and biologically active recombinant human ZP3 (rhuZP3) is still not yet available commercially. As a result, various assay protocols exist that employ biological agonists or inducers of the AR with human follicular fluid (hFF), calcium ionophore (most usually A23187), or progesterone being used most often [1]. Pentoxifylline does not itself induce the human sperm AR, but rather it sensitizes the response to calcium ionophore in cases where the sperm show poor responsiveness to A23187. Unfortunately, hFF is impossible to standardize for long-term or multi-centre use as an agonist in this assay.

Good correlations have been found between the response of human spermatozoa to calcium ionophore and their fertilizing ability [9], and a modification of the original ARIC test (whose practical usefulness has been confirmed by numerous workers) is currently recommended [1].

Specimen

- Liquefied semen collected, ideally, at the laboratory after a three-day period of prior sexual abstinence. A semen examination should be performed on the specimen.

Equipment

See also Appendix 2.

- As for a semen examination
- As for sperm preparation using density gradient centrifugation
- Air displacement pipetters, 10 µl, 200 µl and 1000 µl capacities
- Analytical balance capable of reading to 0.1 mg accuracy
- CO_2 incubator, operating at 6.0% CO_2-in-air if close to sea level. If a CO_2 incubator is not available, then gas the tubes with pre-mixed gas containing 6.0% CO_2, cap them tightly and mix by inversion to equilibrate with the gas, and place the tubes in a 37°C incubator with an air atmosphere.
- Fluorescence microscope equipped with the appropriate filter set for the particular acrosome probe used.

Disposable Materials

- As for semen examination
- As for sperm preparation using density gradient centrifugation
- Falcon #2003 culture tubes
- 0.5 ml Eppendorf tubes

Reagents

1. *A23187 stock:* Dissolve 5 mg of A23187 (Sigma C5149) in 4.775 ml DMSO (Sigma D8779) to give a 2 mM stock solution. Store frozen at -20°C in small aliquots in 0.5 ml Eppendorf tubes. Cover the tubes in aluminium foil to protect the A23187 from exposure to light.
2. *ARIC reagent:* Add stock A23187 to the 'sperm medium' (see below) in a ratio of 1:200, i.e. to give a final concentration of 10 µM A23187 and 0.1% (v/v) DMSO.

3. *Sperm medium:* A bicarbonate-based (not HEPES-buffered) culture medium that supports human sperm capacitation, it should include at least 10 mg/ml HSA (ideally Sydney IVF Sperm Medium, Cook Medical, see www.cookmedical.com/products).
4. *Fixative:* Either 25% v/v glutaraldehyde (e.g. Sigma G6257) or absolute ethanol.

Calibration

None required.

Quality Control

- A positive control sample (i.e. semen from a control donor who has known ARIC response) must be run each time the test is performed.
- Each new batch of probe must be verified by using it in parallel with the previous batch on a positive control specimen.

Procedure

1. Prepare a selected motile population of spermatozoa using a standardized two-layer discontinuous density gradient method (see Chapter 9) in sperm medium at 1×10^6 motile spermatozoa/ml.
2. Label two small Falcon #2003 culture tubes with the patient's name, the Andrology Lab Accession Number and the date, and either 'ARIC control' or 'ARIC'.
3. Transfer 1.0 ml of the washed sperm preparation into each tube.
4. Incubate the tubes loosely capped at 37°C in the CO_2 incubator.
5. Add reagents to the tubes:
   a) To the ARIC control tube add 5 µl of DMSO
   b) To the ARIC test tube add 5 µl of the ARIC reagent
   c) Mix thoroughly but gently; do not vortex
6. Incubate both tubes for a further 15 min in the CO_2 incubator.
7. Remove a small aliquot from each tube and assess for sperm motility before stopping the effect of the ARIC reagent by adding 200 µl of fixative.
   Notes:
   a) Remember to mix each tube thoroughly – but not too vigorously – before taking the aliquots for motility assessment; do not vortex.
   b) Mix the tubes thoroughly again after adding the fixative, gentle vortex mixing is acceptable with fixed spermatozoa.
8. Prepare slides from the fixed sperm suspensions for staining using whichever probe has been selected.
9. Examine the preparations under epifluorescence and assess the proportion of acrosome-reacted spermatozoa according to the appropriate criteria for the probe being used (Figure 7.3). Count at least 100 spermatozoa per slide.

Calculations and Results

1. Calculate the percentage of acrosome-reacted spermatozoa ('AR+ve') in the Control and ARIC populations using the total numbers of spermatozoa counted in the replicate preparations.
   The ARIC value for each specimen is calculated as: ARIC AR+ve % – Control AR+ve %
2. Two types of AR pathology can be defined from ARIC tests: 'AR insufficiency' and 'AR prematurity'.
   a) AR prematurity: >20% of spermatozoa show spontaneous ARs after 3 h incubation under capacitating conditions.
   b) AR insufficiency: <10% ARs inducible by ionophore treatment above the spontaneous background, indicating a likely impairment of fertilizing ability; 10–15% is a grey area, indicating a risk of sperm dysfunction.

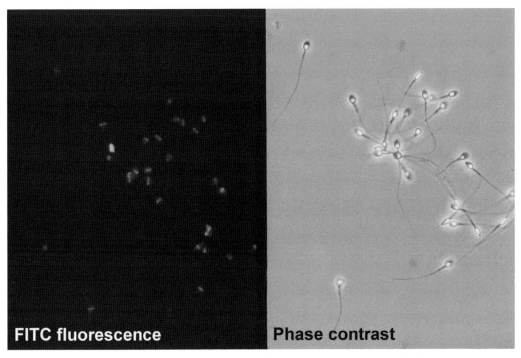

FITC fluorescence　　　　**Phase contrast**

Figure 7.3 Photomicrographs of the same field of spermatozoa following agonist treatment to induce the acrosome reaction under either phase contrast optics (right panel) or epifluorescence for FITC-labelled PNA lectin (left panel). Note the fluorescent labelling over the equatorial segment of the acrosome denoting the acrosome-reacted status.

   c) Normal result: >15% ARs inducible by ionophore treatment above the spontaneous background.
3. If the sperm motility is significantly lower in the ARIC sample compared to the control, then this must be reported as a likely confounding factor for interpreting the results. Sperm death can be confirmed if the AR staining method includes assessment of sperm vitality.

Interpretation Guidelines
1. Approximately 5% of infertility patients have an AR problem, about half AR insufficiency and half AR prematurity [1].
2. Both AR prematurity and AR insufficiency are good indicators of a likely clinical problem: a poor ARIC test result is a strong indicator of poor sperm fertilizing ability at IVF (although a good ARIC result does not necessarily indicate the absence of any problem with the physiological AR). The ARIC score has been reported to be a better predictor of pregnancy during IUI treatment than conventional descriptive semen characteristics [10].
3. Both problems can be treated by ICSI because there is no apparent relationship between AR function and ICSI outcome.
4. Given the overall prevalence of such problems, one cannot propose AR studies as an upfront diagnostic test like semen analysis, although automation of test scoring, and simplified protocols using rhuZP3 might make such testing more amenable to routine clinical use in the future.
5. Extensive studies have demonstrated that the zona-induced acrosome reaction, or 'ZIAR', is an interesting assessment of sperm functional potential [11,12], which has been further correlated with sperm morphology [13,14]. However, the difficulty of running this assay in routine andrology laboratories continues to hinder its wider application and acceptance into routine pre-treatment evaluation.

Notes

The standardized ARIC test protocol provided above is based on the consensus protocol from the ESHRE Special Interest Group in Andrology [1], and has also been promoted by the WHO [15]. Their particular criteria were:

- Spermatozoa must be separated from seminal plasma using a non-deleterious preparation method and suspended in a bicarbonate-based culture medium capable of supporting capacitation, supplemented with at least 10 mg/ml albumin (preferably HSA).
- Preincubate the prepared sperm suspension under capacitating conditions for 3 h. While preincubation is not essential for responsiveness to A23187, it improves reproducibility and allows for the simultaneous assessment of spontaneous acrosome loss (i.e. AR prematurity).
- Assess acrosomal status before and after a rather standard ionophore treatment of 10 μM A23187 for 15 min.
- Given the extensive studies validating various techniques for visualizing the human sperm acrosome, either lectins (e.g. peanut, *Arachis hypogea*, or pea, *Pisum sativum*, agglutinins, i.e. PNA or PSA), monoclonal antibodies, or the triple stain may be employed as probes for the acrosome reaction status of human spermatozoa [16–19]. Replicate (minimum two) slides must be scored for each determination, with at least 100 spermatozoa counted per slide.
- A vitality assessment should be included to differentiate post-mortem acrosomal degeneration or loss from a true acrosome reaction unless the labelling technique gives an 'equatorial segment only' pattern, which is typical of a true AR and rarely seen with degenerative acrosome loss. This information is very important if many spermatozoa die during the ARIC treatment step. Exclusion of the fluorescent dye Hoechst 33258 is preferred over a HOS-type test [16,19].
- As with any bioassay, a positive control sample is mandatory in each assay run, although a negative control is not essential. The positive control need not necessarily be from a proven fertile donor (although this is preferred), but it must be from a man proven to have a normal response in the test. Because cryopreservation alters sperm membranes, fresh semen must be used for the positive control.

Sperm-Zona Pellucida Binding Tests

Background

Sperm binding to the zona pellucida (ZP) is an essential recognition stage in the eutherian fertilization process. After penetrating the cumulus oophorus spermatozoa bind tightly to the zona pellucida through the ZP3 receptors present on the zona pellucida, which induces a signal transduction cascade within the spermatozoon leading to the acrosome reaction. Acrosome-reacted spermatozoa are then considered to bind to another zona protein (ZP2), facilitating penetration of the zona matrix and progression into the perivitelline space. Much of the species-specificity of human fertilization occurs at the level of sperm-zona pellucida interaction, including induction of the physiological acrosome reaction in the fertilizing spermatozoon, which has led to great interest in the development of tests to assess sperm binding to the human zona pellucida [1].

Two types of sperm-zona pellucida binding tests have been described in the literature. The original hemizona assay test (HZA) that makes use of the two halves of a bisected oocyte, one as the test and the other half as the internal control [20,21]. The second type of test, called the competitive sperm-zoa binding test [22], uses intact zonae pellucidae that are exposed to spermatozoa from both the test subject and a control subject to observe sperm binding to the same oocytes. Sperm-zona binding tests assess tight sperm binding to the human ZP as the primary endpoint and have a high predictive value for *in-vitro* fertilization in prospectively designed studies, as well as a high capacity to identify possible male factor cases at risk for failed or poor fertilization, indicating the multiple sperm functions necessary for successful fertilization, of which many can be indicated by abnormal sperm morphology patterns [1,22–25].

Materials: Zonae Pellucidae

1. *Sources:* Zonae pellucidae (ZPs) are from human oocytes and can be obtained from a variety of sources, including the following:

   - Post-mortem derived ovaries: It is important that all applicable ethical and legal guidelines must be followed. Ovarian oocytes can be obtained by macerating ovarian tissue in a Petri dish containing any culture medium used for human IVF. After mincing the tissue, the fluid is examined under a stereozoom microscope and the oocytes, mostly immature prophase I oocytes, are collected by means of a small-bore pipette. Studies have indicated that ovarian age does not influence the sperm binding capacity of the ZP of prophase I oocytes, although the mean numbers of spermatozoa bound to metaphase II oocytes were found to be higher than those for immature prophase I oocytes [26].

   - Inseminated but non-fertilized IVF oocytes: These are oocytes not showing any evidence of either two pronuclei or cleavage at 48–60 h post-insemination. After removal of any remaining cumulus cells by repeated pipetting using a fine glass pipette, they can be transferred into a storage medium, preferably a concentrated salt solution (1 M ammonium sulphate) and stored at 4°C [26].

   - Recycled hemizonae. After the first assay, all bound spermatozoa are removed using a hand-drawn glass micropipette of 90 μm diameter, which is slightly smaller than the size of a hemizona, thereby shearing the spermatozoa from the hemizona surface (although a few spermatozoa whose heads, either partially or entirely, are embedded in the ZP, might remain) [26].

2. *Storage:* ZPs can be stored in several ways, including:

   - Salt storage: A solution of 1.5 M $MgCl_2$, 0.01% polyvinylpyrrolidone (average MW = 40,000, e.g. Sigma PVP-40) and 40mM HEPES buffer. Usually employed as 0.5-ml in an Eppendorf tube containing 10–30 oocytes. Intended for short-term storage of up to 30 days, although most references indicate up to 7 days [21].

   - Ammonium sulphate solution: Usually stored as 15–30 oocytes in 1 ml of a 1 M ammonium sulphate solution in a cryotube for two to eight weeks.

   - DMSO: 2 M DMSO in PBS. 10–30 oocytes in this solution are loaded into a cryopreservation straw and the ends sealed, e.g. Critoseal haematocrit putty (Fisher Scientific, Springfield, NJ, USA) for PETG straws. Straws are immediately frozen at -70°C and can be stored for one to six months before use.

     Note: While all these means of storage reserve the ZP and its receptivity to sperm biding, the cytoplasm of the enclosed oocytes is rendered non-functional, precluding any possibility of their subsequent fertilization.

The Hemizona Assay

Principle

In this technique an oocyte (usually preserved) is bisected prior to use so that the halves can be used for assessing the sperm-zona binding ability of a patient's spermatozoa and the spermatozoa of a matched control in parallel. The bisection of oocytes into the matching hemizonae can be performed using either a micromanipulation technique (preferred) [20], manual cutting under high power stereo-zoom magnification [27,28], or using a laser [29].

Note: After dissection of the oocytes, the residual cytoplasm is removed to eliminate any possibility of inadvertent fertilization [26].

Specimens

- *Sperm preparations:* Two sperm samples are involved in the hemizona assay, one specimen is obtained from a previously tested fertile male whose sperm-zona binding capacity is known (control), and a second semen specimen from the patient whose sperm-zona binding potential is to be evaluated (test). Motile sperm preparations are prepared as described in Chapter 9 and finally resuspended in a bicarbonate-buffered medium capable of supporting sperm capacitation (e.g. IVF medium) and adjusted to a concentration of 0.5×10^6 motile spermatozoa per ml.

- *Zonae pellucidae:* Stored ZPs, obtained and stored by any of the already described techniques, are washed using 4×1-ml changes of the same culture medium as will be used for the assay over a 4 h period of incubation at 37°C. Each oocyte is micro-bisected into two matching hemizonae.

Equipment

See also Appendix 2.

- As for standard semen analysis
- As for sperm preparation using density gradients
- Inverted microscope with 10× and 40× phase contrast objectives and micromanipulation arm
- CO_2 incubator, operating at 6.0% CO_2-in-air if close to sea level. If a CO_2 incubator is not available, then gas the tubes with pre-mixed gas containing 6.0% CO_2, cap them tightly and mix by inversion to equilibrate with the gas, and place the tubes in a 37°C incubator with an air atmosphere.
- Air displacement pipette, 100 µl

Disposable Materials

- As for standard semen examination
- As for sperm preparation using density gradients
- Small and large Petri dishes (Falcon #3001 and #3003)
- Glass Pasteur pipettes
- Conical 15 ml tubes (e.g. Falcon #2095)
- Culture oil

Reagents

Sperm medium: A bicarbonate-based (not HEPES-buffered) culture medium that supports human sperm capacitation. This medium should include at least 10 mg/ml HSA.

Calibration

None required.

Quality Control

The HZA incorporates an internal control by comparing the patient and positive control (sperm donor) results on matched hemizonae.

Procedure

1. For each assay, prepare:
   a) A 60 mm Petri dish with two 50 µl droplets of sperm suspensions, one from the test patient and the other from the control donor, and cover with oil.
   b) Another Petri dish with two 50 µl droplets of medium only under oil.
2. Transfer the matching hemizonae, one into each of the sperm droplets.
3. Co-incubate the spermatozoa and hemizonae at 37°C under an appropriate CO_2-in-air atmosphere for 4 h.
   Note: Put the second dish into the CO_2 incubator to equilibrate alongside the assay dish.

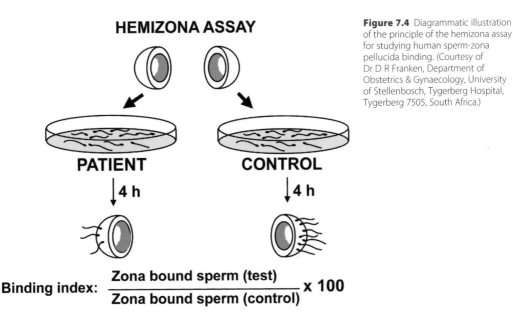

HEMIZONA ASSAY

PATIENT   CONTROL

4 h   4 h

Binding index: $\dfrac{\text{Zona bound sperm (test)}}{\text{Zona bound sperm (control)}} \times 100$

Figure 7.4 Diagrammatic illustration of the principle of the hemizona assay for studying human sperm-zona pellucida binding. (Courtesy of Dr D R Franken, Department of Obstetrics & Gynaecology, University of Stellenbosch, Tygerberg Hospital, Tygerberg 7505, South Africa.)

4. Rinse each hemizona separately using clean medium by gently pipetting 4–6× through a finely-drawn micropipette (100 μm diameter) to dislodge all loosely attached spermatozoa and transfer it into the correct medium droplet in the second dish.
   Note: Ensure that the hemizonae are positioned with their outer surfaces upwards [30].
5. Hold the rinsed hemizonae in the culture medium droplets under oil until examination (within 1 h).
6. Using phase contrast microscopy at 400× magnification, count the number of spermatozoa that are tightly bound to each hemizona (Figure 7.4).

Calculations and Results

The HZA result, the 'hemizona index' or 'HZI' is calculated from the absolute numbers of tightly bound spermatozoa for each of the test and control hemizonae as follows:

$$HZI = \frac{\text{Number of tightly bound spermatozoa for the patient test}}{\text{Number of tightly bound spermatozoa for the control}} \times 100\%$$

Interpretation Guidelines

Clinical studies indicated a cut off value of ≥36% as prognostic for IVF fertilization. With an HZI ≤35%, the chances for poor IVF fertilization *in vitro* are 90–100%, whereas the chances for fertilization are 80–85% with a HZI >35%. The observed false-positive rate is less than 15%. For further information see [26].

Notes

1. *Indirect sperm-zona binding test at IVF*
   The ESHRE consensus workshop on advanced diagnostic andrology recommended that, in cases of total fertilization failure at IVF, the oocytes should be examined for the presence of spermatozoa bound to the zona pellucida [1]. Absence of zona-bound spermatozoa may indicate a sperm-binding defect. Although not as reliable as a sperm-zona binding test, this

procedure will at least provide an indication as for the reason for the failure of fertilization and may be the only source of information, as the performance of sperm-zona binding tests is not readily available in most laboratories, mainly due to lack of oocytes.

2. *Standardization of sperm-zona binding tests*

   The hemizona assay and competitive sperm-zona binding tests both provide highly comparable results confirming that sperm-zona binding tests are good predictors of both *in-vitro* fertilization and non-fertilization results. To better standardize both tests, and make the results even more comparable, the ESHRE consensus workshop proposed the following general guidelines [1]:

   - A protein-supplemented, bicarbonate-based, IVF culture medium should be used to resuspend selected (isolated) motile spermatozoa to a concentration of 100,000–250,000/ml. Patient and control donor preparations must be at the same motile sperm concentration.
   - Co-incubation of spermatozoa and zonae should take place in a drop of culture medium (e.g. 100 μl) under oil for 4 h at 37°C in an appropriate CO_2-enriched atmosphere.
   - After coincubation with the spermatozoa, zonae should be washed thoroughly, after which the number of tightly bound spermatozoa is counted on the entire surface of the (hemi)zona to avoid any skewing of results due to heterogeneous distribution of spermatozoa.
   - Results can be expressed as a percentage index of the test results relative to the control results.
   - Zona intact oocytes intended for binding tests should preferably be stored in a hypertonic salt solution able to preserve the sperm-binding capacity of the zona pellucida for up to at least three months.

The Competitive Sperm-Zona Binding Assay

Principle

The competitive sperm-zona binding assay (CZA) uses intact unfertilized oocytes instead of hemizonae as in the HZA. Immature oocytes can also be used as a source of ZPs as it has been confirmed that such ZPs possess similar biological activity for sperm-ZP binding as those from mature oocytes [31]. Fresh or salt-stored oocytes can be used for the assay [22].

For this method the patient (test) and control (donor) sperm populations are labelled with different fluorochromes and then incubated together with the ZPs to determine their respective abilities to achieve sperm binding to the ZP [22].

Specimens

- *Sperm preparations:* Two sperm samples are involved in the hemizona assay, one specimen is obtained from a previously tested fertile male whose sperm-zona binding capacity is known (control), and a second semen specimen from the patient whose sperm-zona binding potential is to be evaluated (test). Motile sperm preparations are prepared (as described in Chapter 9) in a bicarbonate-buffered culture medium capable of supporting sperm capacitation (e.g. IVF medium) and adjusted to a concentration of 0.5×10^6 motile spermatozoa per ml.
- *Zonae pellucidae:* Stored ZPs, obtained and stored by any of the already described techniques, are washed using 4×1-ml changes of the same culture medium as will be used for the assay over a 4 h period of incubation at 37°C. It is recommended to use four ZPs for each patient being tested.

Equipment

See also Appendix 2.

- As for standard semen examination
- As for sperm preparation using density gradients

- Inverted microscope with 160× or 250× phase contrast magnification
- CO_2 incubator, operating at 6.0% CO_2-in-air if close to sea level. If a CO_2 incubator is not available, then gas the tubes with pre-mixed gas containing 6.0% CO_2, cap them tightly and mix by inversion to equilibrate with the gas, and place the tubes in a 37°C incubator with an air atmosphere.
- Air displacement pipette, 100 μl

Disposable Materials

- As for standard semen examination
- As for sperm preparation using density gradients
- Small and large plastic Petri dishes (Falcon #3001 and #3003)
- Glass Pasteur pipettes
- Glass microcapillary pipettes, inner diameter 250 μm
- Conical 15 ml test tubes (Falcon #2095)
- Culture oil

Reagents

1. *Sperm medium:* A bicarbonate-based (not HEPES-buffered) culture medium that supports human sperm capacitation, it should include at least 10 mg/ml HSA.
2. *PBS+glucose:* Dulbecco's phosphate-buffered saline containing 55 mM glucose. Filter sterilize through a 0.22 μm membrane filter (e.g. Millipore Millex-GV) and store at +4°C for up to one month. Discard if there are any signs of precipitation or cloudiness.
3. *FITC label:* Dissolve 1.0 mg of fluorescein isothiocyanate (FITC, Sigma F7250) in 0.1 ml of a 100 mM aqueous solution of KOH and dilute within 15 s to 5 ml with sterile PBS+glucose. Store at 4°C in a Falcon #2003 tube wrapped in aluminium foil for up to one week.
4. *TRITC label:* Dissolve 0.5 mg of tetramethylrhodamine B isothiocyanate (TRITC, Sigma T3163) in 0.1 ml of a 100 mM aqueous solution of KOH and dilute within 15 s to 5 ml with sterile PBS+glucose. Store at 4°C in a Falcon #2003 tube wrapped in aluminium foil for up to one week.

Calibration

None required.

Quality Control

The assay incorporates an internal control by mixing the differentially fluorescently labelled patient and positive control (donor) spermatozoa and then testing them simultaneously on the same ZPs.

Procedure

1. *Fluorochrome labelling of spermatozoa* (based on [22]). For each sperm preparation:
   a) Centrifuge an aliquot of the washed sperm preparation at 600 *g* for 5 min. Carefully remove and discard the supernatant, then resuspend the pellet in 0.3 ml of the appropriate fluorochrome labelling solution (e.g. FITC for the patient test sample and TRITC for the control donor).
   b) Incubate at 37°C for 15 min.
   c) Centrifuge the sperm suspensions at 600 *g* for 5 min to recover the spermatozoa.
   d) Carefully remove and discard the supernatant, then resuspend the pellet in 10 ml of sperm medium.
   e) Centrifuge the sperm suspensions at 600 *g* for 5 min to recover the spermatozoa.
   f) Carefully remove and discard the supernatant, then resuspend the pellet in sperm medium to a final concentration of 0.1×10^6 motile spermatozoa per ml with fresh sperm medium.

167

2. *Preparation of coincubation drops:*
   a) In a separate Petri dish for each patient being tested, dispense 25 µl droplets of the labelled patient sperm preparation. Prepare one droplet for each ZP to be used in the test.
   b) To each patient sperm drop add 25 µl of the labelled control donor sperm preparation. Change the pipette tip between patients.
   c) Cover the drops with culture oil.
   d) Add a single ZP to each drop. Remember to change the pipette tip between patients.
3. Incubate in a CO_2 incubator at 37°C for 4 h. During this time prepare a small Petri dish with fresh sperm medium for each patient being tested and put these dishes in the incubator adjacent to the test dishes to equilibrate.
4. Rinse each ZP in the appropriate wash dish by vigorous aspiration in and out of a finely drawn glass pipette to dislodge any loosely attached spermatozoa.
5. Transfer each ZP individually, when ready, onto a clean microscope slide and mount it under a square coverslip supported by four small pillars of high vacuum silicone grease at its corners; compress the coverslip to flatten the ZP.
6. Examine the mounted ZP at magnification of 160× to 250× under an epifluorescence microscope using separate filter sets to visualize the FITC (green) and TRITC (red) labelled spermatozoa separately (see Appendix 3). Count the total number of each colour of spermatozoa bound to the ZP.
7. Repeat steps 5 and 6 for each ZP.

Calculations and Results

For each patient test, calculate the total numbers of patient and donor spermatozoa bound to all the ZPs used in that test. The result of each test, the 'sperm-zona binding ratio', is calculated as:

$$\text{Sperm-ZP binding ratio} = \frac{\text{Total number of ZP-bound spermatozoa for the test patient}}{\text{Total number of ZP-bound spermatozoa for the donor}}$$

Interpretation Guidelines

A sperm-zona binding ratio of ≥0.88 can be regarded as a normal value, in which case an IVF fertilization rate of >50% can be expected [22].

Notes

See Notes for the Hemizona Assay (above).

Zona-Free Hamster Egg Penetration Test

Although popular during the 1980s and early 1990s, the 'hamster egg penetration test' ('HEPT') – often referred to in the US literature as the 'sperm penetration assay' ('SPA') – is used in very few laboratories nowadays [1]. Since there is still widespread clinical and patient awareness of the test, a brief overview has been included here. More extensive reviews and detailed laboratory protocols can be found elsewhere [15,19].

The HEPT is an integrated assessment of the ability of spermatozoa to capacitate *in vitro* and undergo the acrosome reaction, which leaves them in a fusogenic state, able to bind to and fuse with the hamster oocyte oolemma. After the sperm head has been incorporated into the oocyte, the nucleus decondenses, and visualization of this 'swollen sperm head' is the test endpoint (Figure 7.5).

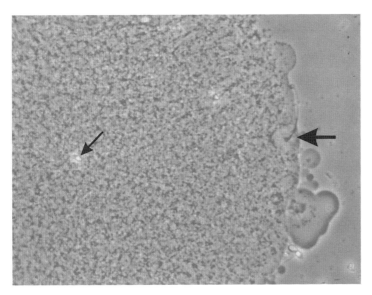

Figure 7.5 Photomicrograph (phase contrast optics) of a zona-free hamster oocyte showing a swollen sperm head (large arrow), denoting that the oocyte had been penetrated during the test. Note the still-attached sperm tail extending in the 12-o'clock direction from the centre of the swollen sperm head. The head of a spermatozoon attached to the oolemma is indicated, for comparison of size, by the small arrow.

Because of substantial intra- and inter-sample heterogeneity in sperm populations, both in the time required for spermatozoa to undergo capacitation and in their susceptibility to undergoing spontaneous acrosome loss, results from protocols that rely on spontaneous ARs will perforce vary according to preincubation conditions. A wide range of protocols were developed employing strategies to induce ARs artificially in more-or-less capacitated sperm populations, including the use of the calcium ionophore A23187 – but with no single one having been generally accepted as providing optimum physiologically meaningful results [1,15,19].

Inconsistent terminology caused substantial confusion in understanding the clinical relevance of the HEPT and very few papers reported prospective studies using clinically relevant endpoints such as the achievement of *in-vivo* conception or *in-vitro* fertilization. False negative results were common in many early studies based on spontaneous ARs, and false positive results were a persistent problem. General interpretation guidelines for HEPT results were not, therefore, possible; each laboratory had to interpret its results according to its own criteria.

The ESHRE Special Interest Group in Andrology therefore concluded that, although its value as a research tool for assessing sperm function is unquestioned, the HEPT was not a frontline clinical diagnostic test [1] – a conclusion since echoed by other authorities [32].

Sperm Survival Assay

Principle

Assessments of human sperm survival *in vitro* are carried out for two purposes:

1) As a bioassay for determining the acceptability of culture media and contact materials in an assisted reproductive technology laboratory [33,34]; or
2) In an attempt to evaluate the longevity of a subject's spermatozoa [35].

While well-validated protocols are available for the former application (see below), the latter application does raise some intriguing physiological questions. The prolonged incubation of human spermatozoa under capacitating conditions results in their capacitation, followed by a high level of spontaneous acrosome reactions due to the lability of the capacitated spermatozoon; and once having undergone the acrosome reaction the spermatozoa die [36]. Consequently, there is a dilemma as to whether a high sperm survival after 24 h incubation is 'good' or 'bad', since in a medium optimized for sperm capacitation, a high proportion of dead spermatozoa after 24 h could be seen as revealing a high physiological response of the man's spermatozoa to the incubation conditions, whereas in a medium that is sub-optimal for sperm capacitation, and/or where the man's spermatozoa respond poorly to the capacitating conditions, a high level of sperm survival would not reflect a 'good' result. However, notwithstanding this discussion, when a sperm survival test (SST) is carried out as part of an IVF treatment cycle under controlled conditions, it can yield useful information [35] – although that information might not necessarily be transferable to another laboratory using a different culture system.

The method provided below for the QC version of the SST is based on a protocol generously provided by Dr Ri-Chen Chiang. It is an optimized method where albumin is omitted from the culture medium so as to increase the sensitivity of the system to spermotoxic substances.

Specimen(s)

Either contact materials or culture media to be tested for sperm toxicity.

Note: The suspension of washed spermatozoa used in the assay is considered to be a reagent (see below), not a specimen.

Equipment

See also Appendix 2.

- As for sperm preparation using density gradient centrifugation (see Chapter 9)
- Air displacement pipetters, 1–20 µl, and 1000 µl
- CO_2 incubator, set at the correct pCO_2 for the sperm medium being used. If a CO_2 incubator is not available, then gas the tubes with a suitable pre-mixed gas, cap them tightly and mix by inversion to equilibrate with the gas; then place them in a 37°C incubator with an air atmosphere.
- For analysis, either:
    - Phase contrast compound microscope configured for andrology
    - CASA instrument (see Chapter 6)
- Laboratory counter

Disposable Materials

- As for semen examination
- As for sperm preparation using density gradient centrifugation (see Chapter 9)
- Sterile small Falcon culture tubes (#2003 or #2054)
- NUNC four-well dishes

Reagents

- A suspension of washed spermatozoa, at a concentration of 5×10^6 motile spermatozoa/ml, prepared using density gradient centrifugation. If cryopreserved semen is used, then swim-up can be used as an alternative sperm preparation procedure (see Chapter 9).
- *Sperm Buffer:* Any suitable HEPES-buffered sperm-washing medium with ≥5 mg/ml HSA.

Calibration

No calibration is required unless the motility assessments are being made using computer-aided sperm analysis (CASA), in which case the standard CASA calibration requirements must be met (see Chapter 6).

Quality Control

Note: All media and contact materials used in the assay must have been tested and certified suitable for assisted-conception use, i.e. non-spermotoxic or have passed the mouse embryo bioassay, and be free of endotoxin.

- *Positive control:* An aliquot of the prepared sperm suspension in sperm buffer must be run in each assay. To be valid, this control must show >70% progressively motile spermatozoa at the end of the 18–24-h assay period. If using cryopreserved spermatozoa, then the requirement is >40%.
- *Negative control:* An aliquot of the prepared sperm suspension in sperm buffer that has been adulterated with formaldehyde, or some other substance toxic to spermatozoa, must be run in each assay. To be valid, this control must have a Sperm Motility Index (SMI, see below) of <0.50 at the end of the 18–24-h assay period.

Procedure: Testing Contact Materials

1. Expose the test material (e.g. a dish or tube) to 0.5 ml of the sperm suspension at 37°C for 5 min.
2. Remove the sperm suspension using a sterile pipette tip and transfer into a sterile small Falcon tube.
3. Incubate the tube at 37°C under an air atmosphere for 18–24 h.

Procedure: Testing Culture Media

1. For each test medium, centrifuge a 500 μl aliquot of the sperm suspension at 500 $g \times$ 5 min.
2. Resuspend the spermatozoa in 500 μl of the test medium and incubate under the appropriate conditions:
   a) *Bicarbonate-buffered media:* Transfer the sperm suspension into a sterile NUNC four-well dish and incubate in a CO_2 incubator (5.0–6.0% CO_2, as appropriate for the medium being tested and adjusted for altitude if necessary, see the manufacturer's recommendations). An oil overlay is not essential if using a Cook K-MINC 1000 mini-incubator.
   b) *HEPES-buffered media:* Transfer the sperm suspension into a sterile small Falcon tube and incubate in an air incubator.
3. Incubate at 37°C for 18–24 h.

Procedure: Assessing Sperm Survival by Sperm Motility

For each of the positive and negative controls and each test sample preparation:

1. Mix the sperm suspension thoroughly and take an aliquot to assess the sperm motility either visually (see 'Wet Preparation' in Chapter 3) or using CASA (see Chapter 6). Assess at least 200 spermatozoa and determine the proportion of spermatozoa showing active forward progression.
   Note: For media that do not contain HSA, see Note 1, below.
2. Repeat the motility assessment.
3. Verify that the two replicate assessments are in agreement (see Chapter 3 and Appendix 5). If not, then repeat the assessment.
4. Calculate the average % progressive motility for each control and test sample.

Calculations and Results

The *Sperm Motility Index* (SMI) is derived by dividing the % progressive motility in the test sample at the end of the incubation period by the % progressive motility in the positive control sample at the start of the incubation period.

1. Verify that the positive and negative controls meet the assay QC criteria. If not, then repeat the entire assay.
2. For each test sample, calculate the SMI as the ratio between the test sample's progressive motility and the positive control's progressive motility. For example:

Test sample: Count A $= 130/200$; count B $= 142/200$; difference $<10\%$ so results are OK
                         Progressive motility $= 272/400 = 68\%$

Positive control: Count A $= 165/200$; count B $= 175/200$; difference $<10\%$ so results are OK.
                         Progressive motility $= 340/400 = 85\%$

SMI $= 68/85 = 0.80$

Interpretation Guidelines

- SMI values <75% are taken to indicate sperm toxicity in the test material.
- Therefore, the SMI result shown in the example above indicates that the test specimen passed the test, i.e. did not show detectable toxicity to human spermatozoa.

Notes

1. Spermatozoa in a test medium that does not contain any HSA will likely show the 'sticking-to-glass' phenomenon. In this case, the post-incubation sample must be diluted with an equal volume of the sperm buffer (ideally containing at least 10 mg/ml of HSA) before analysis.

Hyaluronan Binding Assay

It has been known for over 20 years that mature human spermatozoa express binding sites for the polysaccharide hyaluronic acid, also known as hyaluronate or hyaluronan, and that the ability of human spermatozoa to bind to hyaluronan indicates cellular maturity, viability, unreacted acrosomal status and low sperm DNA fragmentation [37,38]. A commercial Hyaluronan Binding Assay ('HBA'), based on a hyaluronan coated Cell-Vu® slide, was developed (now from Cooper Surgical, Måløv, Denmark). While sperm motility and morphology were highly correlated with HBA scores, and both abnormal sperm morphology and HBA score were significantly related to IVF fertilization rate, the HBA was less significant than normal sperm morphology [39]. Furthermore, no relationship between hyaluronan binding and fertilization, cleavage, good quality embryo, implantation, clinical pregnancy, miscarriages and biochemical pregnancy rates could be found [38]. Consequently, the general conclusion has been that the HBA does not provide additional information for identifying patients with poor IVF fertilization rate.

In a study of sperm populations prepared using a variety of different density gradient products, there were reductions in sperm DNA fragmentation compared to the original semen samples, but no changes in HBA score [40]. These authors also concluded that the clinical significance of the HBA required further investigation.

See Chapter 9, *Sperm Preparation*, regarding a sperm selection device based on hyaluronan binding, the PICSI® Dish, intended for use in conjunction with ICSI.

References

1. ESHRE Andrology Special Interest Group. Consensus workshop on advanced diagnostic andrology techniques. *Hum Reprod* 1996; **11**: 1463–79.

2. Dresdner RD, Katz DF. Relationships of mammalian sperm motility and morphology to hydrodynamic aspects of cell function. *Biol Reprod* 1981; **25**: 920–30.

3. Mortimer ST. A critical review of the physiological importance and analysis of sperm movement in mammals. *Hum Reprod Update* 1997; **3**: 403–39.

4. Mortimer ST, Swan MA. Variable kinematics of capacitating human spermatozoa. *Hum Reprod* 1995; **10**: 3178–82.

5. ESHRE Andrology Special Interest Group. Guidelines on the application of CASA technology in the analysis of spermatozoa. *Hum Reprod* 1998; **13**: 142–5.

6. Mortimer ST. CASA – Practical aspects. *J Androl* 2000; **21**: 515–24.

7. Mortimer D, Kossakowski J, Mortimer ST, Fussell S. Prediction of fertilizing ability by sperm kinematics. Abstract OC-05–043. *J Assist Reprod Genet* 1997; **14(5) Suppl**: 52S.

8. Mortimer D, Mortimer ST. Laboratory investigation of the infertile male. In: Brinsden PR, ed. *A Textbook of In-Vitro Fertilization and Assisted Reproduction*, 3rd edn. London, Taylor & Francis Medical Books, 2005, 61–91.

9. Cummins JM, Pember SM, Jequier AM, et al. A test of the human sperm acrosome reaction following ionophore challenge: relationship to fertility and other seminal parameters. *J Androl* 1991; **12**: 98–103.

10. Makkar G, Ng EH, Yeung WS, et al. The significance of the ionophore-challenged acrosome reaction in the prediction of successful outcome of controlled ovarian stimulation and intrauterine insemination. *Hum Reprod* 2003; **18**: 534–9.

11. Liu DY, Stewart T, Baker HW. Normal range and variation of the zona pellucida-induced acrosome reaction in fertile men. *Fertil Steril* 2003; **80**: 384–9.

12. Liu DY, Baker HW. Disordered zona pellucida-induced acrosome reaction and failure of in vitro fertilization in patients with unexplained infertility. *Fertil Steril* 2003; **79**: 74–80.

13. Bastiaan HS, Menkveld R, Oehninger S, et al. Zona pellucida induced acrosome reaction, sperm morphology, and sperm-zona binding assessments among subfertile men. *J Assist Reprod Genet* 2002; **19**: 329–34.

14. Bastiaan HS, Windt ML, Menkveld R, et al. Relationship between zona pellucida-induced acrosome reaction, sperm morphology, sperm-zona pellucida binding, and in vitro fertilization. *Fertil Steril* 2003; **79**: 49–55.

15. World Health Organization. *WHO Laboratory Manual for the Analysis of Human Semen and Sperm-Cervical Mucus Interaction*, 4th edn. Cambridge, Cambridge University Press, 1999.

16. Mortimer D, Curtis EF, Camenzind AR. Combined use of fluorescent peanut agglutinin lectin and Hoechst 33258 to monitor the acrosomal status and vitality of human spermatozoa. *Hum Reprod* 1990; **5**: 99–103.

17. Cross NL, Morales P, Overstreet JW, Hanson FW. Two simple methods for detecting acrosome-reacted human sperm. *Gamete Res* 1986; **15**: 213–26.

18. Talbot P, Chacon RS. A triple-stain technique for evaluating normal acrosome reactions of human sperm. *J Exp Zool* 1981; **215**: 201–8.

19. Mortimer D. *Practical Laboratory Andrology*. New York, Oxford University Press, 1994.

20. Burkman LJ, Coddington CC, Franken DR, et al. The hemizona assay (HZA): development of a diagnostic test for binding of human spermatozoa to the human zona pellucida to predict fertilization potential. *Fertil Steril* 1988; **49**: 688–93.

21. Franken DR, Oehninger S, Burkman LJ, et al. The hemizona assays (HZA): a predictor of human sperm fertilizing potential in in vitro fertilization (IVF) treatment. *J in Vitro Fertil Embryo Transf* 1989; **6**: 44–9.

22. Liu DY, Lopata A, Johnston WIH, Baker HWG. A human sperm-zona pellucida binding test using oocytes that failed to fertilize in vitro. *Fertil Steril* 1988; **50**: 782–8.

23. Franken DR, Kruger TF, Menkveld R, et al. Hemizona assay and teratozoospermia: increasing sperm insemination concentrations to enhance zona pellucida binding. *Fertil Steril* 1990; **54**: 497–503.

24. Menkveld R, Franken DR, Kruger TF, et al. Sperm selection capacity of the human zona pellucida. *Mol Reprod Dev* 1991; **30**: 346–52.

25. Oehninger S, Coddington CC, Franken DA, et al. Hemizona assay: assessment of sperm dysfunction and prediction of in vitro fertilization outcome. *Fertil Steril* 1989; **51**: 665–70.

26. Franken DR, Oehninger S. The clinical significance of sperm-zona pellucida binding: 17 years later. *Front Biosci* 2006; **1**: 1227–33.

27. Janssen M, Ombelet W, Cox A, et al. The hemizona assay: a simplified technique. *Arch Androl* 1997; **38**: 127–31.

28. Sanchez R, Finkenzeller C, Schill WB, Miska W. Comparison of two methods to obtain hemizonae pellucidae for sperm function tests. *Hum Reprod* 1995; **10**: 2945–7.

29. Edenfeld J, Schöpper B, Sturm R, et al. Application of a 1.48-μm diode laser for bisecting oocytes into two identical hemizonae for the hemizona assay. *Int J Androl* 2002; **25**: 100–5.

30. Franken DR, Burkman LJ, Oehninger SC, et al. Hemizona assay using salt-stored human oocytes: evaluation of zona pellucida capacity for binding human spermatozoa. *Gamete Res* 1989; **22**: 15–26.

31. Liu DY, Liu ML, Garratt C, Baker HWG. Comparison of the frequency of defective sperm-zona pellucida (ZP) binding and the ZP-induced acrosome reaction between subfertile men with normal and abnormal semen. *Hum Reprod* 2007; **22**: 1878–84.

32. Oehninger S, Franken DR, Sayed E, et al. Sperm function assays and their predictive value for fertilization outcome in IVF therapy: a meta-analysis. *Hum Reprod Update* 2000; **6**: 160–8.

33. De Jonge CJ, Centola GM, Reed ML, et al. Human sperm survival assay as a bioassay for the assisted reproductive technologies laboratory. *J Androl* 2003; **24**: 16–18.

34. Claassens OE, Wehr JB, Harrsion KL. Optimizing sensitivity of the human sperm motility assay for embryo toxicity testing. *Hum Reprod* 2000; **15**: 1586–91.

35. Coccia ME, Becattini C, Criscuoli L, et al. A sperm survival test and in-vitro fertilization outcome in the presence of male factor infertility. *Hum Reprod* 1997; **12**: 1969–73.

36. Mortimer D, Curtis EF, Camenzind AR, Tanaka S. The spontaneous acrosome reaction of human spermatozoa incubated in vitro. *Hum Reprod* 1989; **4**: 57–62.

37. Huszar G, Ozenci CC, Cayli S, et al. Hyaluronic acid binding by human sperm indicates cellular maturity, viability, and unreacted acrosomal status. *Fertil Steril* 2003; **79 Suppl** 3: 1616–24.

38. Ye H, Huang GN, Gao Y, Liu DY. Relationship between human sperm-hyaluronan binding assay and fertilization rate in conventional in vitro fertilization. *Hum Reprod* 2006; **21**: 1545–50.

39. Tarozzi N, Nadalini M, Bizzaro D, et al. Sperm-hyaluronan-binding assay: clinical value in conventional IVF under Italian law. *Reprod Biomed Online* 2009; **19 Suppl** 3: 35–43.

40. Lee D, Jee BC. Evaluation of normal morphology, DNA fragmentation, and hyaluronic acid binding ability of human spermatozoa after using four different commercial media for density gradient centrifugation. *Clin Exp Reprod Med* 2019; **46**: 8–13.

Tests of Sperm-Cervical Mucus Interaction

Introduction

For natural conception *in vivo*, spermatozoa must be deposited at the site of insemination around the external cervical os during the peri-ovulatory period, when the cervical mucus is receptive to penetration by spermatozoa (see Chapter 2). The penetration of spermatozoa into the cervical mucus, followed by their migration through the mucus column contained within the cervical canal, are the essential first steps in the complex series of events by which spermatozoa traverse the female tract and reach the site of fertilization in the ampulla of the oviduct [1,2]. Assessment of sperm-cervical mucus interaction remains an integral part of the comprehensive diagnostic work-up of an infertile couple [3], especially in order to achieve a definitive classification of unexplained or idiopathic infertility. Consequently, the most commonly used techniques are described below.

Because this section of the WHO laboratory manual fourth edition is easier to read than in the fifth (2010) edition, and the sixth (2021) edition no longer includes these tests, this chapter continues to refer to the earlier editions of that publication.

The test of *in-vivo* sperm-mucus interaction is the 'post-coital test' ('PCT'), which requires sampling the cervical mucus several hours after intercourse performed during the peri-ovulatory period and examining it for the presence of spermatozoa. While the clinical value of the PCT has long been questioned, when performed robustly and quantitatively, it can provide information of predictive value for fertility [4,5].

In-vitro sperm-mucus interaction tests are derived from two basic techniques: 'slide tests', using apposed drops of semen and mucus under coverslips, and 'tube' (or 'Kremer') tests, where mucus-filled capillary tubes are placed with one end in contact with liquefied semen. Penetration in either system is assessed by counting motile spermatozoa at various distances from the semen-mucus interface at certain times after establishment of this contact [3,4,6].

To be of physiological and clinical relevance, tests must be performed during the periovulatory period, when the oestrogenic mucus is receptive to penetration by spermatozoa. Experimental evidence has demonstrated that results obtained in oestrogen-treated women can provide reliable indications of normal mucus receptivity to sperm penetration [7], but the integration of such hormonal therapy into the routine management of infertile couples is uncommon in the era of assisted conception treatment.

Mucus must be sampled from within the cervical canal. Receptive intracervical mucus will have an Insler score of ≥10/15 and a pH ≥7.0 (see below). Three days of sexual abstinence should be observed prior to the test (either an *in-vivo* PCT or an *in-vitro* test), both to provide optimum semen characteristics and to minimize any 'contamination' of the mucus with spermatozoa from a previous insemination. A complete semen analysis should be performed on the ejaculate used for an *in-vitro* test. If the abstinence is not three days, some tests may need to be repeated because of abnormal findings of uncertain origin.

As with all tests of sperm function, sperm-mucus interaction tests must be commenced as quickly as possible after ejaculation. Normal semen samples are liquefied within 30 min, making it an ideal standard starting time. If liquefaction is retarded then, while tests can be delayed, mucus-penetrating ability might be reduced by the longer exposure of spermatozoa to seminal plasma [8,9]. Although seminal plasma is important for sperm penetration into cervical mucus, sperm motility and vitality both decline markedly with prolonged exposure to seminal plasma.

Sampling Cervical Mucus

Scheduling

The mucous secretion of the cervix is under endocrine control and shows cyclic variations during the menstrual cycle. Around the fertile period, the mucus is being secreted under oestrogenic control and presents as an abundant, clear, watery secretion (when compared to the mucus produced during the luteal and early follicular phases) and is receptive to penetration by progressively motile spermatozoa.

Cervical mucus receptivity to sperm penetration increases over a period of about four days before ovulation and decreases rapidly (within two days) after. Most cycle-length variation occurs in the follicular phase, with the day of ovulation being equivalent to Day 14 of a 'standard' 28-day cycle (Day 1 being the first day of menstruation). A simple method for scheduling cervical mucus assessments is therefore to book the test about 14 days before the next expected onset of menstruation [10], although this is not always the day of maximum receptivity [11] and could lead to false diagnoses of cervical hostility. Abnormal test results must therefore be confirmed by repeat testing in at least one subsequent cycle.

To ensure optimum mucus quality, women can be treated with estradiol for several days before sampling, e.g. 80 μg ethinyl estradiol per day for seven days [7]. This ensures optimum mucus for the tests, the results of which are predictive of fertility, but it might conceal an underlying endocrine disorder that would affect the chances of *in-vivo* conception.

Equipment

- Sterile speculum
- Forceps

Disposable Materials

- Sterile mucus aspiration device, e.g.
  Spirette and *Mucat* catheters from Laboratoire CCD, Paris, France, see www.laboratoire-ccd.com/products/medically-assisted-procreation/huhner-test-accessories/#huhner-test-accessories
  SelectMucus endocervical aspirator, see www.coopersurgical.com/detail/selectmucus-endocervical-aspirator/
- Sterile disposable syringe (e.g. 1-ml or 3-ml)
- Clean microscope slides, 3" × 1" (75 × 25 mm)
- Coverslips, 22 × 22 mm, #1½ or #2 thickness
- Indicator test strips to measure mucus pH, e.g. EMD Merck *colorpHast*® test strips (Merck KGaA, Darmstadt, Germany), Cat.No, 9583–3 for pH 6.5–10.0 and 9582–3 for pH 4.0–7.0
- Sterile cotton swabs or gauze

Reagents

Coverslip support material: This is required to determine the cellular contents of the cervical mucus when performing this component of the Insler score. A mixture of glass beads in silicone grease is used to make the 100 μm fixed-depth preparations [12] although experience has shown that when this material is being prepared for relatively short-term diagnostic use only (up to three months) the preparation protocol can be greatly simplified to merely mixing the pre-washed glass beads (Sigma G4649, 106 μm diameter and finer) with high vacuum silicone grease (e.g. Dow Corning, Midland, MI, USA) in approximate 1:5 proportions. To create a dispenser for the material, remove the plunger from a 5 ml plastic syringe and, using a weighing spatula, fill the syringe barrel with the glass beads/silicone grease mixture. Replace the plunger and expel as much air as possible from the syringe and fit the syringe with a blunt needle, e.g. Monoject™ 202, 18G × 1" (see www.cardinalhealth.com).

Procedure

1. Insert a warmed speculum into the vagina and examine the cervix for the dilation and appearance of the external os, including the amount of mucus extruding from the os.
2. Gently wipe the external os clean using a sterile dry gauze swab.
3. Insert the sampling device about 10 mm into the cervical canal and gently pull back on the plunger to draw mucus into the catheter. Maintain gentle suction and slowly withdraw the catheter from the cervix. If the mucus is very elastic (i.e. high spinnbarkeit), use a pair of forceps to clamp off the open end of the collection catheter to prevent the mucus from pulling back out of the catheter as it is withdrawn from the endocervical canal.

   Note: Collecting mucus into a syringe (e.g. 1 ml tuberculin type) is acceptable for PCTs, but disrupts the mucus ultrastructure and should not be used when collecting mucus for *in-vitro* sperm-mucus interaction testing.
4. Expel the mucus from the catheter onto a clean glass microscope slide.
5. Measure the pH of the mucus.

Assessing Mucus Quality

The Insler Score

This semi-quantitative score is used to assess the quantity and quality of cervical mucus. The original score proposed by Insler and colleagues [13] was based on the four parameters of the appearance of cervical os, mucus quantity, spinnbarkeit, and ferning, but was modified to include mucus cellularity as a fifth parameter and the criteria simplified for more practical application [3,4,14]. Each parameter is scored, assigning a value between 0 and 3, based on the criteria shown in Table 8.1.

Appearance of the cervical os considers the degree of dilation and hyperemia of the external cervical os.

Mucus quantity is assessed at the same time as the cervical appearance and is based on a combination of whether mucus can be seen at the external os and how much mucus can be aspirated from the endocervical canal.

Spinnbarkeit considers the stretchability or elasticity of the mucus and is best measured by placing a small drop of mucus (about 5 mm diameter) on a clean slide. Place a second slide across the first in the form of a '+' sign and spread the mucus evenly between them. Then gently pull the slides apart and measure the length of the mucus thread.

Ferning is then assessed on the same mucus sample as used for the spinnbarkeit determination. Spread the mucus evenly on the slide and allow it to dry before assessing the presence and degree of ferning (crystallization pattern). Detailed counting of the numbers of side branches in the crystallization pattern is unnecessary, it is more important to ensure that the degree of ferning is assessed over the entire preparation rather than concentrating upon a small area which shows, or does not show, ferning. Initially cervical mucus crystallization forms a very fine pattern of ferning, but as the quality of the cervical mucus increases towards the peri-ovulatory period, the ferning pattern becomes more extensive, ultimately showing very strong crystallization with pronounced primary stems that branch into well-defined secondary, tertiary and quaternary stems (see Figure 8.1).

   Note: If necessary, drying of the cervical mucus can be done by gentle heating over an alcohol flame, but this can influence the pattern of crystallization.

Mucus cellularity considers the number of leukocytes (not erythrocytes or epithelial cells) and is assessed as an inverse score by actual counting of the leucocytes. See the calibration procedure under the post-coital test.

Calculating the Insler Score: The five component scores are added together to give a total Insler Score out of 15. A score of 12 or more is considered to indicate good ovulatory cervical mucus, and scores of 10 or 11 indicate adequate ovulatory cervical mucus.

Table 8.1 Criteria for assigning component values for the Insler Score [3,4,13,14]

Criterion			Score
Appearance of the cervical os			
Tightly closed, same pink colour as the surrounding tissue			0
Beginning to open and redden			1
Intermediate between grades 1 and 3			2
Maximally dilated (*ca.* 6 mm diameter)			3
Mucus quantity			
None visible at the external os, and none aspirated	(WHO: 0.0 ml)		0
None visible at the external os, but some aspirated	(WHO: 0.1 ml)		1
Visible at the external os and can be aspirated	(WHO: 0.2 ml)		2
Definite cascade visible at the external os	(WHO: ≥0.3 ml)		3
Spinnbarkeit			
Will not stretch at all			0
Stretches for 1–4 cm before breaking			1
Stretches for 5–8 cm before breaking			2
Stretches for >8 cm before breaking			3
Ferning			
None visible anywhere on the slide			0
Less than half the mucus is starting to fern			1
More than half shows good ferning (1° and 2° stem ferning)			2
All the mucus shows good ferning, with 3° and 4° stem ferning			3
Mucus cellularity (leucocytes)			
Mucus is full of leucocytes:	>20 per 40× field	>1000/mm^3	0
Many leucocytes	11–20 per 40× field	501–1000/mm^3	1
Few leucocytes	1–10 per 40× field	1–500/mm^3	2
No leucocytes at all			3

Note: See the section on the 'Post-Coital Test' for an explanation of the relationship between cells per 40× field and cells/mm^3 (see also [14]).

Cervical Mucus pH

Periovulatory cervical mucus is usually pH 8.0–8.4. The optimum pH range for sperm migration and survival is between 7.0 and 8.5; sperm progression is impaired below pH 6.8, and pH 6.0 is incompatible with sperm vitality. Consequently, acidic mucus may be at least a partial explanation for poor sperm-mucus interaction.

Storing Cervical Mucus

Many workers have reported that frozen cervical mucus can be unreliable and unsatisfactory for use in *in-vitro* testing procedures. Consequently, cervical mucus should only be stored for a few days at +4°C. Seal the ends of the collection catheter with an inert material such as haematocrit tube sealant (*Plasticine* is spermotoxic). Stored mucus must be allowed to re-equilibrate to ambient temperature and its pH and Insler score should be re-assessed before use.

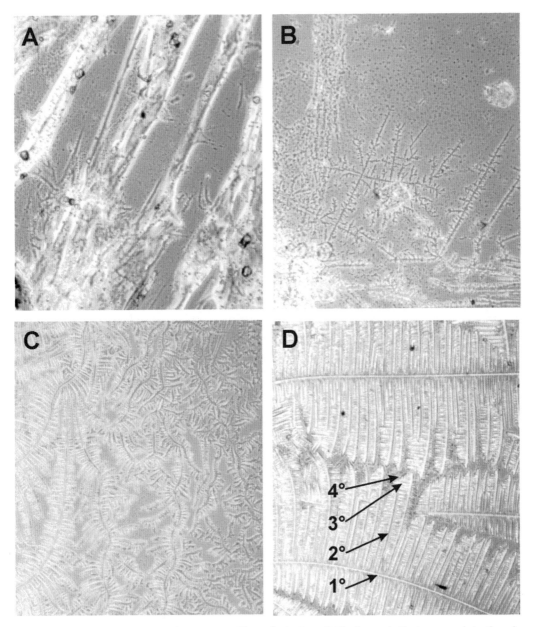

Figure 8.1 Illustration of cervical mucus ferning patterns. (A) = no ferning (score 0); (B) = fine atypical ferning as seen during the early preovulatory stage (score 1); (C) = secondary and early tertiary ferning (score 2); and (D) = extensive tertiary with some quaternary ferning (score 3). 1°, 2°, 3° and 4° denote primary, secondary, tertiary and quaternary levels of branching in the ferning pattern. (Images © David Mortimer PhD.)

Post-Coital Test

Background

The post-coital test (PCT) allows the assessment of sperm-cervical mucus interaction during the peri-ovulatory period under *in-vivo* conditions [15]. Aspirated intracervical mucus is examined under a phase contrast microscope and motile spermatozoa are counted in randomly selected fields. While the PCT evaluates the penetration of spermatozoa from liquefied semen into cervical mucus and their survival within that environment, debate continues as to the true clinical value and significance of the PCT. In cases with suspected sexual dysfunction, a positive PCT can be taken as evidence of an adequate coital technique.

Although anti-sperm antibodies in cervical mucus can cause poor PCTs, technical problems might also be responsible, and caution must be used before attributing a poor PCT to immunologically hostile mucus (if the semen sample was not tested for anti-sperm antibodies). Notwithstanding these issues, many gynaecologists still consider the PCT to be an essential part of an infertile couple's work-up [5], and full-service infertility diagnostic laboratories should be able to offer the procedure.

Principle

The PCT consists of sampling the cervical mucus several hours after intercourse and examining it for the presence of spermatozoa. A PCT must be performed during the peri-ovulatory period, and three days sexual abstinence prior to the 'test intercourse' is strongly recommended to provide optimum semen characteristics and to minimize any 'contamination' of the mucus with spermatozoa from a previous insemination. Although the use of condoms during the follicular phase of the test cycle can facilitate interpretation of the findings, it is unlikely to be practised by infertility patients.

Specimen

Intracervical mucus is obtained, ideally within 12 h after intercourse. Its pH is measured and its quality assessed as described in the section on the 'Insler Score' (see above).

Note: It is very important that each clinic/laboratory should standardize as far as possible the time after intercourse to facilitate comparing results within that clinic/laboratory.

Equipment

See also Appendix 2.
- Microscope configured for andrology with phase contrast optics (10×, 20× and 40× objectives)
- Tally counter

Disposable Materials

- As for semen collection and analysis
- As for cervical mucus collection and assessment

Reagents

- Coverslip support material (see 'Sampling Cervical Mucus', above)

Calibration

Although older reports describe results in terms of cells per high power field or 'HPF' (i.e. a 40× objective), proper quantitative performance of this test requires that the microscope field be calibrated so that numbers of spermatozoa per field can be converted to numbers per unit area (i.e. per $mm^2 \equiv$ per $10^6 \ \mu m^2$), and that glass beads are used to standardize the preparation depth, allowing sperm numbers to be expressed per unit volume (i.e. per $mm^3 \equiv$ per μl: see below). For a 100 μm deep preparation, the field volume for a modern microscope using a 40× objective (numerical aperture or 'NA' 0.65) and widefield oculars will be approximately 0.02 mm^3, so that a traditional count of 10 cells/HPF (non-widefield oculars) will be equivalent to 500 cells/mm^3 [3,14].

The field area of a given combination of objective, intermediate magnification and oculars can be readily calibrated using a micrometer slide to measure the field diameter and then applying simple geometry. For a 'typical' field volume of 0.02 mm^3, with no intermediate magnification, the factor to correct a number of cells per field to per unit volume is ×50. If intermediate magnification is used, then to convert from 1.0× (i.e. no intermediate magnification) to 1.25×, multiply by an additional 1.55; to convert from 1.0× to 1.5×, multiply by an additional 2.23.

If there are very large numbers of spermatozoa in a field then an eyepiece fitted with a reticle (a.k.a. graticule) may be used to delimit small areas of the field. An additional factor is then used to correct for the proportion of the whole field area represented by the fraction of the grid in which the cells were counted; see Figure 8.2 for an illustration of this calculation [3,14].

Quality Control

This is a straightforward observational procedure, but its objective assessment does require the prior calibration of the microscope field size. Quality control aspects relating to the mucus quality assessment are dealt with in the section on 'The Insler Score' (see above).

Procedure

1. Prepare a cleaned microscope slide with four 'posts' of the glass beads/silicone grease mixture arranged in a square pattern with sides of about 20 mm (see Figure 8.3).
2. Place a drop (*ca.* 3 mm diameter) of endocervical mucus in the centre of this square and cover it with a 22 × 22 mm coverslip. Press down gently on the coverslip so that the 'posts' are

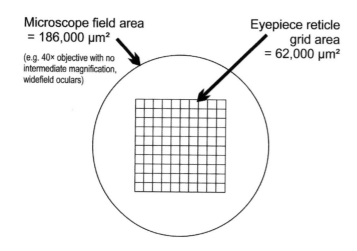

Microscope field area
= 186,000 μm²

(e.g. 40× objective with no intermediate magnification, widefield oculars)

Eyepiece reticle
grid area
= 62,000 μm²

Figure 8.2 Explanation of how to use an eyepiece graticule (or reticle) to subdivide a microscope field of view for easier counting when the field contains many cells.

To convert cells per 100 squares (entire grid), multiply by 3 (i.e. 186,000 ÷ 62,000)

Hence: for cells per 20 grid squares (two rows), multiply by 15

for cells per 10 grid squares (one row), multiply by 30

for cells per 4 grid squares, multiply by 75

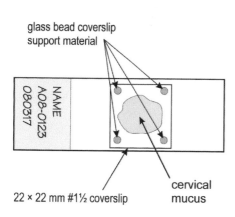

glass bead coverslip
support material

22 × 22 mm #1½ coverslip

cervical
mucus

NAME
AOB-0123
080317

Figure 8.3 The post-coital test. Coverslip set-up to enable quantitation of the numbers of spermatozoa per unit area.

flattened and the coverslip is fixed with a single layer of beads between it and the slide. The mucus drop will spread towards the edges of the coverslip; if it extrudes from under the coverslip another preparation must be made using less mucus to reduce the risk of drying-out artefacts.

3. Microscopic screening of the mucus is performed under a 40× objective using phase contrast optics. Briefly scan the slide to check that the sperm distribution in the mucus sample is more or less uniform.

4. In each of 10 randomly selected fields away from the coverslip edge (fields with air bubbles or large patches of epithelium can be rejected) count the number of spermatozoa according to their motility:

   a) Count the number of progressively motile spermatozoa.

   b) Count all the other spermatozoa present in the same field of view, classifying each one as immotile, non-progressively motile, or 'shaking' (also see the 'Sperm-Cervical Mucus Contact Test', below).

   Note: If there are very large numbers of spermatozoa per field then a part of the field, delimited by an eyepiece reticle or graticule, may be used. Ensure that the microscope field calibration factor allows for the reduced sample area.

Calculations and Results

1. Calculate the average number per field of each type of spermatozoa across the 10 fields. Use the appropriate microscope field correction factor to convert these averages to numbers per unit volume (see 'Calibration', above).

2. Some gynaecologists still disagree with the objective assessment criteria described below (Table 8.2), but they are based upon recalculation from historic clinical series allowing for modern microscope optics and quantitative laboratory methods.

3. According to the average numbers of progressively motile spermatozoa per unit volume, grade the test as shown in Table 8.2.

   Note: If ≥20% of the spermatozoa are shaking, this should be noted on the report. If >50% of the spermatozoa show shaking, then a PCT will always be classified as 'Poor'.

Notes and Interpretation Guidelines

1. A poor or negative PCT does not always denote a negative clinical finding. In such cases the test should be repeated under strictly controlled circumstances.

2. An Insler score of <10 can be considered at least a partial explanation of a poor PCT.

3. Cervical mucus is normally between pH 8.0–8.5; acidic mucus (especially if <7.0) can be at least a partial explanation of a poor PCT.

4. Sperm motility decreases with increasing time *post coitum*. Therefore, a PCT performed after a long post-coital delay that shows many non-progressive spermatozoa (as distinct from shaking spermatozoa) might have been attributed a better result than the number of progressive spermatozoa alone would indicate, had it been performed after a shorter delay.

Table 8.2 Assigning results to the post-coital test [3,14]

No. of spermatozoa per unit volume (per µl)	Test result
None at all	Negative
Present, but <500	Poor
500–999	Average
1000–2500	Good
>2500	Excellent

5. Interpretation of the clinical significance of a PCT must be the responsibility of the physician requesting the test. Such interpretation should always take into account the mucus quality and partner's semen characteristics (and adequacy of coital technique) since low sperm count and particularly poor sperm motility (especially in conjunction with poor sperm morphology), will significantly reduce the quantitative penetration of spermatozoa into mucus.

In Vitro Sperm-Cervical Mucus Tests

Kurzrok-Miller Test

Principle

The Kurzrok-Miller (or 'K-M') test is the oldest *in-vitro* test of sperm-mucus interaction [16]. It consists simply of establishing an interface between a drop of endocervical mucus and fresh liquefied semen under a coverslip.

Specimens

Cervical mucus and semen samples are required (see 'Kremer Test' below for details).

Equipment

See also Appendix 2.
- Phase contrast compound microscope configured for andrology with 10×, 20× and 40× objectives
- Tally counter
- Air incubator
- Humid chamber

Disposable Materials

- As for semen collection and analysis
- As for cervical mucus collection and assessment
- Coverslip support material (see 'Sampling Cervical Mucus', above)
- Sterile gauze swabs 2" × 2" (50 × 50 mm)

Reagents

- Sterile water for injection (for the humid chamber)

Calibration

None required as this test is only interpreted subjectively

Quality Control

The K-M test is an observational technique subject to uncontrollable factors such as the geometry of the semen-mucus interface. If results are reported as described below then the test will have achieved its maximum practicable standardization.

Procedure

1. Prepare a cleaned microscope slide with four 'posts' of the glass beads/silicone grease mixture arranged in a square pattern with sides of about 20 mm (see Figure 8.3 above).
2. Place a drop (*ca.* 3 mm diameter) of endocervical mucus in the centre of this square and cover it with a 22 × 22 mm coverslip. Press down gently on the coverslip so that the 'posts' are flattened and the coverslip is fixed with a single layer of beads between it and the slide. The mucus drop will spread

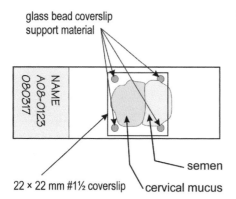

Figure 8.4 The Kurzrok-Miller Test.

towards the edges of the coverslip; if it extrudes from under the coverslip, another preparation must be made using less mucus, to reduce the risk of drying-out artefacts.
3. Place a small drop (about 10 µl) of semen next to the edge of the coverslip. The semen will flow under the coverslip and establish a contact interface with the mucus (see Figure 8.4).
4. Incubate the test in a humidified chamber at 37°C for 20–30 min.
5. Examine the preparation at a magnification of 200× to 250× using phase contrast optics (i.e. using a 20× or 25× objective).

Calculations and Results

Due to the great problems of standardizing the semen-mucus interface, most practitioners only use the K-M test as a qualitative assessment of sperm-mucus interaction. The test is reported according to the following observational criteria.

Normal result: Spermatozoa penetrate into the mucus phase and the great majority (>90%) are motile with definite progression.

Poor result: Although spermatozoa penetrate into the mucus phase, most do not progress further than 0.5 mm (i.e. about 10 sperm lengths) from the semen-mucus interface.

Abnormal result: Spermatozoa penetrate into the mucus phase but rapidly become either immotile or show the 'shaking' pattern of movement.

Negative test: Spermatozoa congregate along the semen side of the interface but none penetrate through the semen-mucus interface; phalanges may or may not be formed.

Notes and Interpretation Guidelines

1. An Insler score of <10 can be considered at least a partial explanation of a poor K-M Test.
2. Cervical mucus is normally between pH 8.0–8.5; acidic mucus (especially if <7.0) can be at least a partial explanation of a poor K-M Test.
3. A prior three-day period of sexual abstinence is advisable as samples produced outside the range of two to four days of abstinence might show impaired mucus-penetrating capacity.
4. Since the exposure of spermatozoa to seminal plasma rapidly impairs their mucus penetrating ability, tests should be set up by 30 min post-ejaculation (see the Introduction to this chapter). All variations from the normal condition should be noted and reported.

Kremer (Capillary Tube) 'Sperm Penetration' Test

Principle

The Kremer sperm penetration test is an *in-vitro* test of sperm-mucus interaction in which a glass capillary tube is filled with cervical mucus and its open end placed in contact with a reservoir of semen [6,8]. Penetration of motile spermatozoa into and along the mucus column is assessed by counting their numbers at various distances from the semen-mucus interface after a set time interval.

The outcome of the test is strongly influenced by the concentration of progressively motile spermatozoa at the semen-mucus interface (i.e. in the semen sample) and has been considered as a test of the proportion of successful collisions between spermatozoa capable of mucus penetration and the interface [17]. Consequently, oligozoospermic samples will most likely produce average to poor results, while oligoasthenozoospermic samples will usually produce abnormal test results. However, such generalizations cannot substitute for performing the test in any but the most extreme male factor cases.

The glass 'sperm penetration meter' devices developed by Dr Jan Kremer, the inventor of this test in the 1960s [6,8] are no longer commercially available. Also, in the method described below, the original round cross-section capillaries have been replaced by rectangular cross-section glass capillaries for easier examination under the microscope. Finally, Kremer's original scoring method, which is rather complicated and hard to standardize, has been replaced by a technique more amenable to routine standardized application [10]; descriptions of Kremer's original assessment scheme are readily available elsewhere [3,14].

Specimens

Mucus: The test must be performed using peri-ovulatory mucus. Intracervical mucus is collected and assessed in terms of its Insler score and pH (see above); if the pH is <7.0 then it can adversely affect the outcome of the test.

Semen: A 50 μl aliquot of liquefied semen is required for each test. It must be taken from a well-mixed ejaculate specimen within 1 h of collection, and preferably at a standard time such as 30 min; see Chapter 3 for details.

Equipment

See also Appendix 2.
- Microscope configured for andrology with phase contrast optics (10×, 20× and 40× objectives)
- Tally counter
- Air incubator operating at 37°C
- Stainless steel iris scissors, sterile
- Rack for the semen reservoir tube (e.g. No.00 BEEM® capsules or 0.5-ml Eppendorf tubes, see below)

Disposable Materials

- As for semen collection and analysis
- As for cervical mucus collection and assessment.
- Glass capillary tubes with rectangular cross-section: 100 × 3 × 0.3 mm rectangular 'Microslide' capillaries (now called 'VitroTubes' from VitroCom, Rockaway, NJ, USA, see www.vitrocom.com/categories/view/69/Miniature-Hollow-Rectangle-Tubing-VitroTubes)
- Tube for use as a semen reservoir, e.g. standard BEEM® electron microscopy embedding capsule, size No.00, or 0.5-ml Eppendorf tubes

Reagents

DTT solution: A 10 mg/ml solution of dithiothreitol (Sigma D0632) in sterile water. Prepare fresh daily and maintain at ambient temperature. Discard any unused portion.

Calibration

Fully objective performance of this test requires that microscope objective fields be calibrated so that numbers of spermatozoa per field may be converted to numbers per unit area (i.e. per mm^2, or per 10^6 µm^2; as described for the PCT, see above). Although there is no dependable method for determining sperm numbers per unit volume within capillary tubes, if the same magnification objective is always used then the third dimension will be constant; for this test, a 20× is preferred due to its greater depth of focus.

The field area of a given combination of objective, intermediate magnification and oculars can be readily calibrated using a micrometer slide to measure the field diameter and then applying simple geometry.

For a modern microscope using a 20× objective (numerical aperture indicated as 'NA' 0.46 on the objective) and widefield oculars (with no intermediate magnification) the field area will be approximately 0.75 mm^2, so the factor to correct a number of cells per field to the number per unit area is ×1.33. If intermediate magnification is used, then to convert from 1.0× (i.e. no intermediate magnification) to 1.25×, multiply by an additional 1.55; to convert from 1.0× to 1.5×, multiply by an additional 2.23.

If there are very large numbers of spermatozoa in a field then an eyepiece fitted with a reticle or graticule may be used to delimit small areas of the field. An additional factor is then used to correct for the proportion of the whole field area represented by the fraction of the grid in which the cells were counted (see the 'Post-Coital Test' section in this chapter for further explanation).

Quality Control

- This is a straightforward observational procedure. Quality control aspects relating to the semen analysis and mucus quality assessment are dealt with under the appropriate tests.
- The field area of each combination of microscope objective, intermediate magnification and oculars must be calibrated to allow calculation of sperm numbers per unit (see 'Calibration', above).
- Due to the marked influence of temperature upon sperm progression, these tests must be run at 37°C. Because changing the incubation time and/or temperature will alter sperm migration along the mucus column, Kremer tests must be run at 37°C for 60 min; shorter times will require completely re-defined criteria for determining the result.

Procedure

1. Prepare the testing device:
   a) Mark a flat glass capillary tube at 10 mm intervals using a fine-pointed indelible (spirit-based) marker pen.
   b) Prepare the semen reservoir by making a slit or hole in its cap (e.g. using a punch plier) sufficient to allow the glass capillary to pass through quite easily.
      Note: Given the very small size of the sperm reservoirs, it is not possible to label them in the normal manner using two unique identifiers, so they must be identified by a sequence number and the specimen identity of this number written on a label attached to the rack.
2. Expel the mucus from the collection catheter onto a clean glass slide; cut trailing mucus using iris scissors. Mucus from the proximal 20 mm of the collection catheter (corresponding more or less to mucus from the endocervical level of the canal) should be used.

3. Aspirate mucus from the slide into the capillary tube using a syringe and tubing manifold. The mucus meniscus should be 20–30 mm from the top of the tube, creating a mucus column of 70–80 mm (exact length is noted to the nearest mm). Mucus trailing from the lower end of the tube is cut with iris scissors after the loading manifold has been removed. Seal the upper end of the tube with haematocrit tube sealant; after sealing the mucus should protrude slightly from the open end of the tube.

4. Before setting up the test, the mucus-filled capillary tube is checked under the microscope for the presence of spermatozoa (phase contrast optics, and at same magnification as will be used for scoring the test). If any spermatozoa are seen, the number in 10 random fields along the length of the mucus column are counted (including classification of their motility) so that the average 'contamination' per field can be used to correct the sperm penetration scores (see 'Calculations', below).

5. At 30 min post-ejaculation, a 50 µl aliquot of the mixed liquefied semen is transferred into the bottom of the semen reservoir tube, which is held upright in a rack, and the cap of the tube closed.
   Note: A complete semen analysis is performed on ejaculate.

6. The open end of the mucus-filled capillary tube is inserted through the slit in the lid of the semen reservoir until its corners rest on the tapered base of the tube. The mucus interface will be immersed 1–2 mm into the semen (see Figure 8.5).

7. Replace the test in the rack and incubate at 37°C for 60 min.

8. After incubation, remove the capillary tube and rinse its open end thoroughly with a freshly prepared solution of DTT to remove residual spermatozoa from the mucus interface and surface of the capillary. Stand the open end of the tube in the DTT solution for 30–60 s to ensure complete removal of any contaminating semen.

9. Assess the depth and degree of sperm penetration into the mucus column under the microscope (phase contrast optics, 20× objective). Count the number of in-focus spermatozoa present in each of three microscope fields at the 10, 40 and 70 mm marks along the tube. Select fields that are mid-way between the upper and lower walls of the capillary, and do not adjust the microscope focus to find additional spermatozoa.

10. Determine the farthest distance travelled along the mucus column by the 'vanguard' spermatozoon.

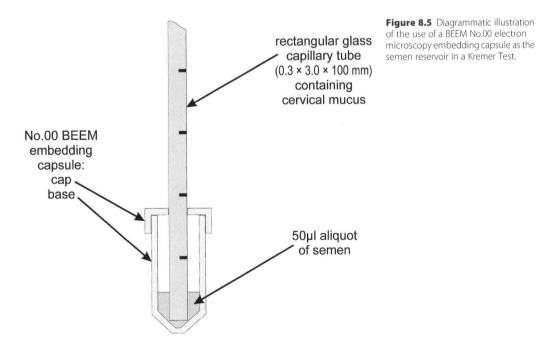

rectangular glass
capillary tube
(0.3 × 3.0 × 100 mm)
containing
cervical mucus

No.00 BEEM
embedding
capsule:
cap
base

50µl aliquot
of semen

Figure 8.5 Diagrammatic illustration of the use of a BEEM No.00 electron microscopy embedding capsule as the semen reservoir in a Kremer Test.

Table 8.3 Criteria for calculating the Sperm Penetration Test score [10]

Spermatozoa/mm^2	Score	Vanguard spermatozoa
0	0	<30 mm
1–30	1	30–39 mm
31–60	2	40–49 mm
61–120	3	50–59 mm
121–200	4	61–69 mm
>200	5	≥70 mm

Table 8.4 Criteria for deriving the result of the Sperm Penetration Test [10]

Total SPT score	Test result
0	Negative
1–8	Poor
9–11	Average
12–15	Good
16–20	Excellent

Calculations and Results

1. For each of the 10, 40 and 70 mm distances along the tube:
   a) Calculate the average number of spermatozoa present per field.
   b) Correct the average number of spermatozoa per field for any 'contaminating' spermatozoa that were present in the mucus at the start of the test.
   c) Convert the corrected number into per unit area (see above) using the appropriate microscope calibration factor.
2. Use these values to calculate the 'Sperm Penetration Test' or 'SPT' score, an empirically derived scheme used to create a semi-quantitative score for this test [9], as shown in Table 8.3.
3. Derive the test result from the calculated total SPT score according to the criteria shown in Table 8.4.

Notes and Interpretation Guidelines

1. An Insler score of <10 can be considered at least a partial explanation of a poor Kremer Test.
2. Cervical mucus is normally between pH 8.0–8.5; acidic mucus (especially if <7.0) can be at least a partial explanation of a poor Kremer Test.
3. A prior three-day period of sexual abstinence is advisable as samples produced outside the range of two to four days of abstinence might show impaired mucus penetrating capacity.
4. Since the exposure of spermatozoa to seminal plasma rapidly impairs their mucus penetrating ability, tests should be set up by 30 min post-ejaculation (see the Introduction to this chapter). All variations from the normal condition should be noted and reported.

Sperm-Cervical Mucus Contact Test

Principle

The sperm-cervical mucus contact (SCMC) test is a slide test whereby spermatozoa and cervical mucus are mixed to establish the presence of ASABs in either the seminal plasma or the cervical mucus [18]. This test is performed by mixing drops of mucus and semen (see Figure 8.6, below).

Specimens

Semen: A 30 μl aliquot of liquefied semen is required for each test. It must be taken from a well-mixed ejaculate specimen within 1 h of collection, and preferably at a standard time such as 30 min; see Chapter 3 for further details.

Mucus: The test must be performed using peri-ovulatory mucus. Intracervical mucus is collected and assessed in terms of its Insler score and pH (see above); if the pH is <7.0 then it can adversely affect the outcome of the test.

Equipment

See also Appendix 2.

- Microscope configured for andrology with phase contrast optics (10×, 20× and 40× objectives)
- Tally counter

Disposable Materials

- As for semen collection and analysis
- As for cervical mucus collection and assessment

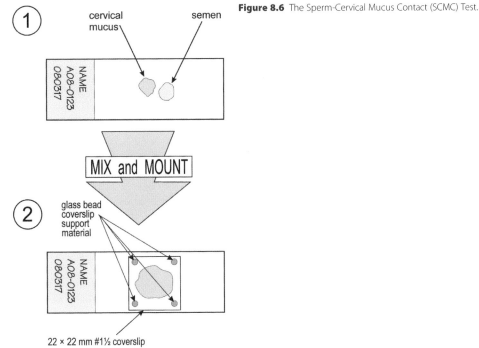

Figure 8.6 The Sperm-Cervical Mucus Contact (SCMC) Test.

Table 8.5 Criteria for assigning the result of the Sperm-Cervical Mucus Contact Test

Shaking spermatozoa	Test result	Ranking
0–25	Negative	(−)
26–50	Positive	(+)
51–75	Positive	(++)
76–100	Highly positive	(+++)

Reagents

None required.

Calibration

None required.

Quality Control

This is a simple, subjective, observational test. Provided that the results are reported as noted in 'Results' then the test will have achieved its maximum practicable standardization.

Procedure

1. Place a 3–5 mm diameter drop of endocervical mucus and a drop (about 25 μl) of liquefied semen side by side on a clean microscope slide and mix gently using a disposable plastic stirring rod or disposable pipetter tip (see Figure 8.6).
2. Cover with a 22 × 22 mm coverslip and press gently to spread the preparation to the edges of the coverslip.
3. Examine immediately under phase contrast optics (200–500× magnification) for a period of 5–10 min. Note the development of any 'shaking' pattern of the movement of motile spermatozoa. Shaking describes a specific pattern of movement whereby the spermatozoa are actively motile but non-progressive; they appear to be stuck to some invisible structure inside the mucus.
4. Count at least 100 spermatozoa, with the aid of a tally counter, recording the progressively motile spermatozoa and the actively shaking motile spermatozoa.

Calculations and Results

1. Calculate the percentage of shaking spermatozoa.
2. The SCMC test is reported according to criteria shown in Table 8.5.

Notes and Interpretation Guidelines

1. Acidic cervical mucus can kill spermatozoa quickly, preventing an SCMC Test from being read.

Crossed-Hostility Testing

Principle

When the result from a homologous sperm-mucus interaction test has been average or worse then a crossed-hostility test ('XHT') should be performed in a subsequent cycle to simultaneously verify the previous cycle's finding, and also evaluate the origin of the problem, i.e. semen or mucus, (see Figure 8.7).

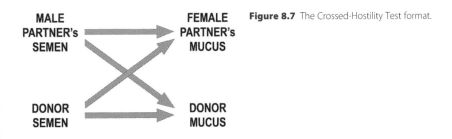

Figure 8.7 The Crossed-Hostility Test format.

However, given the difficulty in obtaining donor mucus, and the current expense of donor semen, XHT format testing is nowadays quite rare.

Specimens

Patient mucus and semen: These are obtained as for the Kremer Test.

Donor mucus: Obtained from a patient receiving artificial insemination treatment. Mucus samples are taken and assessed as per standard procedures (see 'Insler Score', above) and, to be suitable for this test, must have an Insler score of ≥12/15 and a pH ≥7.0. Donor mucus may be stored at +4°C for up to four days before being used. Ensure that stored mucus has re-equilibrated to ambient temperature before use.

Donor semen: Usually cryopreserved donor semen (or fresh 'control donor' semen) with known good mucus-penetrating ability.

Equipment, Disposable Materials and Reagents

All as for the component 'Kremer' and 'Sperm-Cervical Mucus Contact' Tests (see above).

Calibration and Quality Control

As for the component 'Kremer' and 'Sperm-Cervical Mucus Contact' Tests (see above).

Procedure

- Whenever sufficient material is available, the Kremer test method should be used as the basic test. However, if only a limited amount of the patient's mucus is available, then the K-M test can be used instead.
- A 'Sperm-Cervical Mucus Contact Test' (see above) should also be performed on at least the homologous (i.e. patients') sperm-mucus interaction, mucus quantity permitting. If at all possible, SCMC tests should be performed on all four combinations.

Calculations and Results

The results of each component test are derived according to the procedures described for those tests.

Notes and Interpretation Guidelines

While the physician requesting the XHT procedure is solely responsible for interpreting the results of the component tests, the following general guidelines can be established when the interaction of the donor materials was normal.

- If the patient's spermatozoa penetrate neither the partner's mucus nor the donor mucus, then there is probably a male factor problem (e.g. abnormal sperm motility, or anti-sperm antibodies on the sperm surface).
- If neither the patient's nor the donor's spermatozoa penetrate the patient's mucus then there is probably a female factor problem (e.g. abnormal mucus quality, or anti-sperm antibodies in the mucus).
- In some cases, both the above problems may be seen simultaneously. This indicates the likely presence of both male and female factors.

Complementary Tests

The need for donor semen and cervical mucus often makes the routine implementation of crossed-hostility format testing rather impractical. Additional tests can provide essentially similar information to that obtainable from studying the interactions of a man's spermatozoa with donor mucus, and of donor spermatozoa with his partner's mucus. Such protocols can obviate the need for donor mucus and/or donor semen, making a comprehensive assessment of the interaction between a man's spermatozoa and his partner's cervical mucus more practicable in a full-service diagnostic andrology laboratory in the era of assisted conception treatment.

Extended Sperm Morphology Evaluation

This is applicable to both the post-coital and *in-vitro* sperm-mucus penetration tests. Although a strong relationship between motility and cervical mucus penetration has been reported in the literature [10,19], it is also reported that sperm morphology and especially the type of abnormalities is just as strong a predictor of sperm-cervical mucus penetration test outcomes *in vivo* and *in vitro* [20,21]. An extended sperm morphology evaluation that includes an in-depth break-down of the different types of abnormal spermatozoa can indicate expected *in vivo* and *in vitro* sperm-mucus penetration ability. Even though certain types of abnormal spermatozoa might penetrate cervical mucus, an association with fertilizing ability is possible [21].

Testing for Anti-Sperm Antibodies

Including a direct test for anti-sperm antibodies on a patient's spermatozoa and an indirect test on the partner's mucus will greatly facilitate the interpretation of abnormal XHT findings (see Chapter 4 for further information).

Sperm Kinematics

Kinematic analysis of sperm movement using CASA might also help understand the possible origin of a male factor problem (see Chapter 6 for further information) [2].

Cervical Mucus Substitutes

Although there was early interest in the use of bovine cervical mucus as a surrogate medium for human sperm testing, commercial products such as Serono Diagnostics' *Penetrak®* disappeared some years ago.

The ability of spermatozoa to penetrate into, and migrate along, a capillary tube filled with a synthetic medium containing high molecular weight sodium hyaluronate (Sperm Select®, Cooper Surgical, USA) was found to be dependent upon very similar sperm characteristics to those required for human peri-ovulatory cervical mucus [22–24]. However, due to the unavailability of a commercial product that can be used in such tests, the 'Hyaluronate Migration Test' never entered routine practice.

Other substances such as hens' egg white [25] and polyacrylamide gel [26,27] have also been investigated but did not find a place among standardized routine andrology laboratory tests.

References

1. Mortimer D. Sperm transport in the female genital tract. In: Grudzinskas JG, Yovich JL, eds. *Cambridge Reviews in Human Reproduction, Volume 2: Gametes – The Spermatozoon.* Cambridge: Cambridge University Press, 1995, 157–74.

2. Mortimer ST. A critical review of the physiological importance and analysis of sperm movement in mammals. *Hum Reprod Update* 1997; **3**: 403–39.

3. World Health Organization. *WHO Laboratory Manual for the Analysis of Human Semen and Sperm-Cervical Mucus Interaction,* 4th edn. Cambridge: Cambridge University Press, 1999.

4. Mortimer D. *Practical Laboratory Andrology.* New York: Oxford University Press, 1994.

5. Hunault CC, Habbema JD, Eijkemans MJ et al. Two new prediction rules for spontaneous pregnancy leading to live birth among subfertile couples, based on the synthesis of three previous models. *Hum Reprod* 2004; **19**: 2019–26.

6. Kremer J. A simple sperm penetration test. *Int J Fertil* 1965; **10**: 209–14.

7. Eggert-Kruse W, Leinhos G, Gerhard, I, et al. Prognostic value of in vitro sperm penetration into hormonally standardized human cervical mucus. *Fertil Steril* 1989; **51**: 317–23.

8. Kremer J. *The In Vitro Spermatozoal Penetration Test in Fertility Investigations.* MD thesis. Groningen, Rijksuniversiteit te Groningen, 1968.

9. Kremer J, Jager S, van Slochteren-Draaisma T. The 'unexplained' poor post-coital test. *Int J Fertil* 1978; **23**: 277–81.

10. Pandya IJ, Mortimer D, Sawers RS. A standardized approach for evaluating the penetration of human spermatozoa into cervical mucus in vitro. *Fertil Steril* 1986; **45**: 357–65.

11. Makler A. A new method for evaluating cervical penetrability using daily aspirated and stored cervical mucus. *Fertil Steril* 1976; **27**: 533–40.

12. Drobnis EZ, Yudin AL, Cherr GN, Katz DF. Hamster sperm penetration of the zona pellucida: kinematic analysis and mechanical implications. *Devel Biol* 1988; **130**: 311–23.

13. Insler V, Melmed H, Eichenbrenner I, et al. The cervical score: a simple quantitative method for monitoring of the menstrual cycle. *Int J Gynaec Obstet* 1972; **10**: 223–8.

14. World Health Organization. *WHO Laboratory Manual for the Analysis of Human Semen and Sperm-Cervical Mucus Interaction,* 3rd edn. Cambridge: Cambridge University Press, 1992.

15. Moghissi KS. Postcoital test: physiologic basis, technique and interpretation. *Fert Steril* 1976; **27**: 117–29.

16. Kurzrok R, Miller EG. Biochemical studies of human semen and its relation to mucus of the cervix uteri. *Am J Obstet Gynecol* 1928; **15**: 56–72.

17. Katz DF, Overstreet, JW, Hanson FW. A new quantitative test for sperm penetration into cervical mucus. *Fertil Steril* 1980; **33**: 179–86.

18. Kremer J, Jager S. The sperm-cervical mucus contact test. A preliminary report. *Fertil Steril* 1976; **27**: 335–40.

19. Insler VV, Bernstein D, Glezerman M, Misgav N. Correlation of seminal fluid analysis with mucus-penetrating ability of spermatozoa. *Fertil Steril* 1979; **32**: 316–19.

20. Freundl G, Grimm HJ, Hofmann N. Selective filtration of abnormal spermatozoa by the cervical mucus. *Hum Reprod* 1988; **3**: 277–80.

21. Eggert-Kruse W, Reimann-Andersen J, Rohr G, et al. Clinical relevance of sperm morphology assessment using strict criteria and relationship with sperm-mucus interaction in vivo and in vitro. *Fertil Steril* 1995; **63**: 612–24.

22. Mortimer D, Mortimer ST, Shu MA, Swart R. A simplified approach to sperm-cervical mucus interaction using a hyaluronate migration test. *Hum Reprod* 1990; **5**: 835–41.

23. Aitken RJ, Bowie H, Buckingham D, et al. Sperm penetration into a hyaluronic acid polymer as a means of monitoring functional competence. *J Androl* 1992; **13**: 44–54.

24. Neuwinger J, Cooper TG, Knuth UA, Nieschlag E. Hyaluronic acid as a medium for human sperm migration tests. *Hum Reprod* 1991; **6**: 396–400.

25. Eggert-Kruse W, Gerhard I, Tilgen W, Runnebaum B. The use of hens' egg white as a substitute for human cervical mucus in assessing human infertility. *Int J Androl* 1990; **13**: 258–66.

26. Goldstein MC, Wix LS, Foote RH, et al. Migration of fresh and cryopreserved human spermatozoa in polyacrylamide gel. *Fertil Steril* 1982; **37**: 668–74.

27. Urry RL, Middleton RG, Mayo D. A comparison of the penetration of human sperm into bovine and artificial cervical mucus. *Fertil Steril* 1986; **45**: 135–7.

Chapter

9

Sperm Preparation

Background

Spermatozoa in the ejaculate are prevented from undergoing capacitation by decapacitation factor(s) present in the seminal plasma. Seminal plasma also contains one or more factors to which prolonged exposure adversely affect sperm function, including the ability to penetrate cervical mucus, undergo the acrosome reaction *in vitro* and the fertilization process generally [1,2]. Exposure to seminal plasma for more than 30 min after ejaculation can permanently diminish the fertilizing capacity of human spermatozoa *in vitro* [3], and contamination of prepared sperm populations with only trace amounts of seminal plasma (0.01% v/v = 1-in-10,000) can decrease their fertilizing capacity (see Figure 9.1) [4].

Because sperm capacitation is essential for fertilization both *in vivo* and *in vitro*, spermatozoa for clinical procedures such as IUI or IVF (and also for laboratory tests of sperm fertilizing ability) must be separated from the seminal plasma environment not only as soon as possible after ejaculation (allowing for the required wait for liquefaction), but also as efficiently as possible to eliminate decapacitation factor(s), and the spermatozoa must then be suspended in a culture medium capable of supporting capacitation. Consequently, these essential pre-requisites for capacitation dictate the requirements for manipulating spermatozoa to be used for clinical IVF [1,2]. Since ICSI does not depend on sperm fertilizing ability, an effect of prolonged exposure to seminal plasma on perceived sperm function is less likely, but does result in increased sperm DNA damage [5]. However, a short interval between semen collection and processing is definitely beneficial for IUI [6,7], confirming the collection of semen samples at the clinic, and starting processing as soon as possible, as best practice. Apparently contradictory studies in particular must be examined critically in regard to their actual sperm processing techniques, especially the progressive motility in the final washed preparation (expected to be >95% for normozoospermic semen samples), and how fertilization rates compare to international benchmarks [8]. In summary, it is still strongly recommended that all semen samples for ART use be collected at the clinic and processing commenced by 30 min post-ejaculation.

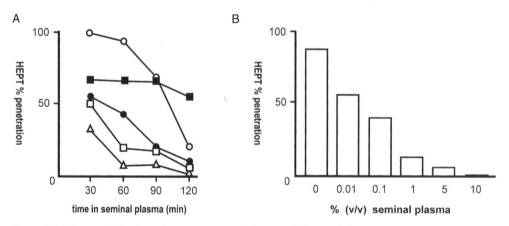

Figure 9.1 Influence of (A) prolonged exposure to seminal plasma and (B) seminal plasma contamination during sperm capacitation on the fertilizing ability of human spermatozoa as assessed using the zone pellucida-free hamster egg penetration test ('HEPT'). Figures redrawn from [3] and [4].

Because the area of sperm preparation methods has been reviewed extensively elsewhere [2,9,10], only an overview of the five basic approaches for sperm preparation is provided here as background to the later section on established 'safe' methods in common current usage.

- Simple dilution and (repeated) washing to remove seminal plasma
- Methods based on sperm migration to separate motile spermatozoa; this includes methods based on microfluidics
- Adherence-based methods to eliminate dead spermatozoa and debris, including selective methods such as magnetically activated cell sorting (MACS) using labelled beads
- 'Selective' washing methods using density gradients to separate motile spermatozoa
- Sperm separation based on their electrophoretic mobility

Simple Washing

Simple dilution of semen with a relatively large volume (typically 5× to 10×) of culture medium and separation of the spermatozoa by centrifugation is the simplest method for washing spermatozoa. Repeated centrifugation (usually two or three times) is often used to ensure removal of contaminating seminal plasma, although it is essential to avoid forces greater than 800 g [11]. This procedure has the great disadvantage that all the spermatozoa, including the dead, moribund and abnormal ones, present in the original semen, remain in the final sperm population, as well as all other cells that were present in the semen, including germ line cells that were sloughed from the seminiferous epithelium and leucocytes of various types.

The presence of large numbers of non-functional gametes in the final preparation could be detrimental by inhibiting capacitation and has been reported to increase the risk of developing anti-sperm antibodies if inseminated into the uterine cavity at IUI [12]. Furthermore, it has been known for more than three decades that if whole semen is centrifuged, the functional potential of the motile cells, even when isolated later, is impaired [13–15]. Centrifuging human ejaculates causes the production of ROS within the resulting pellet, causing irreversible damage to the spermatozoa via peroxidation of sperm plasma membrane phospholipids and via oxidative damage to the sperm chromatin. Indeed, ROS can cause substantial degradation of the sperm DNA while not necessarily affecting their fertilizing ability [16,17].

Consequently, the practice of washing spermatozoa by centrifuging unselected sperm populations is potentially hazardous, and it has been recommended since 1991 that it should be abandoned in favour of known safe practices such as direct swim-up from semen and density gradient centrifugation techniques [18].

Migration-Based Techniques

In-vivo, the potentially functional sperm population is separated from liquefied semen by virtue of their migration into cervical mucus. Sperm migration into the culture medium layer is therefore considered functionally equivalent to the process whereby human spermatozoa escape from the ejaculate and colonize the cervical mucus [19–21], although some differences do exist due to the different rheological characteristics between the culture medium and mid-cycle cervical mucus.

In the original 'swim-up' technique, liquefied semen is layered beneath culture medium (or culture medium is layered over the semen, but the former provides a much cleaner interface). During a subsequent incubation period (15 to 60 min depending on the application) the progressively motile spermatozoa migrate from the semen into the culture medium.

A combined migration-sedimentation technique, designed originally for asthenozoospermic samples, combined swim-up from semen with gravitational settling of spermatozoa from the upper medium layer using special 'Tea-Jondet' tubes [22]. While the method was an interesting approach for dealing with male factor semen samples with very sluggish motility (direct swim-up from semen being preferable for samples with average or better progression), it is rarely used nowadays.

Microfluidics-Based Techniques

Early studies on human spermatozoa swimming in capillaries and channels go back to the 1950s [23] and were the basis for the Kremer Test (see Chapter 8) [24], as well as systems used to test spermicides [25]. However, more recent studies have elaborated the technology from simple channels to ones with flow, to capitalize upon the rheotactic behaviour of spermatozoa [26] and arrays of microchannels to increase the bandwidth of the sperm migration process [27], including the *Zech-Selector* device for clinical ART sperm preparation patented by Josef Zech of Innsbruck, Austria in 2011 [28]. More recent studies have focused on sperm DNA integrity rather than just their motility and morphology of the selected spermatozoa.

There has recently been great clinical interest in such devices, e.g. the *Zymōt ICSI* and *Zymōt Multi* (850 μl) sperm separation devices (Zymōt Fertility, Gaithersburg, MD, USA, see www .zymotfertility.com), which are the same as the *Fertile®* and *Fertile Plus®* devices from Koek Biotechnology (Izmir, Turkey, see www.koekbiotech.com) [29–31]. Reports are encouraging, certainly in terms of the low sperm DNA fragmentation measurements in the processed samples, but the <90% progressive motility results reported in at least some of the samples processed in parallel by DGC raise questions about the patient populations and/or DGC methodology(ies) used. In at least one paper it seems that the post-gradient pellet was washed in the same tube [30]. The high cost of these devices might be a barrier to their widespread adoption in routine practice. It should also be noted that the larger (850 μl) device is not actually a microfluidic device but a DSUS system whose interface has been stabilized by a membrane, a principle that has been around for four decades [32,33].

Direct Swim-Up from Semen

Aliquots of semen are taken as soon as the specimen has liquefied and placed in a series of tubes underneath layers of culture medium. Round-bottomed, not conical, tubes are used to maximize the surface area of the interface between the semen layer and the culture medium, and multiple tubes containing relatively small volumes of semen will increase the total interface area (e.g. sufficient semen to bring the interface to the point of maximum diameter of the tube under 600 μl of culture medium) and hence maximize the yield (Figure 9.2). Tubes can be incubated at an angle of 45° to increase the interface area, but they must then be kept at that angle until after harvesting so as not to risk contaminating the medium layer with seminal plasma as the tube is returned to the vertical. After an appropriate incubation period at 37°C – longer incubations give greater yields (although this should not exceed 60 min) – most of the upper culture medium layer (typically ⅔ or ¾) is removed, taking great care not to aspirate from the interface. This sperm population is then usually washed once by centrifugation and resuspended into fresh culture medium at the desired concentration of motile

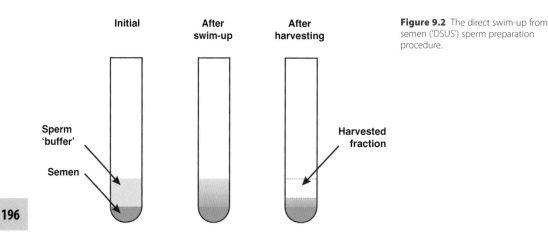

Initial   After swim-up   After harvesting

Sperm 'buffer'

Semen

Harvested fraction

Figure 9.2 The direct swim-up from semen ('DSUS') sperm preparation procedure.

spermatozoa. Keeping a small aliquot of the preparation back while the majority is being centrifuged allows sperm concentration and motility counts to be completed during the centrifugation.

Swim-Up from a Washed Pellet or Sperm Suspension

While these methods have been used successfully in many clinical IVF programmes, especially with non-male factor cases, the established risk of adversely affecting the fertilizing ability of many men's spermatozoa makes it a poor choice in the modern era where IVF is frequently used for couples where there is a significant male factor, and whose chances of successful IVF could be compromised [2,18]. Responsible laboratory management should preclude the continued use of a technique incorporating steps known to cause irrevocable damage to spermatozoa prejudicial to a desired functional endpoint.

Adherence-Based Methods

These methods are based on the fact that dead and moribund spermatozoa are extremely sticky and will attach to glass surfaces even in the presence of relatively high concentrations of protein (the 'sticking-to-glass' phenomenon). Techniques using glass wool columns were quite common in the 1980s, but reports that glass wool could induce damage to the sperm plasma membrane and acrosome [34], and the danger of glass wool fragments in the final sperm population, led to their abandonment, especially for preparing sperm populations to be used for IUI. Methods based on glass beads, while used widely for preparing rodent spermatozoa, saw little use with human spermatozoa. Selective filtration using Sephadex columns was also described, but only limited studies comparing the functional competence of these sperm preparations with techniques such as direct swim-up from semen and density gradients were reported.

Magnetically Activated Cell Sorting

For the last 15 years, magnetically activated cell sorting (MACS) technology has been proposed as a sperm selection technique for use in ART. The technique uses magnetic beads to isolate apoptotic cells (Annexin V-positive) and there have been a plethora of publications investigating its effectiveness [35,36]. Initial experiments were promising [37–39] but subsequent randomized controlled trials did not confirm a significant clinical benefit of the technique, such as improvements in live birth rates [40]. While the technique might be useful in some cases, e.g. high levels of DNA-damaged cells in the ejaculate, even then the data are not clear and there are conflicting reports of its effectiveness [41]. A recent Cochrane review concluded that the evidence for MACS in ART was low, and that there was uncertainty whether MACS (a) improved live birth or clinical pregnancy, or (b) reduced the miscarriage rate per woman or per clinical pregnancy [42].

Sperm Separation by Electrophoresis

This novel approach is based on the principles that the highest quality spermatozoa in an ejaculate also carry the greatest net negative charge and that they can be separated from other electronegative cells, such as leucocytes and immature germ cells, by virtue of their smaller cross-sectional size (Figure 9.3) [43]. A commercial system 'Felix', using a sealed disposable cassette, is anticipated soon (Memphasys Limited, Homebush West, NSW, Australia, see www.memphasys.com.au).

Hyaluronan Binding Selection of Spermatozoa for Intracytoplasmic Sperm Injection

The ability of spermatozoa to bind to hyaluronic acid, and in so doing selecting for mature spermatozoa with anticipated lower levels of DNA fragmentation, was proposed as an approach for 'physiological ICSI' or PICSI [44], leading to the development of the PICSI® Dish (now from Cooper Surgical, Målov, Denmark). Early clinical trials indicated clinical benefit, including that in couples where ≤65% of spermatozoa bound to hyaluronan in the HBA, the use of hyaluronan-bound spermatozoa in ICSI led to a statistically significant reduction in pregnancy loss rate [45].

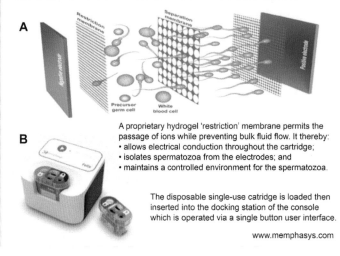

Felix is a simple automated system that efficiently separates the best quality spermatozoa from liquefied semen in about six minutes.

Figure 9.3 Sperm preparation by electrophoresis using the Felix system. Illustration courtesy of Memphasys Ltd, Homebush West, NSW, Australia.

A proprietary hydrogel 'restriction' membrane permits the passage of ions while preventing bulk fluid flow. It thereby:
• allows electrical conduction throughout the cartridge;
• isolates spermatozoa from the electrodes; and
• maintains a controlled environment for the spermatozoa.

The disposable single-use catridge is loaded then inserted into the docking station of the console which is operated via a single button user interface.

www.memphasys.com

However, a large prospective randomized trial of the PICSI® Dish found that, compared to ICSI, PICSI did not significantly improve term livebirth rates, and concluded that wider use of PICSI was not recommended [46].

Selective Washing Using Density Gradient Centrifugation

These methods separate cells based upon their density or specific gravity (i.e. mass per unit volume), and result in cells being distributed throughout a gradient column according to the location in the gradient that matches their density, i.e. at their isopycnic points. Although density gradients can be either continuous, where the density of the material comprising the gradient changes in a smooth manner from its minimum at the top of the gradient to its maximum at the bottom, or discontinuous, where a series of layers of decreasing density are placed one on top of another, the latter have been used almost exclusively for clinical applications with human spermatozoa.

In discontinuous gradients, the interfaces separating the layers create step-wise changes in densities and can become clogged by cells or other materials, retarding – or even preventing – the passage of more dense cells down the gradient. DGC methods were popularized in the early 1980s following the commercialization of colloidal silica that had been coated with polyvinylpyrrolidone – *Percoll®* (Pharmacia Biotech, Uppsala, Sweden), which dominated clinical human sperm preparation until its withdrawal from clinical use by its manufacturer in 1996 [2]. Density gradients for human sperm preparation were also described using other products such as *Nycodenz®*, *OptiPrep™* and *Accudenz®* (all from Nycomed Pharma, Oslo, Norway) [47–49], although the osmotic activity of these molecules required special media for their optimal use.

Mature, morphologically normal human spermatozoa have a density (specific gravity) above 1.12 g/ml, whereas immature and many abnormal spermatozoa have densities between 1.06–1.09 g/ml [50]. The specific gravity of colloidal silica preparations equivalent to 40% and 80% of the original *Percoll®* product is about 1.06 and 1.10 g/ml respectively, therefore only the most mature, normal spermatozoa can penetrate the lower layer of an appropriately formulated density gradient (Figure 9.4).

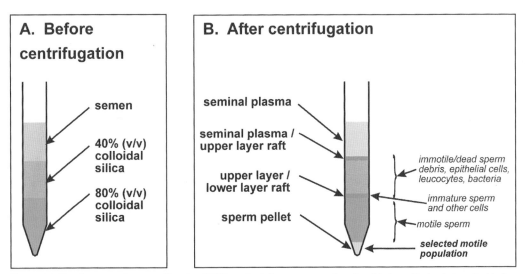

Figure 9.4 The density gradient centrifugation ('DGC') method of sperm preparation. Panel A shows the loaded gradient before centrifugation, while panel B shows the same tube after centrifugation in a swing-out rotor.

Densities of Different Colloidal Silica Density Gradient Centrifugation Products

Several intrinsic properties of colloidal silica make it an ideal density gradient material for sperm preparation. Being a mineral, it allows the formulation of high-density preparation media, but makes no osmotic contribution to the media and, because it is a colloid rather than a solution, it has low viscosity and so does not retard sperm cell sedimentation. The toxic effect of pure colloidal silica is eliminated by coating the particles with a suitable material (e.g. PVP as in *Percoll*®, or covalently bound silane molecules ('silanized silica') as in current human sperm preparation products such as *PureSperm*® (Nidacon International AB, Mölndahl, Sweden, see www.nidacon.com), *ISolate*® (FujiFilm Irvine Scientific, Santa Ana, CA, USA, see www.irvinesci.com) or *Sil-Select*™ (FertiPro NV, Beernem, Belgium, see www.fertipro.com). The physical characteristics of these new colloids are equivalent to *Percoll*® preparations, and their clinical utility is at least as good, if not better [2]. The only real difference is that whereas *Percoll*® was sold as colloidal silica in a weak inorganic buffer solution (requiring it to be used in conjunction with a 10× buffer to make 'isotonic' 90% v/v *Percoll*® colloid), the silanized silica-based products are prepared in an isotonic culture medium ready-to-use.

Unfortunately, this has given rise to a crucial difference between modern density gradient centrifugation (DGC) products that can affect their performance unless used carefully, as in the erroneous comparison and recommendations in the fourth and fifth editions of the WHO laboratory manual [51,52]. While *PureSperm*® was formulated as a direct equivalent of 100% stock *Percoll*® colloid as supplied by the manufacturer, *ISolate*® is produced as an equivalent to 'isotonic' 90% v/v *Percoll*® colloid. Hence comparing a 90% *ISolate*® lower layer with 90% *PureSperm*® would result in *PureSperm*® giving a lower yield – but only because it was actually a 90% colloid-equivalent layer, instead of the 81% colloid in the *ISolate*® lower layer. Likewise, an 80% *ISolate*® lower layer (i.e. 72% colloid-equivalent) would give an even higher yield, but only by allowing less good spermatozoa into the pellet – i.e. ones with a higher ROS-generating capacity [14]. Consequently, proper use of modern DGC products with human spermatozoa requires that manufacturers state the actual colloid concentration, so that a lower layer of 1.10 g/ml can be employed. The protocol provided below is based on an upper and lower layer of correct 40% and 80% colloid respectively, e.g. 40%/80% *PureSperm*® or 45%/90% *ISolate*®.

Risk of Reactive Oxygen Species Using Density Gradient Centrifugation

A low level of heavy metal contamination is inherent in the manufacturing process of colloidal silica products, and while this can lead to evidence of oxidative DNA damage, the effect can be inhibited by

EDTA [53]. This is also the reason why culture media containing iron, such as Ham's F-10, should not be used for sperm preparation [54], even though that medium is still suggested in the WHO Manual [51,52], and is likely the cause of the reported ROS damage in at least one experimental study [49]. In this regard it should be noted that the *PureSperm* family of products were all designed to include EDTA to chelate these ions, protection that will be reduced or lost if culture media not containing EDTA are used to dilute the concentrated colloid and/or used to wash the pellets. The new generation of Origio sperm preparation products also include EDTA for this purpose (Cooper Surgical, Trumbull, CT, USA, see www .fertility.coopersurgical.com).

Osmolarity and Protection against Osmotic Shock

Low osmolarity is another mechanism that can promote the generation of ROS by sperm during washing, and some osmotic shock is inherent in almost all sperm washing protocols, since the seminal plasma at 30 min post-ejaculation is around 340 mOsm, and ART culture media are mostly between 285 and 295 mOsm. Interestingly, the use of a hypertonic density gradient has been reported to produce better sperm preparations [55]. In those experiments, a six-step discontinuous gradient was used, ranging from 335 mOsm in the uppermost layer to 394 mOsm in the bottom layer. The great majority of commercial density gradient media for sperm preparation are formulated to be in the same range as ART culture media. However, when used as a coherent system, the *PureSperm* family of products, as well as the new Origio Gradient Series, will create an intermediate osmolarity of 310 mOsm, reducing the osmotic shock the spermatozoa will experience during processing.

Optimization of Density Gradient Centrifugation Methods

A variety of physical and practical factors affect the optimization of human sperm preparation using colloidal silica-based DGC methods [2,9,10].

Tube Shape and Size and Rotor Type

A more discrete pellet is obtained when a tube is centrifuged in a swing-out rotor rather than a fixed-angle rotor, making it easier to recover the entire pellet when harvesting the gradient. Tube shape affects the area of the bottom of the tube where the pellet is located, hence a more discrete pellet will be formed in a conical tube, again making it easier to recover the entire pellet (Figure 9.5). The cross-sectional area of the tube, i.e. the area of the interface between the layers, will reduce the rate of formation of the 'rafts' that block the gradient, allowing more spermatozoa to reach their isopycnic point – giving higher yields when using larger diameter tubes.

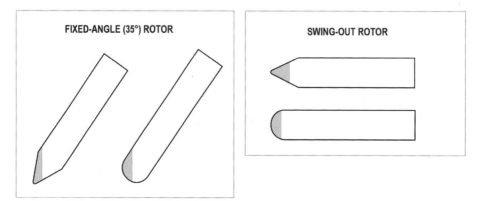

Figure 9.5 The effect of tube shape and centrifuge rotor type on the location and shape of the pellet.

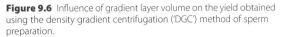

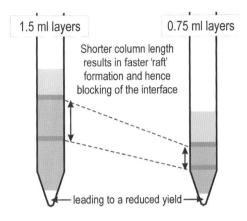

1.5 ml layers   0.75 ml layers

Shorter column length results in faster 'raft' formation and hence blocking of the interface

leading to a reduced yield

Figure 9.6 Influence of gradient layer volume on the yield obtained using the density gradient centrifugation ('DGC') method of sperm preparation.

Layer Number and Volume

Longer column layers (i.e. larger volume layers) also result in higher yields (Figure 9.6), but there is no general benefit to using more than two layers (40% and 80% colloid-equivalent) in routine practice. Very occasionally, for extremely dirty specimens, a third, intermediate layer of 60% colloid can be helpful by slowing/reducing the formation of the 'rafts' at the interfaces between layers, but routinely using three layers unnecessarily increases technical complexity as well as both materials and labour costs.

Centrifugation Time and Speed

Since the earliest work with *Percoll*®, gradients have been centrifuged at 300 g_{max}, it having been found empirically to provide optimum sperm recovery. Various studies during the past 20–25 years have shown no systematic benefit to changing either the centrifugation speed or time for this step. Slower centrifugation speeds (i.e. lower g-force) only serve to reduce the yield, they do not improve sperm quality, and faster speeds do not increase the yield since the method is a true isopycnic separation and by 20 min all the spermatozoa have reached their isopycnic points.

Harvesting Technique

Although some DGC methods and product Instructions-for-Use have described the recovery of the pellet by passing a glass Pasteur pipette straight through the entire gradient, these studies were conducted mostly on research donors or normal fertile men, whose semen samples were reasonably 'clean'. When using DGC with poor quality patient specimens, the 'rafts' that build up at the interfaces can be dragged down with the pipette tip, contaminating the pellet. The standard recommended method is to aspirate downwards from the meniscus, stopping once the raft between the 40% and 80% layers has been removed, leaving clear 80%-layer colloid. Then, using a clean (sterile) Pasteur pipette, the pellet is recovered through the remaining part of the 80% layer, ensuring that it is not contaminated by any of the seminal plasma and raft material that is slowly running down the inside wall of the tube and collecting on the meniscus of the residual 80% layer (Fig. 9.7). Pellets are then transferred to clean centrifuge tubes for washing.

The following incorrect actions will result in contamination of the pellet to a greater or lesser degree, and should not be employed:

- Removing all the bottom gradient layer to reveal the pellet for recovery (mild risk of contamination).
- Recovering the pellet using the same pipette as was used to remove the upper layers (moderate contamination).
- Resuspending the pellet in the gradient tube (certain high-level contamination).

201

Harvesting the pellet

Figure 9.7 The density gradient centrifugation ('DGC') method of sperm preparation: correct harvesting procedure.

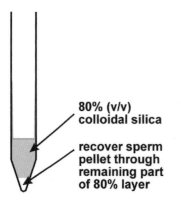

80% (v/v) colloidal silica

recover sperm pellet through remaining part of 80% layer

Such incorrect techniques were used in several published studies and readers should be aware that results reported from such studies may have been compromised, even to the extent of having no practical relevance.

Washing

The second 'wash' centrifugation step needs to be sufficient to recover the great majority of the spermatozoa without exposing them to excessive centrifugal force. For this, the combination of 500 g_{max} × 10 min has been found to be optimal; lower speeds increase the risk of discarding spermatozoa in the supernatant, and neither higher speed nor longer time provides any significant benefit, while speeds higher than 800 g_{max} should be avoided [11]. More than one wash step has not been shown to have any measurable benefit in terms of IVF fertilization rate or embryo quality. Additional washing is inadvisable to reduce exposure to unnecessary centrifugation and avoid the loss of spermatozoa that occurs during each wash step – and hence optimize efficiency and cost-effectiveness.

Post-Gradient Swim-Up

Performing a 'swim-out' or 'sperm rise' migration step following the post-gradient wash step in an attempt to eliminate all remaining immotile spermatozoa from the final preparation is ill-advised because:

- A few immotile spermatozoa in the inseminate have no detectable adverse effect on either fertilization rate or embryo quality; hence a few such spermatozoa are not biologically – or clinically – relevant.
- The time taken for this step greatly increases the overall time for sperm preparation, decreasing laboratory efficiency and increasing costs.
- The vast majority of sperm preparations should have ≫90% progressively motile spermatozoa in the final preparation (typically >95%) if the technique was done properly.* So, in the absence of technical error, a sperm preparation with <85% motility must be seen as an indication of some sperm pathology.

  A recent consensus on IVF Lab KPIs from the ESHRE SIG Embryology and Alpha Scientists in Reproductive Medicine set the competency and aspirational benchmark values for progressive sperm motility in the final washed sperm populations for normozoospermic ejaculates as 90% and ≥95% respectively [8].

'Safe' Methods for Sperm Preparation

Although discontinuous DGC using silane-coated colloidal silica is the current 'gold standard' method for human sperm preparation, direct swim-up from semen with one wash step can also be used safely for semen samples showing good sperm progression. Both these methods can provide sperm populations with selected morphology and also spermatozoa with fewer DNA nicks and better chromatin stability, although DGC seems to be better overall [2,56,57]. A particular importance of this is that, while many ART laboratories prepare their IVF spermatozoa using density gradients, many continue to use simple washing for their ICSI spermatozoa since the attendant risk of ROS-induced sperm dysfunction is considered unimportant. However, men who need ICSI have high levels of abnormal spermatozoa and are hence most susceptible to ROS-induced sperm DNA damage. Moreover, since it is well-established that ROS can cause substantial degradation of the sperm DNA that does not necessarily affect their fertilizing ability [16,17], spermatozoa prepared by simple washing will have an increased risk of contributing a defective genome to the embryo. Indeed, this might underlie the increased developmental failure of ICSI-derived embryos after the eight-cell stage when the embryonic genome is activated [58].

Given that the fundamental principle of medical care is 'primum non nocere' (first, do no harm), clinical scientists participating in the management of ART programmes are obligated to avoid techniques that have known hazards if other, safer, techniques are available. To this end, the following sections provide detailed procedures for human sperm preparation using direct swim-up from semen and density gradient centrifugation techniques.

Which Type of Culture Medium Should Be Used for Sperm Preparation?

Because centrifugation is usually performed under air, rather than a CO_2-enriched atmosphere, DGC preparative techniques should use a zwitterion-buffered medium (e.g. HEPES), often referred to as a 'sperm wash buffer' rather than a bicarbonate-based medium (this is regardless of whatever suggestion might be made by an embryo culture medium company). Swim-up techniques should also be performed in a 'sperm buffer' (and incubated either in an air incubator or else in tightly capped tubes in a CO_2 incubator), as this will prevent premature capacitation. Because sperm capacitation requires the presence of significant concentrations of bicarbonate ions, the final resuspension of sperm populations that are to undergo in-vitro capacitation must be into a bicarbonate-buffered 'sperm wash medium', otherwise their fertilizing capacity will be compromised.

For IUI preparations, a 'sperm buffer' can be employed, as it will be greatly diluted after insemination, and also because if the spermatozoa undergo capacitation in vitro during prolonged incubation prior to insemination, their hyperactivated motility might compromise their ability to traverse the utero-tubal junction [21,59]; although if insemination is to be performed soon after sperm preparation, then a 'medium' can be used safely. Spermatozoa being prepared for ICSI can be processed and resuspended in a 'sperm buffer' since capacitation is irrelevant for fertilization using ICSI.

Protocol: Sperm Preparation Using Direct Swim-Up from Semen

Principle

Sperm migration into a layer of culture medium mimics the process whereby human spermatozoa escape from the liquefied ejaculate and colonize the cervical mucus. Seminal plasma contains decapacitation factors(s) that prevent spermatozoa from undergoing capacitation [2]. Exposure to seminal plasma for more than 30 min after ejaculation can permanently diminish human sperm fertilizing ability [3], and only trace amounts of seminal plasma contaminating prepared sperm populations can decrease their fertilizing capacity [4]. Consequently, spermatozoa for clinical procedures such as IUI or IVF (as well as for laboratory tests of sperm fertilizing ability) must be separated from the seminal plasma environment not only as soon as possible after ejaculation (allowing for the required wait for liquefaction) [6,7], but also as efficiently as possible. Depending on their intended use, the spermatozoa are then suspended in culture media either capable of supporting in-vitro capacitation (e.g. for IVF) or not (e.g. for IUI or ICSI).

Specimen

Liquefied, homogeneous human semen, ideally within 30 min of ejaculation. Longer post-ejaculatory delays, incomplete liquefaction and increased viscosity must be noted on the laboratory and report forms. For other types of specimens and abnormal semen samples, see the section on 'Working with Difficult Specimens' later in this chapter.

Equipment

See also Appendix 2.

- Microscope configured for andrology with phase contrast optics (10×, 20× and 40× objectives)
- Air incubator operating at 37°C
- Centrifuge
- Tally counter
- Syringe+tubing adapter to permit volumetric control of glass Pasteur pipettes
- Rubber bulbs to control glass Pasteur pipettes
- Counting chamber (e.g. Makler Chamber)

Disposable Materials

- Semen collection container
- Sterile serological pipette
- Round-bottom polystyrene 7-ml culture tubes (e.g. Falcon #2003 or #2058)
- Round-bottom polystyrene 14-ml culture tubes (e.g. Falcon #2001 or #2057)
- Conical-bottom polystyrene 15-ml centrifuge tubes (e.g. Falcon #2095)
- Glass Pasteur pipettes

Note: All disposables that will come into contact with spermatozoa that are to be used for either therapeutic or critical testing purposes should be either pre-tested for sperm toxicity or else obtained from a trusted manufacturer, e.g. if a sterile plastic syringe is used during processing then it must be of a brand known not to have any deleterious effects upon spermatozoa [60].

Reagents

- *'Sperm buffer'* culture medium (HEPES- or MOPS-buffered) containing at least 10 mg/ml HSA
- *Sperm washing medium* (bicarbonate-buffered culture medium) containing at least 10 mg/ml HSA
- *IVF medium* (bicarbonate-buffered) containing at least 10 mg/ml HSA

Note: All reagents that are to be used in preparing human spermatozoa for therapeutic purposes must be CE-marked (or equivalent) and certified as pyrogen-free and not having any sperm toxicity. Reagents for IVF and ICSI applications should also be certified as not being embryotoxic.

Calibration

Centrifugation speeds must not be described using rpm values, as these are highly dependent upon the rotational radius of the centrifuge rotor. Also, the g forces are expressed as g_{max} values, calculated for what the spermatozoa would experience at the bottom of the centrifuge tube (not the bottom of the centrifuge bucket). The formula describing the relationship between rotation speed, rotational radius and g-force is:

$$g = 0.0000112 \times r \times N^2 \quad or \quad N = \sqrt{[g/(0.0000112 \times r)]}$$

where: g = the maximum g-force achieved at the bottom of the tube
r = the rotational radius (cm)
N = the rotational speed (rpm)

Quality Control

- All specimen containers and processing/preparation tubes must be labelled with two identifiers, e.g. the subject's name and the specimen's laboratory reference or ID number. Temporary analytical preparations (e.g. sperm motility slides) can be identified using the specimen's laboratory reference or ID number only.
- Washed sperm preparations from normozoospermic semen specimens should show at least 90%, and ideally ≥95%, progressive motility [8].

Procedure

1. Label the following tubes with the subject's name and specimen ID number:

   2 × round-bottom 14-ml culture tubes (more tubes can be prepared if a higher yield is required)

   1 × conical-bottom 15-ml centrifuge tube

   1 × round-bottom 7-ml culture tube (this will be for the final sperm preparation)

2. Using aseptic technique, place 0.6 ml of sperm buffer into the bottom of each tube and place in the incubator to warm to 37°C before use.

3. Using a sterile glass Pasteur pipette, carefully underlay well mixed, liquefied semen into the bottom of each tube under the sperm buffer; the interface should be sharp and clearly visible (see Figure 9.2). Approximately 300 μl will be required to fill the hemispherical bottom part of the tube; adding more semen than this will not improve the yield.

4. Cap the tube and place upright in the rack (see Note #1). Transfer the rack to the incubator for 20–30 min at 37°C.

5. Using a clean, sterile glass Pasteur pipette, remove the upper ⅔ of the sperm buffer layer (*ca.* 400 μl). Take great care not to disturb the sperm buffer:semen interface. If the semen layer is disturbed, then the preparation should be discarded.

6. Transfer the aspirated upper layer material to the 15-ml centrifuge tube.

7. Repeat steps #5 and #6 for the other tube, transferring the aspirated upper layer material to the same 15-ml centrifuge tube.

8. Add 6 ml of sperm buffer to the sperm suspension and mix gently.

9. Cap the tube and centrifuge at 500 g_{max} for 10 min.

10. Using a clean glass Pasteur pipette, aspirate the supernatant almost to the pellet.

11. Resuspend the pellet in a suitable volume of the final sperm preparation medium (see Note #2), mixing gently by aspirating in and out of the Pasteur pipette. The volume of medium to use will depend on the size of the pellet and the desired final sperm concentration.

12. Analyse the sperm concentration and motility, e.g. using a Makler Chamber (see Note #3).

13. Adjust the sperm concentration, if necessary, by adding more of the final sperm preparation medium. Transfer the final sperm preparation into the 7-ml culture tube.

14. Hold the specimen at the appropriate temperature (see Note #1) until required.

Calculations and Results

Use the concentration and sperm motility results to calculate the concentration of progressively motile spermatozoa in the final preparation (see also Note #3) and, using the preparation volume, the total number of such spermatozoa in the final preparation.

Interpretation Guidelines

None, this is a preparative technique only (but see the section on 'The Trial Wash' later in this chapter)

Notes

1. Tubes can be incubated at an angle of 45° to increase the interface area, but they must then be kept at that angle until after harvesting, so as not to risk contaminating the medium layer with seminal plasma as the tube is returned to the vertical.

2. Each migration tube should be harvested separately, and the individual preparations combined only after verifying that they contain very high proportions of motile spermatozoa (typically >90–95% motile [53]) and are not contaminated with debris or other cellular elements from the semen fraction.

3. The final sperm preparation medium will vary according to the intended use of the sperm preparation and the likely delay prior to its use. The principle here is to prevent premature sperm capacitation and sperm senescence that will occur when sperm are incubated for prolonged periods at 37°C, especially in a medium that support sperm capacitation *in vitro*. For example:

   IUI: It is recommended that a sperm buffer be employed as it will prevent premature sperm capacitation should there be a prolonged delay before insemination (the zwitterion will be greatly diluted after insemination and have no adverse effect on the spermatozoa). Hold the sperm preparation at ambient temperature (ideally in a styrofoam box to protect it from light and cold draughts). If insemination is to be performed more-or-less immediately after sperm preparation, then a bicarbonate-buffered medium at 37°C in a CO_2 incubator can be used safely.

   IVF: A bicarbonate-buffered medium capable of supporting sperm capacitation (e.g. IVF medium) should be used. However, if there will be a long delay before IVF insemination, then the prepared spermatozoa could be resuspended in a sperm buffer and held at ambient temperature until about 2 h beforehand and then washed into fertilization medium and incubated in a CO_2 incubator for the final 90 min before inseminating the oocytes.

   ICSI: Spermatozoa being prepared for ICSI can be processed and resuspended in a sperm buffer since capacitation is irrelevant for fertilization using ICSI. Again, the preparation should be held at ambient temperature (ideally in a styrofoam box to protect it from light and cold draughts) until the ICSI dish is prepared.

4. If a small, known volume of the resuspended pellet preparation is kept back while the remainder is being washed (e.g. 100 µl from the total specimen), the sperm concentration and motility can be determined during the centrifugation step. The washed pellet could then be resuspended into a specific volume to give the desired concentration of progressively motile spermatozoa.

See also the section on 'Working with Difficult Specimens' later in this chapter for information relevant to this part of the SOP.

Protocol: Sperm Preparation Using Density Gradient Centrifugation

Background

Seminal plasma contains decapacitation factors(s) that prevent spermatozoa from undergoing capacitation [2]. Exposure to seminal plasma for more than 30 min after ejaculation can permanently diminish human sperm fertilizing ability [3], and only trace amounts of seminal plasma contaminating prepared sperm populations can decrease their fertilizing capacity [4]. Consequently, spermatozoa for clinical procedures such as IUI or IVF (as well as for laboratory tests of sperm fertilizing ability) must be separated from the seminal plasma environment not only as soon as possible after ejaculation (allowing for the required wait for liquefaction) [6,7], but also as efficiently as possible. Depending on their intended use, the spermatozoa are then suspended in culture media either capable of supporting *in-vitro* capacitation (e.g. for IVF) or not (e.g. for IUI or ICSI).

Principle

Mature, morphologically normal human spermatozoa have a density (specific gravity) above 1.12 g/ml, whereas immature and many abnormal spermatozoa have densities between 1.06–1.09 g/ml [46]. Therefore, if they are centrifuged on a density gradient whose bottom layer has specific gravity of 1.10 g/ml (equivalent to 80% v/v of the original Percoll® colloidal silica product), only the most mature, normal spermatozoa will penetrate this layer and form a pellet.

Specimen

Liquefied, homogeneous human semen, ideally within 30 min of ejaculation. Longer post-ejaculatory delays, incomplete liquefaction and increased viscosity must be noted on the laboratory and report forms. For other types of specimens and abnormal semen samples, see the section on 'Working with Difficult Specimens' later in this chapter.

Equipment

See also Appendix 2.
- Microscope configured for andrology with phase contrast optics (10×, 20× and 40× objectives)
- Air incubator operating at 37°C
- Centrifuge
- Tally counter
- Syringe+tubing adapter to permit volumetric control of glass Pasteur pipettes
- Rubber bulbs to control glass Pasteur pipettes
- Counting chamber (e.g. Makler Chamber)

Disposable Materials

- Semen collection container
- Sterile serological pipette
- Round-bottom polystyrene 7-ml culture tubes (e.g. Falcon #2003 or #2058)
- Conical-bottom polystyrene 15-ml centrifuge tubes (e.g. Falcon #2095)
- Conical-bottom polystyrene 50-ml centrifuge tubes (e.g. Falcon #2074) – for retrograde urine

Note: All disposables that will come into contact with spermatozoa that are to be used for either therapeutic or critical testing purposes should be either pre-tested for sperm toxicity or else obtained from a trusted, reliable manufacturer, e.g. if a sterile plastic syringe is used during processing then it must be of a brand known not to have any deleterious effects upon spermatozoa [60].

Reagents

- Density gradient colloid (silane-coated colloidal silica). See the discussion (above) regarding the correct colloid concentrations to be used for different manufacturers' products (also Note #1).
- 'Sperm buffer' medium for diluting the 100% density gradient colloid
- Sperm washing medium
- *Upper layer:* 40% v/v colloid diluted using sperm buffer, either prepared by mixing 20 ml of stock 100% colloid and 30 ml of sperm buffer or purchased as a ready-made product (see Note #1).
- *Lower layer:* 80% v/v colloid diluted using sperm buffer, either prepared by mixing 40 ml of stock 100% colloid and 10 ml of sperm buffer or purchased as a ready-made product (see Note #1).

Note: All reagents that are to be used in preparing human spermatozoa for therapeutic purposes must be CE-marked (or equivalent) and certified as pyrogen-free and not having any sperm toxicity. Reagents for IVF and ICSI applications should also be certified as not having any embryo toxicity.

Calibration

Centrifugation speeds must not be described using rpm values, as these are highly dependent upon the rotational radius of the centrifuge rotor. Also, the g forces are expressed as g_{max} values, calculated for what the spermatozoa would experience at the bottom of the centrifuge tube (not the bottom of the centrifuge bucket). The formula describing the relationship between rotation speed, rotational radius and g-force is:

$$g = 0.0000112 \times r \times N^2 \quad or \quad N = \sqrt{[g/ (0.0000112 \times r)]}$$

where: g = the maximum g-force achieved at the bottom of the tube
r = the rotational radius (cm)
N = the rotational speed (rpm)

Quality Control

- All specimen containers and processing/preparation tubes must be labelled with two identifiers, e.g. the man's name and the specimen's laboratory reference or ID number. Temporary analytical preparations (e.g. sperm motility slides) can be identified using the specimen's laboratory reference or ID number only.
- Washed sperm preparations from normozoospermic semen samples should show at least 90%, and ideally ≥95%, progressive motility [8].

Procedure

1. Label the following tubes with the subject's name and specimen ID number:

    3× conical-bottom 15-ml centrifuge tubes (two for the gradients, one for the wash)

    1× round-bottom 7-ml culture tube

2. Using a sterile Pasteur pipette, place the upper layer (1.5 ml or 2.0 ml) into each of the 15 ml conical tubes. Then, carefully add the lower layers underneath the upper layers. A clear interface should be visible between the two layers. See Figure 9.4A 'before centrifugation'.

    Alternatively, the lower layer can be placed in a tube first and the upper layer added on top, but this approach often results in a less sharp interface between the two layers than using the under-layering method.

3. Carefully overlay liquefied semen onto each (maximum volume is the same as the volume of the upper gradient layer). Cap the tubes tightly.

4. Centrifuge at 300 g_{max} for 20 min in a swing-out rotor with sealed buckets.

5. For each gradient:

    a) Using a sterile glass Pasteur pipette, carefully aspirate from the meniscus downwards to remove the seminal plasma, upper interface 'raft', upper (40%) layer and the lower interface 'raft'; leave most of the lower (80%) layer in place. Discard the aspirated material. See Figure 9.4B 'after centrifugation'.

    b) Using another clean, sterile glass Pasteur pipette, remove the soft pellet from the bottom of the gradient by direct aspiration (maximum 0.5 ml) from the bottom of the tube beneath the lower (80%) layer. See Figure 9.7. Tip: Blow one or two small bubbles as the pipette tip passes through the meniscus to minimize contamination with residual material from the upper layers of the gradient.

    c) Transfer the pellet to a single clean conical tube.

6. Repeat steps 5a–c for the other gradient.

7. Resuspend the pellets in 5 to 10 ml of sperm buffer and mix gently. Cap the tube.

8. Centrifuge at 500 g_{max} for 10 min.

9. Aspirate the supernatant with a sterile Pasteur pipette and resuspend the pellet in 1 to 3 ml of fresh sperm buffer or IVF medium. Transfer to a small round-bottom culture tube, then:

a) For IUI or DI (sperm resuspended in sperm buffer) leave the sample at ambient temperature in a styrofoam box on the bench until it is collected by the nurse for insemination; or

b) For IVF, (sperm resuspended in IVF medium) equilibrate the loose-capped tube in a CO_2 incubator for 30 min then cap it tightly and place it in the dark at room temperature (i.e. in a cupboard in the embryology laboratory); or

c) For ICSI, cap the tube tightly and place in a 37°C incubator.

10. Assess the concentration and motility of the washed sperm preparation using a Makler chamber (if available, computer-aided sperm analysis (CASA) can be used).

   • Even though there will be some (perhaps even 10%) immotile or dead spermatozoa in the final preparation, this is not a problem and there is no need to perform any further preparation (e.g. swim-up) as it will have no benefit and could compromise sperm function or survival.

   • On occasions, a washed sperm preparation in culture medium might contain a high proportion of hyperactivated cells that, although very vigorous, may present little progression. In such cases the motility report should state the percentages of progressive and hyperactivated cells, as well as the total motility.

Calculations and Results

Use the concentration and sperm motility results to calculate the concentration of progressively motile spermatozoa in the final preparation (see Note #2) and, using the preparation volume, the total number of such spermatozoa in the final preparation.

Interpretation Guidelines

Typically, none, as this is a preparative technique only (but see the section on 'The Trial Wash' later in this chapter). However, if an IUI or IVF sperm preparation shows such reduced motility, serious consideration should be given to switching the treatment modality to ICSI, and almost certainly switching if there is <80% motility. Obviously, this is best established during a pre-treatment 'diagnostic' sperm preparation or 'trial wash', rather than discovering it on the day of treatment – although an aberrant preparation might arise due to an intervening problem with the man (e.g. a bout of febrile illness).

Notes

1. An optimum density gradient for separating mature, normal human spermatozoa requires that the bottom gradient layer have a density of 1.10 g/ml, equivalent to 80% v/v of the original *Percoll*® colloid product. Consequently, products for which the manufacturer does not state the actual colloid concentration might not be able to be employed reliably for optimal sperm preparation.

2. If a small, known volume of the resuspended pellet preparation is kept back while the remainder is being washed (e.g. 100 µl from the total specimen), the sperm concentration and motility can be determined during the centrifugation step. The washed pellet could then be resuspended into a specific volume to give the desired concentration of progressively motile spermatozoa.

Also see the section on 'Working with Difficult Specimens' later in this chapter for information relevant to this part of the SOP.

Evaluating a Sperm Preparation Method

The usefulness or applicability of a sperm preparation technique should be considered in terms of both the quantity and quality of the spermatozoa obtained in the final preparation.

Quantitative Aspects

Here we are usually only concerned with spermatozoa showing progressive motility, since non-progressive spermatozoa have negligible functional competence under any circumstances other than ICSI.

Relative yield is the proportion of progressively motile spermatozoa submitted to a preparative procedure that are present in the final preparation:

$$\text{Yield} = (v \times c \times pm\%)/(V \times C \times PM\%) \times 100\ \%$$

where: v = final preparation volume

c = sperm concentration in the final preparation

pm% = prepared sperm population progressive motility

V = volume of semen used

C = sperm concentration in the semen

PM% = progressive motility in the semen.

Absolute yield is the total number of progressively motile spermatozoa that could be obtained were the whole ejaculate to be used (an allowance usually being made for losing an aliquot of semen used for semen analysis purposes, e.g. 0.3 ml). Note that the progressive motility and Yield are each divided by 100 to convert the percentage values back into fractions.

$$\text{Absolute yield} = (V - 0.3) \times (PM\%/100) \times (\text{Yield}/100)$$

Qualitative Aspects

The quality of the prepared sperm population is also of vital importance, especially when creating embryos, and includes not only considerations of both sperm fertilizing ability and sperm DNA integrity, but also the yield purity (e.g. the reduction or elimination of infectious micro-organisms such as bacteria and viruses) [2].

Dealing with Atypical Semen Specimens

Highly Viscous Samples

It can be extremely difficult to obtain good yields of motile spermatozoa from highly viscous samples, but do not 'needle' viscous semen through a 19G or 22G needle as the high shear forces exerted upon the spermatozoa can damage them [61]. Instead, dilute the semen with a 1–2× volume of sperm buffer (i.e. a medium that is not based on a bicarbonate buffer, so that it can be used safely under an air atmosphere) and mix gently using a sterile Pasteur pipette before loading onto the gradient. If the sample does not disperse within 2 min of pipetting, incubate at 37°C for 10 min and then mix further. Once the sample has been successfully diluted it can be loaded onto the gradients as usual.

'Dirty' Specimens

With semen samples that are heavily contaminated with particulate debris or contain high numbers of other cells, the 'rafts' at the interfaces between either the seminal plasma and 40% layer or the 40% and 80% layers might form too quickly, and/or be too dense, and block the gradient, drastically reducing the sperm yield. To avoid this problem:

a)   Only process part of the ejaculate; and/or

b)   Load less semen onto each gradient, perhaps dividing the sample over four gradients instead of two; and/or

c)   Use longer columns of colloid, e.g. 3 ml per layer; and/or

d)   When loading the semen onto the gradient, mix it gently with the upper one-fifth of the upper layer; and/or

e)   Prepare a three-step gradient using layers of 40%, 60% and 80% colloid (but do not use a lower layer of >80% colloid as it will reduce the sperm yield unnecessarily).

Cryopreserved Specimens

Cryopreserved spermatozoa are in a highly hypertonic medium (due to the cryoprotectant medium) and hence will suffer extreme osmotic shock upon entering the upper layer of a density gradient, and hence decrease their specific gravity – causing them to be too buoyant to pass through the density gradient (and also causing impaired sperm function). Therefore, cryopreserved sperm specimens must be diluted with a relatively large volume of 'isotonic' medium prior to loading onto the gradients. For spermatozoa cryopreserved using a traditional TEST-yolk-glycerol cryoprotectant medium, a 10× dilution works well, but with many egg-yolk-free cryoprotectant media, a 5× dilution is sufficient. The thawed specimen should be diluted slowly (drop-wise) with constant gentle mixing over a period of at least 10 min. Note that the maximum volume that can be loaded onto a single gradient is based on the original semen component, i.e. if semen was diluted 1:1 with a cryoprotectant medium, and then diluted 5× after thawing, 1 ml of the original semen is now contained in 12 ml of diluted material, making it very hard to overload a gradient. If the total volume did exceed the maximum volume that could be loaded onto a pair of gradients, the diluted post-thaw material could be centrifuged at 500 g_{max} × 10 min and, after removing and discarding the supernatant, the pellet resuspended in 1–2 ml of fresh medium (still, ideally, sperm buffer), and then loaded onto a pair of gradients. This procedure is sub-optimal, but relatively safe because the cells that generate ROS during centrifugation do not survive the freezing and thawing process.

Poor-Quality Specimens

An increased yield can be obtained from most samples, but especially low concentration ones and ones with low sperm motility, if slightly less dense layers are used, e.g. 72% and 36% colloid. However, this is only achieved by recovering less dense, and hence less good quality, spermatozoa, and should only be used as a last resort. Whatever spermatozoa can be recovered from a standard 40/80 gradient will always be the best available from the specimen.

Retrograde Ejaculate Urine Specimens

In the case of retrograde ejaculation, the semen does not pass out to the exterior through the urethra ('antegrade ejaculation') but passes back into the bladder. Various protocols exist for managing these cases (see Chapter 3), but after the retrograde ejaculate urine specimen has been concentrated by centrifugation (e.g. 500 g_{max} × 10 min in one or more 50 ml polystyrene conical tubes) and resuspended into a small volume of a 'sperm buffer', the material can be layered over one or several two-step (40%/80%) density gradients and processed as though it were a normal semen sample.

Surgically Retrieved Sperm Specimens

In the case of sperm suspensions obtained from the epididymis (or after homogenization of testicular tissue), it might be necessary to separate all the spermatozoa from the other cells, etc. This can be most easily achieved by centrifuging the material through a single column of 40% colloid, using the standard conditions of 300 g_{max} × 20 min. After carefully removing most (e.g. ¾) of the supernatant, the pellet is recovered through the remaining ¼ of the layer using a clean, sterile glass Pasteur pipette. See also Chapter 11.

Infectious Ejaculates

To minimize the risk of transmission of infectious agents, DGC can be used in conjunction with a special insert inside the gradient tube(s) to ensure separation between the semen and the pellet during harvesting (see Figure 9.8) [62]. The outer chamber of the *ProInsert* device is used for loading the density gradient layers, while the central channel is only used for retrieving the sperm pellet (using a special

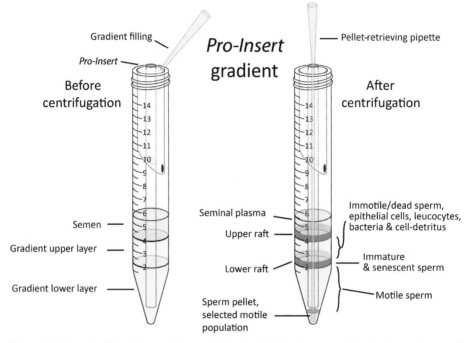

Figure 9.8 Illustration of the *Pro-Insert* device to minimize the risk of viral carry-over during density gradient centrifugation ('DGC') preparation of spermatozoa. Illustration courtesy of Nidacon International AB (Mölndahl, Sweden).

pipette supplied with the device), so the pellet should never come into contact with the semen. This technique has been validated for HIV-positive semen samples [62,63], as well as for minimizing bacterial contamination in the final washed sperm preparation [64].

Protease treatment can also be incorporated into the process to destroy the virus [62,65]. The protease can be included in the gradient layers and then eliminated during the washing step. Additionally, a protease inhibitor could be used in conjunction to increase protection of the spermatozoa from prolonged action by the protease: e.g. protease in the upper gradient layer and inhibitor in the lower layer, or protease in the gradient layers and inhibitor in the washing buffer, although the latter approach might well require a second washing step to remove the inhibitor from the final preparation.

The Trial Wash

Many laboratories perform an initial sperm preparation, sometimes comparing two or more alternative methods, during diagnostic workup, to establish the suitability of a subject's semen for particular treatment modalities. Most commonly this involves at least a DGC preparation and hence the often-used term of 'Trial Wash'. Based on the yield found during the Trial Wash, including extrapolation from the aliquot processed to what would have been obtained had the entire ejaculate been processed, the suitability of semen specimens for IUI or IVF can be ascertained.

In cases where too few spermatozoa can be obtained in the final washed preparation to permit IVF, then a need for ICSI is established – indeed this is one of the few situations where a *real* need for ICSI can be identified. Observed low results on a basic semen analysis are not considered sufficient grounds for such a decision [8,66].

In cases where the washed sperm population shows poor progressive motility, a Trial Wash can reveal what might otherwise have been an unexpected poor preparation on the day of ART treatment, perhaps necessitating conversion from IVF to ICSI. In some cases, despite apparently 'good' semen quality at a basic semen analysis, the spermatozoa do not respond well to being washed. As noted already <80% progressive motility in a final sperm preparation carries a significant risk of possible sperm dysfunction. Hopefully, this finding was due to biology and not as a result of a poor technical procedure. The Vienna Consensus on fresh ART cycle KPIs has established the competence and aspirational benchmark values for progressive motility in a final sperm preparation as >90% and ≥95% respectively [8].

Selecting a Sperm Preparation Method

Selecting an appropriate sperm preparation method for clinical or research use requires consideration of the following perspectives:

- Relative simplicity and rapidity of a method, for reasons of laboratory efficiency.
- Cost of the materials (and equipment) required for the method.
- Any risk of iatrogenic damage inherent in the method, balanced against the level of protection from iatrogenic damage that the method affords.
- General applicability of a method, i.e. the range of semen qualities relative to what is seen by the laboratory for which the method will provide adequate yields of motile spermatozoa for the intended form of treatment or experimental design.

Any method being considered must employ optimized technique, and staff must be trained in its proper performance. Failure to observe all protocol details, including correct product selection and matching (as already discussed in this chapter), can result in reduced yields as well as iatrogenic damage to the spermatozoa [18,53]. Claims by some vendors in marketing materials and representations that any and all centrifugation will damage spermatozoa need to be balanced against experimental evidence from properly designed and executed DGC studies as well as historically widely successful clinical outcomes.

Defining 'acceptable yield' relates to the ultimate use of the prepared sperm population: e.g. IUI might require 5×10^6 motile spermatozoa in a 100 μl volume for insemination, whereas IVF uses only about 80,000 motile spermatozoa per droplet or well, even if oocytes are inseminated as a group. 'Heavy insemination' as a form of IVF for men with moderate male factor (up to 500,000/ml: [67]) has largely been replaced by ICSI as a more reliable way to ensure a good fertilization rate.

Because of the risks of potentially severe detrimental effects upon the spermatozoa, methods involving any centrifugal washing of semen that result in the pelleting of unselected spermatozoa (e.g. 'swim-out' or 'sperm-rise') have been contra-indicated since the late 1980s [13,14,18].

Direct swim-up from semen ('DSUS') remains the simplest technique for obtaining populations of highly motile spermatozoa and has been recommended by the WHO for >30 years. It can be a very rapid procedure when working with normal semen samples but the most widely applicable and practical method for preparing motile sperm populations from both normal and abnormal semen samples is DGC. Although the results can be disappointing with asthenozoospermic samples, whatever population of spermatozoa is obtained does represent the good quality spermatozoa that were present in the ejaculate.

Processing Multiple Samples

Risk management purists assert that only a single semen specimen should be processed by a scientist at any one time, always using a separate centrifuge and workstation for each specimen. However, in a busy clinical laboratory this is frequently not just impracticable but impossible, as it would require unrealistic numbers of staff and centrifuges. Due process mapping and analysis reveals that proper observance of a carefully designed process, in conjunction with a formal risk assessment, can permit the 'safe' processing of more than one sample at a time, provided that the following are ensured [68]:

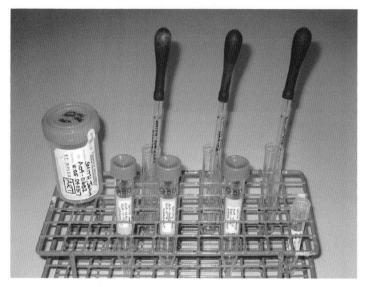

Figure 9.9 An example of a system to minimize the risk of cross-contamination between sperm specimens being processed in parallel. All the tubes, etc., for a given specimen are placed in a single rack so that even if two specimens are being centrifuged together, they are each harvested and resuspended separately. Note that the semen collection jar is labelled with the man's name and the andrology lab reference number (A04-0682) as well as the date and time of collection. Each tube and pipette are labelled with the name plus both the andrology lab number and the oocyte retrieval case number (R04-0179) as identifiers, along with the date and the purpose of each item. There is no label on the rack because it is the identity of each of the individual items that must be verified at each stage of the process; if there was a large label on the rack there would be a tendency for the operator to read only that when going to work on a sample. Reproduced from [58] with permission.

- Each specimen is allocated to a separate tube rack (see Figure 9.9).
- All disposable materials are labelled using at least two unique identifiers, one of which must be a number (since the human brain innately 'completes' sequences of letters as words), and perhaps also using a colour-coding scheme.
- All the disposable material to be used for a specimen are held together in a defined working area, such as a plastic box or tray.
- Racks and trays are *never* labelled, only tubes, so as to ensure their proper re-identification at every step.
- Pipettes should be labelled for each specimen and organized in such a way that they cannot be confused between specimens being processed in parallel, e.g. they can be held in a second rack in the tray alongside the tube rack.
- Only one specimen is actually worked on at any point in time, i.e. only one rack or tray is in a scientist's 'active' work area at a time, and a scientist *never* has tubes belonging to more than one sample open at a time.
- Multiple samples may be centrifuged together so long as there is an established procedure for verification of each tube's identity afterwards, before it is opened.
- Each re-identification step should be documented and, if possible, witnessed.

References

1. Yanagimachi R. Mammalian fertilization. In: Knobil E, Neill JD, eds. *The Physiology of Reproduction*, 2nd edn. New York: Raven Press, 1994, 189–317.

2. Mortimer D. Sperm preparation methods. *J Androl* 2000; **21**: 357–66.

3. Rogers BJ, Perreault SD, Bentwood BJ, et al. Variability in the human-hamster in vitro assay for fertility evaluation. *Fertil Steril* 1983; **39**: 204–11.

4. Kanwar KC, Yanagimachi R, Lopata A. Effects of human seminal plasma on fertilizing capacity of human spermatozoa. *Fertil Steril* 1979; **31**: 321–7.

5. Tvrdá E, Arroyo F, Gosálvez J. Dynamic assessment of human sperm DNA damage I: the effect of seminal plasma-sperm co-incubation after ejaculation. *Int Urol Nephrol* 2018; **50**: 1381–8.

6. Punjabi U, et al. Time intervals between semen production, initiation of analysis, and IUI significantly influence clinical pregnancies and live births. *J Assist Reprod Genet* 2021; **38**: 421–8.

7. Yavas Y, Selub MR. Intrauterine insemination (IUI) pregnancy outcome is enhanced by shorter intervals from semen collection to sperm wash, from sperm wash to IUI time, and from semen collection to IUI time. *Fertil Steril* 2004; **82**: 1638–47.

8. ESHRE Special Interest Group of Embryology and Alpha Scientists in Reproductive Medicine. The Vienna consensus: report of an expert meeting on the development of ART laboratory performance indicators. *Reprod Biomed Online* 2017; **35**: 494–510 and *Hum Reprod Open* 2017; hox011. https://doi.org/10.1093/hropen/hox011

9. Mortimer D. Sperm recovery techniques to maximize fertilizing capacity. *Reprod Fertil Devel* 1994; **6**: 25–31.

10. Mortimer D. *Practical Laboratory Andrology*. New York: Oxford University Press, 1995.

11. Jeulin C, Serres C, Jouannet P. The effects of centrifugation, various synthetic media and temperature on the motility and vitality of human spermatozoa. *Reprod Nutr Dévélop* 1982; **22**: 81–91.

12. Friedman AJ, Juneau-Norcross M, Sedensky B. Antisperm antibody production following intrauterine insemination. *Hum Reprod* 1991; **6**: 1125–8.

13. Aitken RJ, Clarkson JS. Cellular basis of defective sperm function and its association with the genesis of reactive oxygen species by human spermatozoa. *J Reprod Fertil* 1987; **81**: 459–69.

14. Aitken RJ, Clarkson JS. Significance of reactive oxygen species and antioxidants in defining the efficacy of sperm preparation techniques. *J Androl* 1988; **9**: 367–76.

15. Selley ML, Lacey MJ, Bartlett MR, et al. Content of significant amounts of a cytotoxic end-product of lipid peroxidation in human semen. *J Reprod Fertil* 1991; **92**: 291–8.

16. Aitken RJ, Gordon E, Harkiss D, et al. Relative impact of oxidative stress on the functional competence and genomic integrity of human spermatozoa. *Biol Reprod* 1998; **59**: 1037–46.

17. Aitken RJ. Free radicals, lipid peroxidation and sperm function. *Reprod Fertil Devel* 1995; **7**: 659–68.

18. Mortimer D. Sperm preparation techniques and iatrogenic failures of in-vitro fertilization. *Hum Reprod* 1991; **6**: 173–6.

19. Katz DF, Morales P, Samuels SJ, Overstreet JW. Mechanisms of filtration of morphologically abnormal human sperm by cervical mucus. *Fertil Steril* 1990; **54**: 513–16.

20. Mortimer D. Sperm transport in the female genital tract. In: Grudzinskas JG, Yovich JL, eds, *Cambridge Reviews in Human Reproduction, Volume 2: Gametes – The Spermatozoon*. Cambridge: Cambridge University Press, 1995, 157–74.

21. Mortimer ST. A critical review of the physiological importance and analysis of sperm movement in mammals. *Hum Reprod Update* 1997; **3**: 403–39.

22. Tea NT, Jondet M, Scholler R. A 'migration-gravity sedimentation' method for collecting motile spermatozoa from human semen. In: Harrison RF, Bonnar J, Thompson W, eds, *In Vitro Fertilization, Embryo Transfer and Early Pregnancy*. Lancaster: MTP Press Ltd., 1984, 117–20.

23. Botella-Llusiá J. Measurement of linear progression of the human spermatozoon as an index of male fertility. *Int J Fertil* 1956; **1**: 113–30.

24. Kremer J. A simple sperm penetration test. *Int J Fertil* 1965; **10**: 209–14.

25. Kricka LJ, Nozaki O, Heyner S, et al. Applications of a microfabricated device for evaluating sperm function. *Clin Chem* 1993; **39**: 1944–7.

26. Zhang B, Yin TL, Yang J. A novel microfluidic device for selecting human sperm to increase the proportion of morphologically normal, motile sperm with uncompromised DNA integrity. *Anal Methods* 2015; **7**: 5981.

27. Nosrati R, Vollmer M, Eamer L, et al. Rapid selection of sperm with high DNA integrity. *Lab Chip* 2014; **14**: 1142.

28. Ebner T, Shebl O, Moser M, et al. Easy sperm processing technique allowing exclusive accumulation and later usage of DNA-strandbreak-free spermatozoa. *Reprod Biomed Online* 2011; **22**: 37–43.

29. Yetkinel S, Kilicdag EB, Aytac PC, et al. Effects of the microfluidic chip technique in sperm selection for intracytoplasmic sperm injection for unexplained infertility: a prospective, randomized controlled trial. *J Assist Reprod Genet* 2019; **36**: 403–9.

30. Gode F, Bodur T, Gunturkun F, et al. Comparison of microfluid sperm sorting chip and density gradient methods for use in intrauterine insemination cycles. *Fertil Steril* 2019; **112**: 842–8.

31. Quinn MM, Jalalian L, Ribeiro S, et al. Microfluidic sorting selects sperm for clinical use with reduced DNA damage compared to density gradient centrifugation with swim-up in split semen samples. *Hum Reprod* 2018; **33**: 1388–93.

32. Hong CY, Chaput de Saintonge DM, Turner P. A simple method to measure drug effects on human sperm motility. *Br J Clin Pharmacol* 1981; **11**: 385–7.

33. Mortimer D, Leslie EE, Kelly RW, Templeton AA. Morphological selection of human spermatozoa in vivo and in vitro. *J Reprod Fertil* 1982; **64**: 391–9.

34. Sherman JK, Paulson JD, Liu KC. Effect of glass wool filtration on ultrastructure of human spermatozoa. *Fertil Steril* 1981; **36**: 643–7.

35. Said TM, Land JA. Effects of advanced selection methods on sperm quality and ART outcome: a systematic review. *Hum Reprod Update* 2011; **17**: 719–33.

36. Vaughan DA, Sakkas D. Sperm selection methods in the 21st century. *Biol Reprod* 2019; **101**: 1076–82.

37. Said TM, Grunewald S, Paasch U, et al. Advantage of combining magnetic cell separation with sperm preparation techniques. *Reprod BioMed Online* 2005; **10**: 740–6.

38. Dirican EK, Özgün OD, Akarsu S, et al. Clinical outcome of magnetic activated cell sorting of nonapoptotic spermatozoa before density gradient centrifugation for assisted reproduction. *J Assist Reprod Genet* 2008; **25**: 375–81.

39. Polak de FE, Denaday F. Single and twin ongoing pregnancies in two cases of previous ART failure after ICSI performed with sperm sorted using annexin V microbeads. *Fertil Steril* 2010; **94**: 351–8.

40. Romany L, Garrido N, Motato Y, et al. Removal of annexin V-positive sperm cells for intracytoplasmic sperm injection in ovum donation cycles does not improve reproductive outcome: a controlled and randomized trial in unselected males. *Fertil Steril* 2014; **102**: 1567–75.

41. Hasanen E, Elqusi K, ElTanbouly S, et al. PICSI vs. MACS for abnormal sperm DNA fragmentation ICSI cases: a prospective randomized trial. *J Assist Reprod Genet* 2020; **37**: 2605–13.

42. Lepine S, McDowell S, Searle LM, et al. Advanced sperm selection techniques for assisted reproduction. *Cochrane Database Syst Rev* 2019; **7**: CD010461.

43. Fleming SD, Ilad RS, Griffin AM, et al. Prospective controlled trial of an electrophoretic method of sperm preparation for assisted reproduction: comparison with density gradient centrifugation. *Hum Reprod* 2008; **23**: 2646–51.

44. Parmegiani L, Cognigni GE, Bernardi S, et al. 'Physiologic ICSI': hyaluronic acid (HA) favors selection of spermatozoa without DNA fragmentation and with normal nucleus, resulting in improvement of embryo quality. *Fertil Steril* 2010; **93**: 598–604.

45. Worrilow KC, Eid S, Woodhouse D, et al. Use of hyaluronan in the selection of sperm for intracytoplasmic sperm injection (ICSI): significant improvement in clinical outcomes – multicenter, double-blinded and randomized controlled trial. *Hum Reprod* 2013; **28**: 306–14.

46. Miller D, Pavitt S, Sharma V, et al. Physiological, hyaluronan-selected intracytoplasmic sperm injection for infertility treatment (HABSelect): a parallel, two-group, randomised trial. *Lancet* 2019; **393**: 416–22.

47. Gellert-Mortimer ST, Clarke GN, Baker HWG, et al. Evaluation of Nycodenz and Percoll density gradients for the selection of motile human spermatozoa. *Fertil Steril* 1988; **49**: 335–41.

48. Sbracia M, Sayme N, Grasso J, et al. Sperm function and choice of preparation media: comparison of Percoll and Accudenz discontinuous density gradients. *Androl* 1996; **17**: 61–7.

49. Smith TT, Byers M, Kaftani D, Whitford W. The use of iodixanol as a density gradient material for separating human sperm from semen. *Arch Androl* 1997; **38**: 223–30.

50. Oshio S, Kaneko S, Iizuka R, Mohri H. Effects of gradient centrifugation on human sperm. *Arch Androl* 1987; **17**: 85–93.

51. World Health Organization. *WHO Laboratory Manual for the Analysis of Human Semen and Sperm-Cervical Mucus Interaction*, 4th edn. Cambridge: Cambridge University Press, 1999.

52. World Health Organization. *WHO Laboratory Manual for the Examination and Processing of Human Semen*, 5th edn. Geneva: World Health Organization, 2010.

53. Aitken RJ, Finnie JM, Muscio L, et al. Potential importance of transition metals in the induction of DNA damage by sperm preparation media. *Hum Reprod* 2014; **29**: 2136–47.

54. Gomez E, Aitken J. Impact of in vitro fertilization culture media on peroxidative damage to human spermatozoa. *Fertil Steril* 1996; **65**: 880–8.

55. Velez de la Calle JF. Human spermatozoa selection in improved discontinuous Percoll gradients. *Fertil Steril* 1991; **56**: 737–42.

56. Sakkas D, Manicardi GC, Tomlinson M, et al. The use of two density gradient centrifugation techniques and the swim-up method to separate spermatozoa with chromatin and nuclear DNA anomalies. *Hum Reprod* 2000; **15**: 1112–16.

57. Tomlinson MJ, Moffatt O, Manicardi GC, et al. Interrelationships between seminal parameters and sperm nuclear DNA damage before and after density gradient centrifugation: implications for assisted conception. *Hum Reprod* 2001; **16**: 2160–5.

58. Shoukir Y, Chardonnens D, Campana A, Sakkas D. Blastocyst development from supernumerary embryos after intracytoplasmic sperm injection: a paternal influence? *Hum Reprod* 1998; **13**: 1632–7.

59. Shalgi R, Smith TT, Yanagimachi R. A quantitative comparison of the passage of capacitated and uncapacitated hamster spermatozoa through the uterotubal junction. *Biol Reprod* 1992; **46**: 419–24.

60. de Ziegler D, Cedars MI, Hamilton F, et al. Factors influencing maintenance of sperm motility during in vitro processing. *Fertil Steril* 1987; **48**: 816–20.

61. Knuth UA, Neuwinger J, Nieschlag E. Bias to routine semen analysis by uncontrolled changes in laboratory environment – detection by long-term sampling of monthly means for quality control. *Int J Androl* 1989; **12**: 375–83.

62. Loskutoff NM, Huyser C, Singh R, et al. Use of a novel washing method combining multiple density gradients and trypsin for removing human immunodeficiency virus-1 and hepatitis C virus from semen. *Fertil Steril* 2005; **84**: 1001–10.

63. Fourie JM, Loskutoff N, Huyser C. Semen decontamination for the elimination of seminal HIV-1. *Reprod Biomed Online* 2015; **30**: 296–302.

64. Fourie J, Loskutoff N, Huyser C. Elimination of bacteria from human semen during sperm preparation using density gradient centrifugation with a novel tube insert. *Andrologia* 2012; **44 Suppl 1**: 513–17.

65. Fourie J, Loskutoff N, Huyser C. Treatment of human sperm with serine protease during density gradient centrifugation. *J Assist Reprod Genet* 2012; **29**: 1273–9.

66. Mortimer D, Mortimer ST. The case against intracytoplasmic sperm injection for all. In: Aitken J, Mortimer D, Kovacs G, eds, *Male and Sperm Factors that Maximize IVF Success*. Cambridge: Cambridge University Press, 2020, 130–40.

67. Wolf DP, Byrd W, Dandekar P, Quigley MM. Sperm concentration and the fertilization of human eggs in vitro. *Biol Reprod* 1984; **31**: 837–48.

68. Mortimer ST, Mortimer D. *Quality and Risk Management in the IVF Laboratory*, 2nd edn. Cambridge: Cambridge University Press, 2015.

Sperm Cryopreservation

Cryobiology Basics

The main objective of cryopreservation of cells is to maintain their viability and functionality over extended periods of sub-zero storage. Cryopreserved cells are stored at −196°C (in liquid nitrogen). At this temperature, neither the phenomenon of diffusion nor sufficient latent thermal energy exist for chemical reactions to occur. Difficulties of cryopreservation do not arise from exposure to low temperatures *per se* but rather from the cooling and warming processes. There are different cryopreservation methods, which depend on the speed of exposure of the spermatozoa to cryoprotectant molecules, the cryoprotectant concentration, and the rate of temperature reduction, which includes slow freezing (0.5–10.0°C/min), relatively slow freezing or rapid freezing (50–2500°C/min), and ultrarapid freezing or vitrification (approximately 10,000–700,000°C/min).

Physical Principles of Freezing and Vitrification

Freezing is the phase transition of liquid becoming a solid by lowering the temperature to below its melting temperature (Tm). Freezing is the reorganization of water molecules into ice crystals, the formation of which first requires nucleation. The classic theory says that stable ice nucleation forms by random clustering of water molecules. Therefore, nucleation is a statistical occurrence by its nature: the more water molecules present, the higher the chances of nucleation occurring. For this reason, the chances of ice nucleation occurring is directly correlated with the volume of the sample. Freezing requires nucleating factors which will induce ice crystal growth, either spontaneously as the temperature reduces, or deliberately by an abrupt, usually local, reduction in temperature, leading to what is referred to as seeding. Once ice nucleation has occurred, the very small (harmless) ice crystals propagate at a very high velocity until larger (harmful) ice crystals form; this velocity is inversely correlated with viscosity [1,2].

Vitrification is the solidification of a solution into a solid glass-like state without forming any ice crystals (Figure 10.1). However, most authors consider vitrification of a solution to be the formation of a solid glass-like state without the expansion of very small ice crystals; in this case the intracellular water undergoes an extreme increase in viscosity without forming large intracellular ice crystals. The temperature at which this occurs is called the glass transition temperature (Tg). The probability of vitrification is a direct function of the cooling rate and viscosity of the liquid and an inverse function of the volume. In general, it requires high viscosity, high cooling rates and a small sample volume. Increasing the viscosity or cooling rate, or decreasing the volume, will all increase the probability of vitrification.

When the temperature decreases and viscosity increases, the Tm of a solution also decreases (it is more difficult to solidify). However, the Tg of a solution increases at the same time (it is easier to vitrify). In other words, with large amounts of exogenous thickeners (high viscosity), the Tg is high and therefore a relatively moderate cooling rate is necessary to reach the Tg (equilibrium vitrification). Conversely, by increasing the cooling rate (10^4–10^{6o}C/min), such high viscosities are not required, and with certain cells such as human spermatozoa (see below), the Tg can be reached without needing high concentrations of solutes (kinetic vitrification).

Thawing is the opposite of freezing: the melting of large ice crystals. Since in vitrification there is no large ice crystal formation, this term should not be used to refer to the warming of a previously vitrified system, but simply warming. During the warming of a vitrified solution, the transition from glass state to

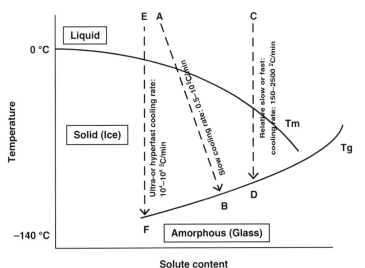

Figure 10.1 Schematic phase diagram comparing three mechanisms for cell vitrification (adapted from [83]). (A-B) Slow freezing. The solute concentration changes dynamically during freezing of extracellular ice and the liquid phase becomes more and more concentrated. When Tg is reached, the cells are vitrified in the inter-ice channels that are surrounded by ice. (C-D) Equilibrium vitrification. This method requires high concentrations of cryoprotective agents (CPAs), which elevate the viscosity of the milieu and prevents the formation and/or growing of both intracellular and extracellular ice. (E-F) Kinetic vitrification. This occurs intracellularly at a much lower concentration of the CPA, or even without permeating CPA, and requires much higher cooling rates to prevent ice formation inside the cells. The ice can still be formed outside the cells but it has no time to cause any osmotic damage to the cells, as kinetic vitrification occurs in a fraction of a second. Due to the special characteristics of spermatozoa, kinetic vitrification can be carried out with a relatively slow cooling rate. Tm = melting temperature; Tg = glass transition temperature.

liquid state is known as devitrification, during which only very small ice crystals are formed. However, if the warming temperature is slow, large harmful crystals are produced and the process is known as recrystallization. Therefore, the formation of ice nucleation (and thus the possibility of large crystal formation) takes place at two points. During cooling, ice growth will be limited by the small number of nuclei which form at higher temperatures where the growth rate is significant. Nucleation continues and accelerates during cooling (crystallization), until the glass transition temperature for water is exceeded. At these temperatures, the nuclei have already formed, but they are too cold to grow. During warming, nucleation resumes when the temperature range close to the Tg is passed again. Consequently, both the nuclei created during cooling and those created during warming are in the solution. This means not only that many more nuclei are present during warming than during cooling, but also that during warming vastly more nuclei will be present at temperatures that favour rapid ice growth (recrystallization). Hence the warming rates required to avoid recrystallization are found to be far higher than the cooling rates [3].

Some authors consider that in order for a cell cryopreservation technique to be called vitrification, vitrification has to take place in the internal and external medium, so they do not consider it correct to refer to procedures which only involve the vitrification of the intracellular medium as sperm vitrification [3].

Cryobiology of the Spermatozoon

Many of the advances made in cryobiology stem from experimentation with spermatozoa, due, among other reasons, to the ease of demonstrating their survival. The spermatozoon presents several characteristics which are necessary to highlight when analysing its behaviour in freezing and vitrification.

A key factor for survival in freezing is that all the regions of a cell are in the same stage (temperature). When the volume is large (e.g. an oocyte), the outer region may have different temperatures to the more central region. The small size of the spermatozoon means it has a greater capacity of diffusion in the intracellular temperature. But in addition to volume, the shape has an influence on the surface of the cell, which will determine the entry and exit of molecules during freezing and the transmission of the temperature to the cell interior. Thus, when the surface:volume ratio is low, the exchange of temperature and solutes will be slower than when this ratio is high. The elliptical form of the spermatozoon means this ratio is much higher than for oocytes (4.8 vs 0.03).

The movement of water across a cell's plasma membrane will depend on the physical factors already mentioned, but also on the plasma membrane's permeability to water and solutes. Considering plasma membrane hydrophobicity, mechanisms other than simple diffusion are required to allow water transport across the plasma membrane in certain cell functions. Aquaporins (AQPs) are a family of ubiquitous integral transmembrane proteins which allow the passive transport of water through cell membranes. Moreover, some AQPs also facilitate the transport of small solutes such as glycerol (aquaglyceroporins). The 'SuperAQPs' group are found specifically in the membrane of intracellular organelles and regulate organelle volume and intra-vesicular homeostasis, while being involved in both water and glycerol transport. These three kinds of AQPs have been identified in human sperm cells. The presence of these channels facilitates the entrance and exit of water and permeating cryoprotective agents (CPAs) [4].

As already noted, the more water molecules present in a cell, the higher the chances of nucleation occurring. The water content of spermatozoa, estimated from their osmotically inactive volume, is only 23–60%, lower than the 80% water that cytoplasm usually contains [3]. The composition of the sperm cytoplasm is rich in molecules (proteins, polymers, sugars and nucleotides) which act by increasing the internal viscosity and therefore hindering ice formation. Another factor which hinders ice formation is the presence of solid surfaces, whose organization of local water structure tends to inhibit ice formation. The special compartmentalized structure of the spermatozoon means that many water molecules are in contact with solid surfaces (plasma membrane, organelle membranes and cytoskeleton) which hinders ice formation during freezing.

These characteristics mean that the spermatozoon quickly becomes dehydrated, and it is difficult for the little water which remains inside to form crystals, achieving a glassy state inside the spermatozoon during slow freezing [5], although not in the external medium. These cryobiological characteristics allow the cooling rate to be achieved easily and produce sperm vitrification without needing to use permeating CPAs, even when using relatively large volumes (0.5 ml).

Cellular Responses to Freezing and Thawing

Cold Shock or Chilling Damage (from 37°C to 0°C)

Cold shock is the damage to cells caused by their sensitivity to the cooling rate, and it results from lipid phase transition effects and ionic imbalances such as calcium loading. Chilling sensitivity is damage arising from cells' sensitivity to a specific temperature or temperature range. Lipids can exist in an ordered rigid state (gel) or in a more flexible and relatively disordered state (fluid). The transition from one state to another takes place over a certain temperature range. This temperature depends on the composition of the fatty acids that compose the membrane. Most membranes of eukaryotic cells have a melting temperature between 0°C and 15°C. The transition phase of a plasma membrane does not occur simultaneously in all of its phospholipids and therefore there is a co-existence of domains in both fluid and gel states during the transition. This situation produces defects in the packing of membranes (mechanical shearing) and conformational changes in membrane topography that give rise to non-linear kinetic responses in some enzymes. These changes are associated with a greater permeability of solutes through the membrane [6].

Ice Formation (0°C to –130°C)

The existence of solutes in the water produces a decrease in the freezing (cryoscopic) point to between –10°C and –15°C and, as a result, the crystallization of water occurs at lower temperatures than the freezing point of pure water (0°C). When temperatures are this low, the sample is supercooled. In this situation, the onset of ice formation is random. To avoid this problem, in many protocols ice formation is provoked in the extracellular medium by means of an abrupt reduction in temperature ('seeding') – thus the system is guaranteed to be in phase change, and ice is present. Ice formation can be induced in many ways, but typically by touching the specimen with a small object that is at a lower temperature than that of the phase change. Seeding is important because, during the crystallization process, a sample releases sufficient heat (latent heat of fusion) to cause a sharp increase in temperature, and consequently the sample temperature does not decrease in tandem with the fall in the chamber temperature. In fact, the sample temperature can remain static for two to three minutes before resuming its decrease [6].

The formation of ice in the extracellular medium removes water from this compartment and this triggers a solvent flow across the semi-permeable membrane towards the region with a higher concentration of solutes. As a result, formation of ice in the extracellular medium provokes cellular dehydration [7].

Thawing

During the thawing process, the osmotic changes that take place are the opposite of what occurred during freezing: as frozen water changes state (solid to liquid), the concentration of solutes in the extracellular medium is progressively reduced and the cell hydrates in order to compensate for the difference in concentration between the extracellular and intracellular compartments. Fast rewarming rates are required for optimal cell recovery due to the formation and growth of small intracellular ice crystals while the cell is between the ice transition point of water (about −132°C) and the melting point of the material. In addition, as the post-thaw temperature increases the lipids and proteins of the plasma membrane undergo structural rearrangements.

Cryodamage

When cell survival is plotted as a function of the cooling rate, the curve produced is a characteristic inverted U-shape (Figure 10.2). In order to clarify this effect of cooling on survival rates, the 'two-factor' hypothesis proposes two different mechanisms to account for cellular damage during the cryopreservation process: ice production and osmotic stress.

Intracellular Ice Formation

Once extracellular ice formation has begun, along with the corresponding cellular dehydration, events in the intracellular space depend on the cooling rate. If freezing occurs too quickly, the cell will not be able to dehydrate efficiently, and the remaining water will form intracellular ice – and the more ice formed within the cell, the lower the chance of cellular survival [8].

Osmotic stress is active at low cooling rates and is related to the mechanical cellular deformation caused by the reduction in size originating from the intense process of dehydration, and by prolonged cellular exposure to high concentrations of electrolytes. This mechanism is known as the 'solution effect' [7]. Two complementary theories exist to explain the phenomenon of osmotic stress during the cryopreservation process:

- The hypothesis of high ion concentrations attributes the cause to the interaction between the high ion concentrations in the extracellular medium and the membrane proteins [6].
- The hypothesis of minimum cellular volume relates the effect of dehydration caused during the concentration of solutes and cellular death with the return of isotonic conditions after the freezing process (osmotic shock). As the cell volume decreases during freezing (by dehydration) the compression of the cytoplasmic contents increases the resistance of the cell to further loss of volume, and when this physical resistance is exceeded an irreversible change in permeability is caused [9].

In summary, when lower cooling rates are used, cellular damage is caused by high extracellular solute concentrations and by high cooling rates causing intracellular ice formation. There is an optimal cooling range, referred to as the 'transition zone', for each cell in which these damaging conditions are minimized, and hence when there will be maximum probability of cell cryosurvival (Figure 10.2). Although the universal validity of this principle has been verified, each cell type

221

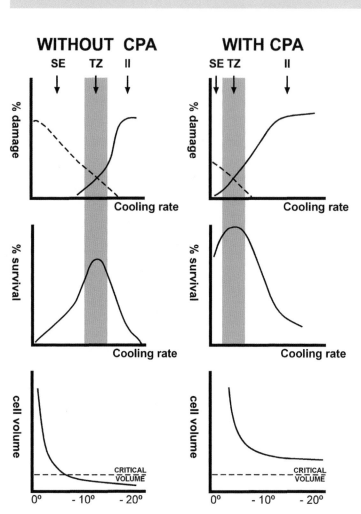

Figure 10.2 Cryodamage, survival and cell volume changes during cryopreservation with and without CPA. II = intracellular ice; SE = solution effect; TZ = transition zone.

requires its own optimized cryopreservation protocol, based on the cell's biophysical properties [10]. In fact, it has been shown that the special cellular characteristics of spermatozoa make osmotic stress the cause of most of the damage they suffer during freezing [5].

During the cryopreservation of human spermatozoa, mainly the osmotic stress causes significant physiochemical damage in the intracellular structures and membranes, which produces ROS (oxidative stress). But in addition to this endogenous ROS production, there is exogenous ROS production in other abnormal spermatozoa, leukocytes and cytoplasmic remnants present in the semen [11]. These endogenous and/or exogenous ROS cause membrane lipid peroxidation; a decrease in sperm motility; induce death-related processes in cells; mitochondrial and acrosomal damage; DNA alteration; and alteration to the cytoskeleton [2,12].

Recrystallization

As discussed already, all biological material must be stored below the glass transition temperature of water (about −132°C) in order to stop all biological activity. At higher temperatures, longevity is reduced to a matter of weeks or months. Glass transition of an already frozen aqueous solution does not occur suddenly at −132°C, it is a progressive phenomenon between this temperature and −90°C. Therefore, at −80°C there is a great risk of substantial change having occurred. At this temperature, warming energy is returned to the system, permitting molecules to resume their natural orientation, and very small ice crystals are formed.

Cryoprotective Agents

In addition to achieving suitable cooling rates, optimizing cellular viability requires alteration of the physicochemical behaviour of the aqueous environment in which cryopreservation takes place. For this reason, CPAs are added to the cryopreservation medium – substances that are very hydro-soluble and low in cytotoxicity, and which lower the eutectic point (i.e. the freezing/melting point) of the solution. Cryoprotectants can be divided into permeating and non-permeating agents, depending on their permeability through the cell membrane.

Permeating Cryoprotective Agents

These are low molecular weight molecules which pass through the cell membrane, most commonly glycerol, 1,2-propanediol, dimethyl sulphoxide and ethylene glycol. Although the cell is permeable to these agents, their permeabilities are not of the same magnitude as that of water.

Non-Permeating Cryoprotective Agents

These are substances of much higher molecular weight than permeating CPAs and are most effective when employed in a high-speed freezing process. Since these molecules do not penetrate the cell, they are not actually cryoprotectants themselves, but act as such by promoting fast cellular dehydration, and are usually used in association with permeating CPAs. The most commonly used non-permeating CPAs are sucrose, glucose, dextrose, dextran, polyvinylpyrrolidone (PVP), raffinose, trehalose, lactose and hydroyethyl starch.

Cryoprotective agents can be added or removed either in a single step, which reduces the time of cellular exposure to the CPA, or step-wise, so as to gradually increase/decrease the concentration of the CPA in the medium, which reduces the osmotic stress on the cell to be frozen or thawed and can avoid exceeding the cells' critical volume limits [13]. The optimum approach is usually determined empirically.

The Benefits of Cryoprotective Agents

Although CPAs are commonly used in cryopreservation, their protection mechanisms are not completely known, but the following physical mechanisms certainly act to promote cellular survival: dilution of electrolytes, decreasing water concentration; increasing viscosity, 'salt buffering' effect; and stabilization of the cell membrane by means of electrostatic interactions [2].

Harmful Aspects of Cryoprotective Agents

There are two main harmful effects of CPAs:

- *Toxicity:* Permeating CPAs are chemical substances that are not normally found in the cell and are effectively poisoning the cell [6]. However, as cell metabolism slows, the toxic effects are markedly diminished, unless very high concentrations are used at relatively high temperatures (around 0°C).
- *Osmosis:* Addition of CPAs exerts osmotic stress on the cell caused by the increased osmolarity of the medium. The cells initially dehydrate to compensate for the osmotic pressure (cell shrinkage) but then, as the permeating CPA enters the cells, the cells return to their original isotonic volume. Upon removal of the permeating CPA by dilution of the post-thaw specimen, water enters the cells quickly, due to the osmotic gradient, and the CPA leaves the cells more slowly; hence, the cells swell before equilibrium is restored. These cell volume excursions (shrinkage and swelling) can be extensive enough to cause irreversible cell damage if the cell exceeds either or both of its critical volume limits (Figure 10.3) [5].

Vitrification

Generally speaking, vitrification involves extremely high cooling and warming rates to prevent intracellular big ice crystal formation. The advantage that the increase in cooling and warming rates offers during vitrification is that less cryoprotectant is needed, reducing the toxic and osmotic damage so that the passage through the critical temperature zones (from +15°C to −5°C) will be fast and the damage due to

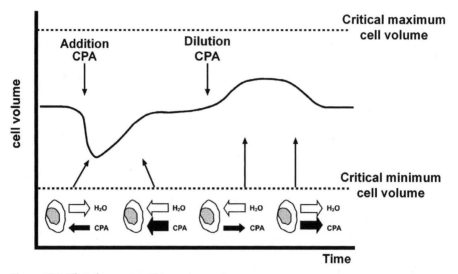

Figure 10.3 Effect of permeating CPA on volume cell.

freezing reduced [12]. This means that if the sample is ultra-fast cooled (immersing small volume samples directly into LN2), high concentration of permeable CPAs is not necessary to achieve a vitrified state, therefore avoiding their toxicity. This methodology, combined with non-permeating substances, has been called 'permeating cryoprotectant-free sperm vitrification' and has been successfully applied to human spermatozoa [14]. A wide variety of sperm vitrification protocols have been reported, both with and without permeating CPAs [15].

Recently, good sperm survival rates in large volumes (up to 0.5 ml) have been achieved after vitrification with a relatively slow cooling rate (150–250°C/min) by using trehalose and butylhydroxy-toluene, a synthetic analogue of vitamin E, without permeating CPAs and increasing the warming rate (42°C) [12,16,17].

It is currently accepted that a wide range of cooling rates can be used for human sperm vitrification, given the specific characteristics of the spermatozoon [15].

Cryopreservation Methods

Background

Although human semen cryobanking can be generally divided into the two broad areas of autoconservation and donor banking, there are many permutations for their clinical application (Table 10.1). Enabling human spermatozoa to survive cryopreservation depends on various factors (Table 10.2). Although the bibliography on the subject is vast [10,18,19], there is no universally accepted method as many are capable of achieving at least satisfactory results. Moreover, given the high degree of variability between men in sperm cryosurvival rates, it is difficult to compare studies and identify the best method of cryopreservation [20–22].

At present, apart from purely biological and technical aspects, other practical factors affect the choice of protocol to be applied in freezing spermatozoa. For example, government regulations require, if possible, the use of a commercially available cryopreservation medium (CPM) and supplements that conform to pharmaceutical standards. In addition, there must be traceability regarding all laboratory activities affecting cryopreserved cells, including the temperature at which

Table 10.1 Applications of sperm cryobanking

Area of activity	Applications
Donor spermatozoa	• To prevent the transmission of hereditary or infectious disease in a heterosexual couple • Insemination for single women • Insemination for lesbian women
Autoconservation	• Pre-vasectomy (fertility 'insurance') • Fertility preservation: before chemotherapy, radiotherapy or orchidectomy, e.g. cancer, autoimmune diseases • Gender reassignment • Testicular biopsy/epididymis • Washed semen from men carrying infectious diseases • Difficulty in the collection of semen, e.g. retrograde ejaculation, erectile dysfunction, psychological problems • Unavailability of the male on the day of the ART • Patients with progressive loss of the seminal quality, e.g. Y-chromosome microdeletions, mosaic Klinefelter syndrome • As a backup for patients with severe oligozoospermia or cryptozoospermia undergoing ICSI • Occupational hazards, sports, death risk (e.g. military) • Post-mortem storage, e.g. desire of the family in case of unexpected death of the male (epididymal aspirations or testicular biopsy specimens)
Research	• Clinical research • Basic biology research • Fundamental cryobiology research

Table 10.2 Factors affecting the optimization of human sperm cryopreservation

Biological factors	Within-subject variability: • Sexual abstinence • Season Between-subject variability: • Genetic factors • Seminal fluid quality • Seminal quality
Technical factors	Cryopreservation medium Addition/removal of cryoprotectants Cooling rate Packaging Storage Thawing

the cells are kept, which means that freezing systems must be fitted with temperature monitoring and recording equipment.

Biological Factors Affecting Sperm Cryopreservation

Various biological factors have been related to within- and between-subject variability of sperm cryopreservation, including sexual abstinence, seasonality, composition of the seminal fluid and genetic factors. Also, although there is a relationship between pre-freeze and post-thaw sperm motility, it is not possible to predict exactly the survival rates of spermatozoa after thawing from the standard semen parameters. Subfertile sperm samples are more susceptible to freezing and thawing injuries than are fertile samples, and epididymal and testicular spermatozoa are more susceptible to cryopreservation injury than are ejaculated spermatozoa [10,23].

225

Technical Factors Affecting Sperm Cryopreservation

The protocols for adding and later eliminating cryoprotective agents consist of one or more stages in which the cells are immersed in a medium containing cryoprotectants of a given composition, for a given period of time, at a given temperature – each of which must be specified at each stage of the process. Consequently, the number of permutations in a method for a particular cell will preclude empirical evaluation of all possible protocols, making the use of theoretical models fundamental to the development of a freezing protocol – notwithstanding the effect of biological variability that can lead to conflicting results [6].

Cryopreservation Media

The permeating CPA most commonly used in sperm cryopreservation is glycerol, although experimental models have shown that higher sperm survival rates can be achieved using ethylene glycol [13,18]. Sucrose and glucose are the non-permeating CPAs most often used. Sperm cryopreservation media may also contain the following components:

- *Agents that interact with the plasma membrane:* Various substances have been shown to be capable of changing lipidic composition of the cellular membrane, improving its fluidity: lecithin, egg yolk, milk, cholesterol and albumin. Other substances with lipophilic properties, such as methyl-ß-cyclodextrin (a derivative of a cyclic oligomer of glucose) and amphipathic compounds, such as glycine, betaine, proline and trehalose, are thought to interact directly with membrane lipids and proteins, altering their phase transition behaviour and hydration state [24]. Long chain alcohols (e.g. lauryl alcohol) have also been used.

- *Chelating agents (e.g. EDTA, citrate):* During cryopreservation, there is poor control of the intracellular concentration of calcium, hence the inclusion of EDTA and citrate in semen diluents can exert beneficial effects via chelating calcium and decreasing its concentration gradient across the sperm plasma membrane. However, EDTA and other metallic ion chelaters might also act by inhibiting lipid peroxidation.

- *Antioxidants:* These are used in order to protect spermatozoa from the endogenous and exogenous ROS produced during cryopreservation. Oxidative stress has been reduced by neutralizing ROS through enzymatic, non-enzymatic, plant-based antioxidants or reductants. Many antioxidants are used in commercial cryopreservation media: vitamins C and E, taurine, hypotaurine and inositol [25,26]. Other agents that prevent lipid peroxidation, such as butylated hydroxytoluene, glutathione and dithiothreitol have been reported to provide protection against peroxidation during cryopreservation, with improvements in post-thaw motility and acrosomal integrity.

- *Buffers:* Many cryopreservation media (CPMs) include glycine, sodium citrate, TRIS or zwitterionic buffers such as HEPES or TES to buffer the pH. Cryoprotectant media based on PBS are not recommended because they provide very poor pH buffering at lower temperatures and because of the 'solute effect', involving the transport of a large quantity of sodium ions across the cell membrane [21].

- Adenosine (as an inhibitor of spontaneous acrosome loss), glutamine (as a source of nitrogen), and antibiotics (gentamicin) have also been included in commercial CPMs [27].

Cryopreservation Media Formulations

Since research into sperm CPMs began, many combinations of components have been used, including: glycerol-egg yolk-citrate (GEYC); HEPES-Tyrode's medium with glycerol and sucrose, glucose, glycine and HSA (HSPM); zwitterion-combination TES-TRIS-sodium citrate-egg yolk-glycerol (TESTCY); a combination TES-TRIS-egg yolk-glycerol (TYG) [19]; and, more recently, MOPS-buffered media. Table 10.3 lists several commercial sperm CPM products.

Table 10.3 Composition of some CE-marked (or equivalent) commercial sperm cryopreservation media

Product	Egg yolk	HSA (w/v)	Glycerol	Sugars	Buffer	Other components	Dilution (sperm+ medium)
Sperm Cryopreservation Buffer (Cook Medical)	-	4 mg/ml	+	glucose sucrose	HEPES	gentamicin glycine	1+2
SpermCryo All-round (Gynotec)	-	0.4%	+ 26.7%	glucose sucrose	HEPES		3+1
Quinn's Advantage Sperm Freeze (SAGE)	-	10 mg/ml	+	sucrose	HEPES	phenol red, gentamicin, EDTA, glutamine	1+1
Spermstore (Gynemed)	-	0.4%	+ 15%	dextrose sucrose	HEPES	glycine	1+0.7
Freezing Medium-TYB (Irvine)	20%	-	+ 12%	fructose	TES-Tris	gentamicin sulfate	1+1
Sperm Freezing Medium (Life Global)	-	3.95 mg/ml	+ 15%	dextrose sucrose	HEPES	glycine gentamicin	1+0.7
Cryosperm (Origio)	-		+	glucose raffinose	HEPES	gentamicin, taurin,e glycine, l-glutamine	1+1
Sperm Freezing Medium (Origio)	-	10 mg/ml	+ <20%	glucose sucrose	HEPES	gentamicin, synthetic serum replacement	1+1
Sperm CryoProtec (Nidacon)	-	-	+ 20%	glucose	HEPES	-	3+1
SpermFreeze Solution (Vitrolife)	-	+	+		MOPS	cholesterol gentamicine	1+1
SpermFreeze (FertiPro)	-	4 mg/ml	+ <20%	dextrose sucrose	HEPES	glycine	1+0.7
SpermFreeze SSP (FertiPro)	-	4 mg/ml	27%	glucose sucrose	HEPES	glycine	3+1
Arctic Sperm Cryopreservation Medium (FujiFilm Irvine Scientific)	-	20 mg/ml	+ 28%	sucrose glucose	HEPES MOPS	glycine, hypotarurine, ascobic acid, inositol, alanyl-glutamine, adenosine	3+1
Sperm Freeze SF1 (Kitazato)	+	-	+	trehalose	TRIS	glycine, lauryl alcohol, tocopherol, gentamicin	1+1
Sperm Freeze with HSA SF3 (Kitazato)	-	+	+	trehalose	TRIS	glycine, lauryl alcohol, tocopherol, gentamicin	1+1

Which Cryopreservation Medium Should Be Used?

In the modern era, in which quality and traceability are the cornerstones of good laboratory practice, 'good manufacturing practice' (GMP) standards must be applied to the preparation of all CPMs. Consequently, GMP documentation and product validation requirements will clearly preclude in-house media preparation except under the most rigorous conditions. Moreover, the components used

227

to make in-house media are usually classified as 'for *in vitro* use only', and freshly prepared media should be checked periodically with known donor spermatozoa, so both preparation and quality control testing time must be taken into account [28].

As already noted, it is very difficult to establish which CPM is the best, although zwitterion buffers are superior to other buffer systems such as citrate, glycine or phosphate [21]. While CPMs with egg yolk seem to achieve higher survival rates than media without [21,29], egg yolk is of animal origin and therefore could introduce microbial agents, such as avian influenza or other, as-yet-unknown, infectious diseases. For this reason, CPMs without egg yolk are to be preferred in the modern andrology laboratory [28].

Whenever spermatozoa are to be cryopreserved, it might be necessary to try various CPMs in order to establish which is best suited for the individual case [29]. Even then, some men, despite having apparently normal pre-freeze and post-thaw sperm quality (and even when their fresh semen is of proven fertility), fail to achieve pregnancies when their cryopreserved spermatozoa are used for insemination [19,30].

Addition/Removal of Cryopreservation Media

It is important to take human sperm sensitivity to shrinkage and swelling into account in cryopreservation techniques in order to increase cryosurvival rates. The human spermatozoon can swell to only 110% of its original isosmotic volume, while it can shrink to 75% of this value and still retain ≥90% of its original motility [13,18]. Consequently, one of the most important aspects is slow CPA addition and removal [31], and most protocols involve a drop-wise addition, with continual mixing for several minutes when adding CPA (freezing) or culture media (thawing) when frozen spermatozoa are to be washed (see Tables 10.4 and 10.5). Rapid dilution can severely damage cryopreserved spermatozoa.

Table 10.4 Table to guide the rate of cryopreservation media addition to semen or washed sperm suspensions (a drop is assumed to be ~30 µl). For samples with fractional ml volumes always err on the slow side, e.g. for a 2.7 ml sample use the column for 2 ml

Time (min)	Starting volume of semen/sperm preparation (ml)				
	1	2	3	4	5
0	1 drop	1 drop	1 drop	1 drop	1 drop
0.5	1 drop	1 drop	1 drop	1 drop	1 drop
1	1 drop	1 drop	1 drop	1 drop	1 drop
1.5	1 drop	1 drop	1 drop	1 drop	1 drop
2	1 drop	2 drops	2 drops	2 drops	2 drops
2.5	2 drops	3 drops	3 drops	3 drops	3 drops
3	2 drops	3 drops	4 drops	4 drops	4 drops
3.5	2 drops	4 drops	5 drops	5 drops	5 drops
4	2 drops	4 drops	6 drops	6 drops	6 drops
4.5	2 drops	4 drops	6 drops	7 drops	7 drops
5	2 drops	4 drops	6 drops	8 drops	8 drops
5.5	2 drops	4 drops	6 drops	8 drops	9 drops
6	2 drops	5 drops	7 drops	9 drops	10 drops
6.5	2 drops	5 drops	7 drops	9 drops	11 drops
7	2 drops	5 drops	7 drops	10 drops	12 drops
7.5	2 drops	5 drops	8 drops	10 drops	12 drops
8	3 drops	6 drops	8 drops	10 drops	13 drops
8.5	3 drops	6 drops	9 drops	11 drops	14 drops
9		6 drops	9 drops	11 drops	14 drops
9.5			9 drops	12 drops	15 drops
10				12 drops	16 drops

Table 10.5 Table to guide the rate of adding diluent medium (ideally sperm buffer) to thawed samples of semen or washed sperm suspensions (a drop is assumed to be ~30 μl). For samples with fractional ml volumes always err on the slow side, e.g. for a 2.7 ml sample use the column for 2 ml

Time (min)	Starting volume of thawed sample (ml)				
	1	2	3	4	5
0	1 drop	1 drop	1 drop	1 drop	1 drop
0.5	1 drop	1 drop	1 drop	1 drop	1 drop
1	1 drop	1 drop	1 drop	1 drop	1 drop
1.5	1 drop	1 drop	1 drop	1 drop	1 drop
2	1 drop	2 drops	2 drops	2 drops	2 drops
2.5	2 drops	3 drops	3 drops	3 drops	3 drops
3	2 drops	3 drops	4 drops	4 drops	4 drops
3.5	2 drops	4 drops	5 drops	5 drops	5 drops
4	2 drops	4 drops	6 drops	6 drops	6 drops
4.5	2 drops	4 drops	6 drops	7 drops	7 drops
5	2 drops	4 drops	6 drops	8 drops	8 drops
5.5	2 drops	4 drops	6 drops	8 drops	9 drops
6	2 drops	5 drops	7 drops	9 drops	10 drops
6.5	2 drops	5 drops	7 drops	9 drops	11 drops
7	2 drops	5 drops	7 drops	10 drops	12 drops
7.5	2 drops	5 drops	8 drops	10 drops	12 drops
8	3 drops	6 drops	8 drops	10 drops	13 drops
8.5	3 drops	6 drops	9 drops	11 drops	14 drops
9		6 drops	9 drops	11 drops	14 drops
9.5			9 drops	12 drops	15 drops
10				12 drops	16 drops

After dilution with the CPM, semen should be packaged and cooled immediately, as the exposure of human spermatozoa to cryoprotectant prior to freezing should be less than 10 min in order to achieve optimal cryosurvival rates. The deleterious effects appear to be greater when HSPM is used rather than TEST-yolk medium [32].

Control of Cooling and Warming Rates in Cryopreservation

Diverse methods for freezing can be defined, but which temperature control system is best remains an open question [19,31]. Nonetheless, it is crucial to ensure the fulfilment of the intended freezing rate, and so a sensor with a data logger and software to monitor the cooling rate, if not already incorporated into the system, is strongly recommended.

Programmable Freezing Systems

This type of freezing system allows cells to be frozen gradually, without abrupt temperature changes, providing more time for the cells to become dehydrated and so reducing the damage caused by the formation of intracellular crystals. Such systems also make it possible to carry out seeding at a given temperature, although seeding during normozoospermic semen cryopreservation has not been shown to confer any significant improvement in cryosurvival rates [31,33].

Static Vapour Phase Cooling

In this method a stable temperature gradient is established in the vapour phase above a quantity of liquid nitrogen, held within an insulated container, usually a large cylindrical stainless steel dewar. Straws are placed at predetermined heights above the liquid phase for predetermined periods to achieve the necessary cooling curve. Problems with this method include the abrupt rate of temperature decrease, poor reproducibility of cooling rates, and increased variability between straws from the same semen sample. Consequently, this method is not recommended from a cryobiological standpoint, especially when trying to cool bundles of straws or several cryotubes in the neck of a cryostorage dewar [32,34]. Special devices have been specifically developed for this procedure (e.g. Cryofloater, NidaCon International AB, Mölndal, Sweden) or a commercial freezing rack can be used.

Mechanically Assisted Vapour Phase Cooling

Such cooling systems cause liquid nitrogen vapour to flow around the samples at a controlled rate so that a desired cooling rate can be achieved. Freezing protocols must be established empirically.

Vitrification

The method is quick and simple, taking only a few seconds, and does not require special freezing equipment. Its success depends on the right combination of volume and CPA(s), although the cooling rates achieved (ranging from 150°C/min for 0.5-ml straws to >20,000°C/min for microdrops or the Cryotop device) are not sufficient to prevent intracellular big ice crystal formation, and the results achieved are not satisfactory [35]. In order to obtain the high cooling and warming rates needed for successful sperm vitrification, in most protocols the volume in which the cells are contained must be very small, only a few microlitres, which greatly limits the number of spermatozoa that can be vitrified. However, recently a system that permits sperm vitrification in larger volumes of up to 0.5 ml in a cryostraw has been developed [12,16]. The loaded and sealed straw is immersed horizontally into LN2, allowing uniform contact between the device and cryogenic agent that allows an immediate cooling of the specimen, making this an aseptic procedure; the straw can also be sealed inside another, larger straw for storage.

In order to try to reduce the Leidenfrost effect (boiling LN2 on the cooled surface forms a heat-insulating vapour layer surrounding the biological sample or device), the device should be shaken or stirred gently once submerged in liquid nitrogen [1].

Flash-Freeze Technique (Ultra-Rapid Freezing)

This is the situation where spermatozoa in straws or naked microdrops are immersed directly into liquid nitrogen with no CPAs present at all, sometimes called 'quench freezing'. Cooling rates can exceed 2,500°C/min for 0.25-ml straws, but nevertheless these rates are not sufficient to prevent intracellular ice formation, and the results achieved are not satisfactory in terms of sperm function, but spermatozoal or seminal plasma components can be examined biochemically after thawing.

Thawing

In general, it is considered that fast warming rates are required for optimal sperm recovery. This has been attributed to the possibility that small intracellular ice crystals formed in some cells during freezing can grow during a slow re-warming process, producing the somewhat counter-intuitive concept of freezing during warming. As explained already, the 'danger zone' is between the ice transition point of water (about −132°C) and the melting point of the specimen. Only if warming is sufficiently fast (e.g. in a water bath at 37°C or 40°C) to prevent the growth of such ice crystals can this phenomenon be avoided [34,36].

Many labs that use straws use a 30°C water bath to reduce possible temperature-dependent toxicity of the permeating CPAs; in such a situation, stirring of the straw within the water is essential to reduce the formation of a boundary zone of cooler water around the straw.

It is very difficult, if not impossible, to achieve an adequate warming rate through the danger zone with cryotubes [31].

Vitrification

There is currently no commercially available medium for vitrification of human spermatozoa. The components used in the protocols are often described as 'for *in vitro* use only' [37,38], or for use in combination with regular sperm-freezing media [39,40].

The sperm vitrification protocols which do not use permeating CPAs seem to have better performance than those which do include them [40], probably due to the greater osmolality control when they are not present. Isomolar vitrification media (300–396 mOsm/l) can be obtained if only non-permeating CPAs are used, however, osmolalities of 600–1000 mOsm/L are usually reached when permeating CPAs are used [15].

Packaging Alternatives

Devices for Slow-Freezing Spermatozoa

Over the years, four main types of packaging container have been used for human spermatozoa:

- Glass ampoules – although these have been strongly discouraged for many years for reasons of safety due to their fragility.
- Plastic screw-top 'cryovials' or 'cryotubes', primarily the *CryoTube*® range of products (Nalge Nunc International, Rochester, NY, USA). These are made from polypropylene with either polypropylene or polyethylene screw caps. Different types have either external or internal screw threads, so that the cap screws either into or onto the outside of the cryovial respectively. Tightening the cap compresses a silicone O-ring seal that is supposed to make the cryovial air- and watertight.
- Plastic straws or 'paillettes' were invented by Cassou [41] and commercialized by his company, Instruments de Medicine Veterinaire ('IMV': L'Aigle, France). Although originally made from polyvinyl chloride (PVC), they were replaced by straws made from polyethylene terephthalate glycol (PETG) in 1998, because PVC straws could not be sterilized by irradiation without compromising their mechanical integrity. Since Cassou's patent expired, plastic straws have also become available from other companies, e.g. Minitüb GmbH (Tiefenbach, Germany).
- Most recently, straws have been made from an ionomeric resin that confers substantial advantages in terms of mechanical strength at cryogenic temperatures and impermeability to viruses. These are the CBS™ *High Security Straws*, sometimes referred to as 'CBS straws', from CryoBioSystem (L'Aigle, France) [42]. When used in conjunction with their thermal welding device, the SYMS sealer (several generations of models are available), they are guaranteed leakproof, and the seals secure up to pressures of 150 kg/cm^{-2}. These straws also use a special filling nozzle to prevent contamination of the outside of the straw with the specimen (a major source of contamination in cryotanks, see [43]) and have both internal and external secure identification options [31].
- There is also the CBS™ *High Security Tube*, which can replace the plastic screw-top cryotubes. It is also thermosealed and eliminates concerns related to possible cross-contamination.

Devices for Sperm Vitrification

As previously explained, the probability of vitrifying a sample is inversely correlated with the volume, which is why it is usually necessary for the volume the cells are contained in to be very small, meaning that very few cells can be vitrified [6]. This protocol is based on microdrops or using devices such as the electron microscopy grid, open-pulled straw, Cryoloop, Cryotop, Cryotip, SpermVD, Cell Sleeper or Cryopiece devices [44], all of which are directly immersed in liquid nitrogen to achieve cooling and warming rates >22,000°C/min and avoid the formation of large intracellular ice crystals. CBS straws can be used for the large volume vitrification protocol.

Selecting the Right Packaging Device

Straws are widely used for packaging human semen, especially in Europe, although plastic cryovials are also used in many laboratories, especially in the USA. Beyond some clinicians' desire (perceived need?) for larger volume specimens, there are significant technical aspects to the 'straws *vs* cryovials' debate, which include issues concerning the cooling and warming rates as well as biocontainment, issues that are tightly interconnected because both are governed by the physical characteristics of the packaging systems. The major points are summarized below, but for more extensive discussions of issues in the straws *vs* cryovials debate, readers are referred to the review by Mortimer [31].

Fecundity Rates Post-Thaw

Although there have been no reliable prospective trials comparing the relative fertility of human spermatozoa frozen in straws *vs* cryovials, it has been argued that there might be as much as a six- to eight-fold higher post-thaw fecundity for sperm frozen in straws [31].

Achievement of Intended Cooling/Warming Rates

Simple physics dictates that the larger radius of cryovials will impede heat transfer, resulting in uneven heat exchange throughout the sample, but nevertheless in a substantial lag between the programmed rate in the controlled-rate freezer and the actual cooling rate achieved inside a cryovial [33]. Similarly, the contents of a cryovial will thaw more slowly and less uniformly when removed from cryostorage than those of a straw, even if immersed in a 30°C water bath. This poses a significant problem, since rapid thawing is required for optimum cryosurvival [31,34]. Figure 10.4A shows that while specimens packaged in all sizes of straws (IMV 0.5 and 0.25 ml and CBS 0.5 ml High Security Straws) experience very similar cooling curves, material packaged in Nunc 1.8 ml cryovials will experience cooling that is considerably delayed behind the programmed curve. Figure 10.4B reveals magnified differences between straws and cryovials when warming at 37°C – but this rapid warming rate of straws does require caution when handling specimens outside the cryogenic storage tank for brief periods (e.g. during cryobank audits): a 0.25-ml straw will warm to -80°C within 15 s in air at room temperature [45].

Effective Sealing

There are very serious concerns regarding leakage of liquid nitrogen into cryovials [46,47], and Nunc documentation [48] clearly states that storing cryovials immersed in LN2 is not advised. This liquid nitrogen represents not only a risk of specimen contamination but can also cause the container to explode when it expands rapidly – by a factor of almost 700× – upon warming when removed from the cryogenic storage tank. For storage under such 'extreme' conditions, *CryoTube*® vials must be correctly sealed in Nunc *CryoFlex*™ tubing – but cryobanks rarely do this as the *CryoFlex* tubing hinders attachment of cryovials to canes [49]. Poor sealing can also affect PVC or PETG straws, unless great care is paid to ensuring that an air space is left in the straw to allow for the expansion of the specimen as it cools, and that a proper seal has been achieved [31]. However, the thermal soldering technique employed with the CBS ionomeric resin straws does ensure a secure seal.

Fragility at −196°C

PVC and PETG straws are very fragile at −196°C and are easily broken if lateral force is exerted upon them (e.g. attempted bending as a straw is placed into or removed from a storage unit). The CBS *High Security Straws* cannot be broken, even at cryogenic temperatures, without extreme bending.

Risk of Cross-Contamination

The isolated report in 1995 of a cluster of six cases of acute Hepatitis B virus infections among patients undergoing cytotoxic treatment [50] – even though it was later established as having been due to the use of a low quality type of blood bag packaging – gave rise to extensive concern over the risk of cross-contamination of specimens during cryostorage. There has since been much debate regarding this issue and, while the risk of cross-contamination cannot be ignored as being 'theoretical', it is certainly

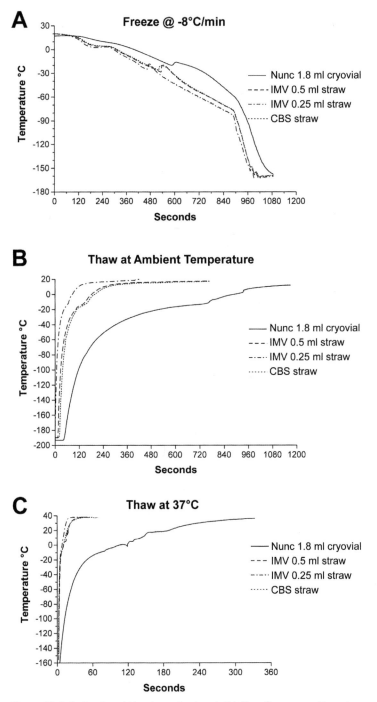

Figure 10.4 Cooling (panel A) and warming (panels B & C) profiles measured by a thermocouple inside various packaging systems. Note the much slower warming rate at ambient temperature compared to 37°C. Figure reproduced from [30] with permission.

unquantifiable [51], precluding robust risk analysis of its real likelihood. Consequently, anyone working in human sperm cryobanking needs to understand its basis and be able to take all practical steps to minimize the risk of its occurring, with the CBS™ *High Security Straw* and *High Security Tube* (properly sealed using the SYMS device) being the safest packaging methods for ensuring biocontainment of cryobanked specimens [31,52,53].

In addition, many vitrification protocols are based on direct contact between spermatozoa and the liquid nitrogen, and with such open devices the vitrified sample is in constant contact with the liquid nitrogen, creating a theoretical risk of cross-contamination. Several systems offer at least clean LN2, e.g. the *Elan 2* (MMR Technologies, San Jose, CA, USA) which produces clean LN2, the *Nterilizer*® (Nterilizer, Bologna, Italy) which sterilizes LN2 using ultraviolet light [54], and the *Veriseq*® (Linde Gas, Schiedam, Holland) which filters gaseous nitrogen and liquefies it to produce sterile LN2. Creating sterile liquid air has also been proposed (it having the same temperature as LN2) by liquefying following air filtration (the *CLAir* benchtop device, FertileSafe, Nes Ziona, Israel). However, some authors have questioned the efficacy of these sterilization methods, suggesting the impossibility of LN2 sterilization [55]. It should also be remembered that when small numbers of spermatozoa are being vitrified, ICSI needles are used to place them into a sterile cryoprotectant, which reduces the potential risk of viral contamination. Furthermore, a packaging system where one straw is sealed inside a second straw allows sperm vitrification with a very low probability of contamination, since the cryopreserved specimen does not come into contact with the liquid nitrogen [12].

Sperm Cryopreservation Procedure

Principle

Large changes in one or more of the technical factors discussed above (temperature, CPA concentration, etc.) would significantly affect the cryosurvival rate, but even small variations could influence the final result, and so it is necessary to take meticulous care in following sperm cryopreservation protocols. In donor sperm banks, what is important is not just the sperm survival rate but also the homogeneity between different aliquots of sperm, so that a given concentration of mobile spermatozoa per vial can be ensured; small differences in several factors may be responsible for non-uniformity between aliquots from the same ejaculate [32].

This example protocol employs CBS™ *High Security Straws* (CryoBioSystem, L'Aigle, France) since they are the most secure and reproducible form of packaging currently available.

Equipment

See also Appendix 2.
- Freezing system: either a controlled rate freezer (programmable) or mechanically assisted vapour phase freezer [19]
- Aspiration device for filling straws
- System for sealing straws (e.g. *SYMS*, CryoBioSystem, L'Aigle, France)
- Water bath
- Dry bath (block warmer)
- Air incubator operating at 37°C
- Microscope configured for andrology with phase contrast optics (10×, 20× and 40× objectives)
- Cryogenic storage tanks
- Straw-handling forceps (NordicCell, Copenhagen, Denmark; see www.nordiccell.com)
- Label printer
- Liquid nitrogen supply vessel
- Counting chamber (e.g. Makler Chamber)

Disposable Materials

- Straws and filling nozzle*
- Inventory system items (as appropriate): visotubes, goblets, canes, flags
- Self-adhesive labels
- Semen collection container*
- Glass Pasteur pipettes*
- Round-bottom polystyrene 14-ml culture tubes* (e.g. Falcon #2001 or #2057)
- Sterile gauze
- Instrument to cut straw: suture scissors (e.g. Cat.No. R50.000 from Rocket Medical, Watford, UK)

*Note: All disposables that come into contact with spermatozoa that are to be used for either therapeutic or critical testing purposes should be either pre-tested for sperm toxicity or else obtained from a trusted manufacturer, e.g. if a sterile plastic syringe is used during processing then it must be of a brand known not to have any deleterious effects upon spermatozoa.

Reagents

- Cryoprotectant medium, e.g. *Sperm CryoProtec* (Nidacon International AB, Göteborg, Sweden)

  Note: *Any CPM used in cryopreserving human spermatozoa for therapeutic purposes must be CE-marked (or equivalent) and certified as pyrogen-free and not having any sperm toxicity.*

- Hypochlorite solution
- Sterile water
- Liquid nitrogen

Calibration

Scheduled examinations of controlled-rate freezers must be performed by qualified individuals or companies who can certify that the unit is functioning according to specification, and who can provide service, repairs and parts authorized by the unit's manufacturer. A reference thermometer should be calibrated annually (or otherwise as per manufacturer's recommendation) by an accredited calibration laboratory (e.g. the National Institute of Standards and Technology in the USA).

Quality Control

Sample Identification

All specimen containers and processing/preparation tubes must be labelled with two identifiers, e.g. the subject's name and the specimen's laboratory reference or ID number. Temporary analytical preparations (e.g. sperm motility slides) can be identified using the specimen's laboratory reference or ID number only. Each straw must be identified individually using a unique straw code. In the EU the 'Single European Code' or 'SEC' unique identifier for tissues and cells is required.

Cross-Contamination

Potentially contaminated parts of the controlled-rate freezer and workstation can be cleaned with ethanol or non-corrosive decontamination fluids.

Temperature

Room temperature sensor, water bath, refrigerators, freezers for storage reagents and temperature sensors for the freezing system and tank should be checked quarterly using a calibrated thermometer. All results and calibration dates must be recorded. Freezers for reagent storage and cryotanks, if possible, should be equipped with a continuous automatic recording system (data logger) and alarms set to respond when temperatures rise; the alarm system should sound during regular working hours and be attached to a telephone notification system outside normal working hours. The temperature curve for each sperm cryopreservation run must be stored for purposes of traceability. Shipping tanks should be fitted with a temperature data logger.

Water Baths

Water baths should be filled with distilled water and cleaned with a disinfectant solution (e.g. 70% alcohol or 10% sodium hypochlorite solution) weekly [56].

Reagents

CPM must be stored as per manufacturer's recommendations and used before its expiry date. This date should be checked before each use of the CPM. Quality control performed by, or on behalf of, the manufacturer will usually be summarized in a Certificate of Analysis for each batch of CPM that will record biological (bioassay), chemical and physical test data; these certificate must be kept on file (ideally electronically as PDF files) [28].

Internal Quality Control

Sample of known donor semen should be frozen and thawed to test equipment function, or to test any new material or commercial cryopreservation medium. New methods should be evaluated using known donor semen specimens. For internal QC semen analysis see the section on 'Quality Control' in Chapter 12.

External Quality Control of the Sperm Donor

High variability between sperm banks has been described [57]. There are three components to EQA in a sperm bank:

- One laboratory can arrange a cross-over proficiency testing programme with another sperm bank, so that straws of frozen semen can be tested by both laboratories
- General EQA programmes for semen analysis
- An EQA programme for bioassay (see the section on 'External Quality Assessment' in Chapter 12).

Homogeneity among Straws from the Same Donor

Within-individual variability in sperm cryopreservation means it is necessary to check every specimen cryopreserved for a given donor. In a commercial sperm bank, it is also very important to guarantee homogeneity among the straws from a sperm donor. A possible strategy is to test the sperm concentration in the test thaw sample; this must be within ± 10% of half the original semen sperm concentration (assuming a 1+1 CPM dilution); otherwise, it would suggest poor mixing of the semen and cryoprotectant. Batches where this condition is not met can show substantial variability in sperm cryosurvival among straws [19]. Another strategy is to randomly test a certain number of straws before starting the delivery of samples from a sperm donor, in order to ensure the required homogeneity (acceptance sampling plan) [58]. If donors do not meet the requisites of the proposed acceptance sampling plan, they should not be included in the distribution schedule. Nevertheless, if they could be used within the same sperm bank at the assisted reproduction centre, any poor-quality straws found could be replaced immediately.

Cryostorage Vessel

The cryotank alarm system should not just rely on temperature measurements, but also include the liquid nitrogen level, since the drop in this will occur prior to the fall in temperature and it is more likely to prevent thawing of the samples. Thermal cameras, tank weight or pressure measurements can be used for detecting liquid nitrogen dewar failure (see Chapter 13).

Specimen

Liquefied, homogeneous human semen, ideally within 30 min of ejaculation. Longer post-ejaculatory delays, incomplete liquefaction and increased viscosity should be noted on the laboratory and report form. For other types of specimens and abnormal semen samples, see the section on 'Dealing with Atypical Semen Specimens' in Chapter 9.

As well as the standard procedure for freezing sperm, it is also possible to freeze prepared sperm samples (as described in Chapter 9, 'Sperm Preparation') using a cryopreservation medium that does not contain egg yolk; these may be used for insemination directly after freezing, with no need for further processing (IUI-ready) [31]. Although IUI-ready samples are regularly prepared as part of sperm-sample freezing procedures in sperm banks, this could also be done when preparing samples from patients who will carry out AIH cycles and who for professional or other reasons cannot be present when the insemination is performed, or from patients who have an infectious disease, due to a delayed virological study, or for safety reasons. There is no generalized view as to the technique that should be used for processing IUI-ready samples before freezing or whether this processing prior to freezing has an effect on cryosurvival rates [59–61].

Testicular/epididymal sperm samples can be cryopreserved using the standard semen freezing or sperm vitrification protocols [44,62]. When mature spermatozoa are identified after dissecting testicular tissue or in the epididymal aspirated, the homogenate or the aspirated are diluted with the CPM. When there are very few spermatozoa, proceed as described in Note 5.

Procedures

Note: For safety reasons, whenever liquid nitrogen is being handled, full cryogenic protective equipment must be worn (see Chapter 15).

A. *Freezing Phase*

1. Have the subject collect the semen specimen in a sterile, labelled container (preferably by masturbation).
2. While the specimen liquefies (no longer than 30 min), prepare the programmable freezer (check the freezing ramps and transfer liquid nitrogen to the system) and allow the CPM to warm to room temperature.
3. As soon as the ejaculate is liquefied, perform a basic semen analysis, either manually or using CASA (see Chapter 3 or 6, as appropriate).
4. Measure out the volume of semen sample to be cryopreserved (e.g. using a wide-bore sterile pipette) and transfer it to the bottom of a clean container.
5. Calculate the number of *High Security Straws* that will be required, taking into account the dilution with CPM recommended by the manufacturer, e.g. 1+1 or 3+1 (Table 10.3).
6. Label the straws and the storage units (e.g. visotubes) by the appropriate identification code(s). Choose an appropriate colour (visotube, straw, flag, etc.) and attach self-adhesive labels with the identification code.
   Note: Straws must be identified individually. In this way, if two insemination doses are removed from the bank and thawed at the same time there is no chance of their being confused. The classical 'bar code' method using lines drawn on each straw using a fine-pointed spirit-based marker pen [19] is no longer recommended.
7. Add the CPM slowly, drop-wise, with continuous gentle swirling to ensure complete mixing (see Table 10.4). This step should take up to 10 min so that an efficient osmotic balance may be achieved with no abrupt alterations in cellular osmolarity.
8. When the mixture is homogeneous the straws can be filled. Each straw is connected to a suction device (e.g. a 1-ml syringe with tubing adapter or a vacuum pump) and the semen + CPM mixture is drawn up the straw, leaving a 10 mm air space at the entry (filling) end. The outside of the straw must not be allowed to come into contact with either the semen or the sides of the container, e.g. fill using a filling nozzle.
9. Seal the ends of each straw by thermal pulse sealing (*SYMS* device).
10. Disinfect the outside of each straw using hypochlorite solution, followed by rinsing with sterile water and drying.

11. Transfer the straws into the freezer racking system of the programmable freezing system and start the programmed freezer cycle. The following generic cooling curve without seeding is provided as an example:

- *Ramp 1*: Reduce the temperature from room temperature (*ca.* 22°C) to +4°C at a moderate cooling rate of –5°C/min. The spermatozoa become dehydrated but the time is very limited.
- *Ramp 2*: Reduce the temperature from +4°C to –80°C at a rapid cooling rate of –10°C/min. In this ramp, there is no seeding and the sperm suspension begins to solidify.
- *Ramp 3*: 'Free fall' from –80°C to –160°C. 'Free fall' denotes uncontrolled cooling, i.e. a cooling rate as fast as the system being used can achieve. The freezing protocol must cool to below –160°C to minimize the risk of recrystallization damage during transfer from the freezing machine into liquid nitrogen.
- *Ramp 4*: Finally, reduce the temperature from –160°C to –196°C by plunging the straws into liquid nitrogen. This must be done very rapidly.

12. Immerse the previously identified visotube into liquid nitrogen in a transfer dewar until the bubbling stops.

13. Using forceps, rapidly transfer the straws of frozen semen into the visotube (which is full of liquid nitrogen).

14. To check cryosurvival, set aside one straw for assessment of post-thaw sperm motility (either immediately or later).

15. Place the visotube of straws in the appropriate storage location (tank and canister number, container level) in the bank.

16. Make out an Index Card for the straw identification codes, semen sample identification code (ID number), date of freezing, storage location and the semen analysis laboratory reference number.

17. Record all information in a logbook or using specialized software.

B. *Checking Post-Thaw Motility*

18. Thaw out the test straw by transferring it into a water bath at 30–37°C for 10 min.

19. Sanitize the outside of the straw so that the straw can be opened without risk of contamination. Wipe the semen end of the straw with sterile hypochlorite solution, rinse with sterile water and dry with sterile gauze. Cut the air-bubble end of the straw, insert it into a tube, and then cut the other end (just below the filter) and allow the contents of the straw to run out into the tube. The ends of the straw must be cut with a sterile device, e.g. disposable suture scissors (scalpel blades are not recommended as there is a significant risk of injury).

   Note: Upon thawing, the outside of all straws or cryotubes will be contaminated with whatever organisms were present in the liquid nitrogen, even if vapour storage was used. Therefore, all cryostorage units should be disinfected after thawing before opening.

20. Assess the quantitative and qualitative sperm motility and determine the total sperm concentration.

C. *Thawing Phase: For Insemination or Other Purposes*

21. Identify the location of the desired straws in the cryobank and confirm against the laboratory records and patient/donor records. Record how many straws are to be thawed and how many remain.

22. Remove the straws from the visotube and thaw quickly by placing in 30–37°C water bath for 10 min.

23. Sanitize and open without risk of contamination (see step 19).

24. Evaluate the qualitative and quantitative aspects of sperm concentration and motility.

25. Process the thawed sample as described in Chapter 9 'Sperm Preparation – Dealing with Atypical Semen Specimens – Cryopreserved Specimens'. See Table 10.5 to guide the slow addition of medium (ideally sperm buffer) to the post-thaw sample.

   Note: 'IUI-ready' samples can be used directly with no need for prior processing.

Cryopreservation Results

The adequacy of semen cryopreservation can be evaluated in several ways [9].

1. *Cryosurvival factor (CSF),* which is calculated as:

$$\text{CSF} = \frac{\% \text{ motile spermatozoa post-thaw}}{\% \text{ motile spermatozoa pre-freeze}} \times 100$$

2. *Concentration and number of progressively motile spermatozoa per straw post-thaw.* Use the post-thaw sperm concentration and motility to calculate the concentration of progressively motile spermatozoa post-thaw per straw and, using the straw volume, the total number of such spermatozoa in the straw post-thaw. The number of motile spermatozoa required is dependent on the intended use of the contents of the straw, ranging from donor intracervical insemination to patient ICSI. This parameter is used to classify the straw and to guarantee homogeneity among the different samples from the same donor (see 'Quality Control', below).

3. *Suitability for use after thawing.* Based on the CSF and motility, a CSF value ≥50% together with a sperm motility of ≥30% motile with ≥25% progressively motile after thawing is considered optimum [63]. To determine the minimum number of progressively motile spermatozoa after thawing, per straw, it should be borne in mind that the greater the concentration of spermatozoa, the lower the proportion of motile spermatozoa that will be necessary to achieve the minimum motile count per straw (although lower motility can indicate lower overall sperm quality). A method to relate the concentration and motility observed in a straw after thawing, taking analytical variation into account, has been described previously [58].

- *Auto cryopreservation:* As the quality of cryopreserved semen stored by patients before cancer treatment is often poor, the only therapeutic option might be assisted fertilization. In this case, straws containing just a few motile spermatozoa are often sufficient to give acceptable fertilization rates using ICSI. As very few spermatozoa are required for assisted conception, it is wise to freeze only a small number per straw (e.g. 40,000) so as to maximize the number of fertilization attempts per semen specimen [30].

- *Donor sperm:* A minimum number of progressively motile spermatozoa post-thaw must be determined for each sperm donor bank in order to decide whether cryopreservation is feasible.

  - *Straws for intracervical insemination (ICI):* Although ICI achieves a lower rate of pregnancies than does intrauterine insemination (IUI) the multiple pregnancy rates are much lower. Therefore, it has been proposed that for some women it might be appropriate to perform six cycles of ICI and then IUI [64]. Some studies have recommended a minimum of 4 to 5 $\times 10^6$ progressively motile spermatozoa per straw post-thaw [22,23,64].

  - *Straws for IUI:* A straw containing less than the generally accepted minimum of 4×10^6 motile spermatozoa can be used for IUI, as this process involves the removal of seminal plasma and the concentration of spermatozoa prior to insemination.

  - *Straws for IVF:* The number of motile spermatozoa per straw of cryopreserved donor semen does not correlate with either fertilization rates or pregnancy rates in IVF, reflecting the highly selected nature of the spermatozoa stored.

  - *Second chance sperm donor:* Although the inter-sample variability in a sperm donor is high [21,22], and an aberrant preparation might arise due to an intervening problem with the donor (e.g. a bout of febrile illness), a very small percentage of donors are allowed a second opportunity when the first sperm donor cryopreservation produces borderline unacceptable results [22,58].

Notes

1. *Repeat freezing for patients or donor.* When freezing subsequent specimens for a patient or donor, it is always advisable to review the test-thaw results from previous specimens in order to avoid any past problems affecting the processing of the current specimen.

2. *Highly viscous samples.* It can be extremely difficult to obtain good mixing of the semen and cryoprotectant. A needle must not be used. Dilute and pipette the sample with sperm buffer in autoconservation; if the sample does not disperse within 2 min of pipetting, incubate at 37°C for 10 min and then mix further. Also refer to Chapter 3 regarding viscous semen samples.

3. *Centrifuging before cryopreservation.* Any centrifuging of the sample that involves the formation of a pellet containing all of the spermatozoa in the sample can lead to sperm damage (see 'Safe Methods for Sperm Preparation' in Chapter 9). Therefore, it is necessary to avoid centrifugation to concentrate high volume/low count specimens in order to obtain the requisite minimum of progressively motile spermatozoa, e.g. $<60 \times 10^6$/ml. Techniques of sperm preparation should be used with these samples.

4. *Refreezing.* Valuable samples (e.g. from cancer patients, testicular sperm) can be refrozen [65].

5. *Very few spermatozoa.* Different techniques have been described as a vehicle for the storage of very few or single human spermatozoa, including human, mouse or hamster zonae pellucidae [44,62]. The use of zonae pellucidae implies a potential contamination of the spermatozoa with infectious or foreign genetic material, and the use of human zonae is especially problematic given their limited availability. Consequently, this approach cannot be recommended.

6. *Fragility of cryopreserved spermatozoa.* Due to the very high osmolarity of cryoprotectant media, and the damage sustained by spermatozoa during freezing and thawing, great care must be taken when handling post-thaw specimens (also see Chapter 9).

Sperm Vitrification Procedures

Most sperm vitrification protocols are carried out either with spermatozoa isolated by micromanipulation or prepared sperm populations [44,62]. The following procedures are for spermatozoa that are free of seminal plasma.

Vitrification Protocol A [17]

Reagents

Base medium ('GBd')

Sydney IVF Gamete Buffer (Cook Medical, see www.cookmedical.com) or sperm wash medium with 1% w/v dextran (Irvine Scientific, Santa Ana, CA, USA)

Vitrification solution

GBd with 0.25 M sucrose
To prepare 1 ml of vitrification solution mix 0.5 ml of GBd and 0.5 ml of a 0.5 M aqueous sucrose solution (MP Biomedicals, Catalogue # 152584).

Specimen

A washed sperm suspension in GBd (see Chapter 9 for sperm washing methods).

Vitrification Procedure

1. Immediately after preparation, centrifuge the sperm suspension at 250 $g \times$ 5 min.
2. Aspirate and discard the supernatant then resuspend the pellet in freshly prepared vitrification solution to a concentration of 5×10^6 motile spermatozoa per ml.

3. Label the required number of packaging devices.

4. Package 100 µl of sperm suspension into 0.25-ml straws, leaving an air space at each end.

5. Insert each straw inside a 0.5 ml CBS™ *High Security Straw*, one end of which has already been sealed.

6. Working one by one, immerse a straw horizontally into LN2, gently move the straw once it has been submerged for 10 s.

7. Transfer all the vitrified straws into the cryostorage dewar.

Warming Procedure

1. Prepare a round-bottom culture tube (e.g. Falcon #2003) with 3 ml GBd and equilibrate to 37°C as a 'thaw tube'.

2. Remove the straw from the LN2 using forceps, grasp the straw as far away as possible from where the vitrified medium is located. Never touch the specimen with your hand.

3. Immerse in a 42°C water bath for 5 s.

4. Sanitize the outside of the straw so that it can be opened without risk of contamination: dry the straw with a paper tissue and then wipe the straw with sterile hypochlorite solution; rinse with sterile water and dry with sterile gauze.

5. Cut the air-space end of the outer straw and insert the cut end into the top of the prewarmed 'thaw tube'.
   Note: The ends of the straw must be cut with a sterile device, e.g. disposable suture scissors; a scalpel blade is not recommended due to the significant risk of injury.

6. Then cut the other end (just below the filter) and shake the straw so that the inner straw falls to the bottom of the tube.

7. Expel the contents of the 0.25-ml straw into the GBd medium using a modified pipette tip.

8. Gently mix for 10 s.

9. Incubate the sperm suspension at 37°C in a CO_2-in-air incubator for 10 min.

10. Centrifuge at 380 g × 5 min.

11. Aspirate and discard the supernatant then resuspend the pellet in IUI or IVF medium.

Vitrification Protocol B [66]

Reagents

Vitrification solution

Dissolve 10 mg/ml HSA in double-distilled water (i.e. 1% w/v) and add 0.5 M sucrose (e.g. 1.71 g in 10 ml).

Specimen

A washed sperm suspension in preferred medium (see Chapter 9 for sperm washing methods).

Vitrification Procedure

1. Immediately after processing, dilute the sperm suspension 1:1 with the vitrification solution (final sucrose concentration of 0.25 M).

2. Maintain at ambient temperature for 5 min.

3. Label the required number of CBS™ 0.5-ml High Security Sperm Straws (with the cotton-PVA powder plug) and mark them with a line 10 mm from the fixed plug.

4. Using a filling nozzle, aspirate the sperm suspension up to the line and then detach the nozzle while continuing the suction (this will ensure a large-enough air space inside the straw to prevent it rupturing when immersed into LN2); the liquid column will reach the PVA plug and cause it to seal.

5. Seal the straw at both ends using the SYMS heat sealer.

6. Working one by one, hold at the cotton-PVA powder-plug end using forceps and immerse it horizontally into LN2; gently move the straw once it has been submerged for 8 s.
7. Transfer all the vitrified straws into the cryostorage dewar.

Warming Procedure

1. Remove the straw from the LN2 using forceps, grasping the straw at the cotton-PVA powder plug end.
2. Immerse in a 42°C water bath for 20 s.
3. Sanitize the outside of the straw so that it can be opened without risk of contamination: dry the straw with a paper tissue and then wipe the straw with sterile hypochlorite solution; rinse with sterile water and dry with sterile gauze.
4. Cut the air-space end of the straw, insert it into a round-bottom culture tube (e.g. Falcon #2003), then cut the straw just below the filter and allow the contents to run out into the tube.
   Note: The ends of the straw must be cut with a sterile device, e.g. disposable suture scissors; a scalpel blade is not recommended due to the significant risk of injury.
5. Process as per the protocol for slow frozen samples.

Sperm Cryobank Organization

Various factors influence the organization of a sperm cryobank (see Figure 10.5). An excellent short monograph on operating a successful cryopreservation facility is available from Planer [67].

Sample Storage Location

For this purpose, various parameters are employed, including the location (each storage tank and canister should be sequentially numbered, e.g. Tank 1, Canister 5), canister level, the shape of the visotube, a combination of colours (e.g. visotube, flag, straw) and a straw code. Radio frequency identification (RFID) tags and barcodes can also be used [68].

Canister

This is a cylindrical container that is hung by a rod (its handle) from the mouth of the cryotank, such that its contents (goblets) are submerged in the liquid nitrogen. The different canisters (the number depends on the capacity of the nitrogen tank) are numbered to specify the location of cryopreserved specimens.

Canister Level

Depending on the tank design, canisters may be short (5" or 13 cm) or tall (11" or 28 cm). Visotubes can be placed directly inside the short canisters, but with tall ones, the use of plastic goblets allows each canister to be divided into upper (U) and lower (L) levels.

Goblet

This is a large (e.g. 35 or 65 mm) plastic cup into which visotubes are placed. Goblets are available in a range of colours.

Visotubes

These are plastic tubes that hold groups of straws, typically only from a single specimen. They can be different shapes (round, triangular, hexagonal, polygonal), different diameters (7.1, 9.2, 10, 12 and 13 mm diameter), and are available in a range of colours.

Cryocane

This is an aluminium rod to which cryovials, cryotubes or visotubes (of straws) can be attached. They have fixed positions and remain firmly in place during storage in liquid nitrogen. Cryocanes can be

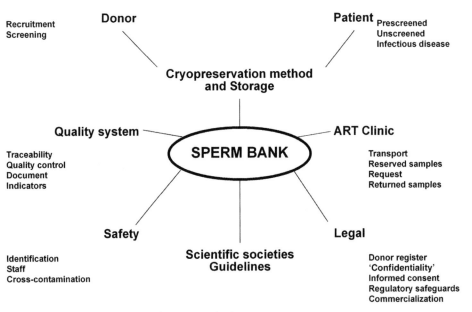

Figure 10.5 Organizational aspects of a sperm cryobank.

numbered or identified by coloured tabs, and self-coloured canes are also available. If re-using a cryocane, make sure that it still grips the devices tightly. Cardboard or transparent plastic sleeves are also available for cryocanes to prevent accidental dislocation of devices, although use of sleeves decreases the number of cryocanes that will fit in a canister. Cryocanes can be cut short to allow their storage within goblet-based inventory systems or tanks that have short (5") canisters.

Cryo-Cassettes

The straws are safely secured inside the cassettes (rectangular or wedge-shaped in cross-section), making it impossible for the straws to float inside the storage bank. Cryo-cassettes have coloured caps and can also be written upon; they incorporate a lifter to facilitate straw insertion or removal.

Cryoflex

A heat shrinkable protective tubing providing extra safety when storing biological samples in cryotubes when immersed in liquid nitrogen.

Storage Box

Cardboard storage box for 100 cryotubes.

Flag

Aluminium or plastic rods which are wider at the top, for labels or colours. Flags can be inserted into visotubes or goblets. The use of paper sticky labels as 'flags' is not recommended due to their fragility at cryogenic temperatures.

Labels

Any labels used must be validated for use at cryogenic temperatures, e.g. Brady labels which have dedicated printing systems (see www.bradyid.com). When straws are used for vitrification, the label must adhere to the end away from the specimen, otherwise use a thermal straw printer to label the devices before loading them.

More commonly used inventory systems are explained in Figure 10.6. While these examples relate to smaller mobile cryotanks, they can be scaled up for use with larger vessels which can have four, some even five, layers of goblets. In four- (or five-) layer systems the layers can be described as top, upper, (middle), lower and bottom. Custom racking systems that allow easy access to multiple layers of goblets in the larger vessels can be obtained from Lifestart Solutions Ltd (Ashford, UK, see www .lifestartsolutions.com), see Figure 10.7.

Samples and Tank Types

To facilitate cryobank management and reduce the possibility of cross-contamination in a sperm bank, there should be different types of tanks corresponding to the origin of the samples. All subjects

CRYOTANK INVENTORY LOCATION SYSTEMS

Heirarchy level		Explanation	Example
1°	CRYOTANK	The cryogenic storage dewars, identified using letters	E
2°	CANISTER	Typically 6 or 10 × 11" canisters per tank, numbered (+ tank ID)	E04
3°	STORAGE UNIT	**Cryocanes** with cryovials (*up to 17 canes per 67mm Ø canister*)	E04–15
		Cryocanes with 2 visotubes (Upper/Lower) for straws, with only 1 case per visotube (*up to 28 canes per 67mm Ø canister*)	E04–15L
		Cryo-cassettes for straws (straws from 1 specimen per cassette) (*up to 37 cryo-casettes per 70mm Ø canister*)	E04–15
4°	SUB- UNITS	**CBS daisy goblets**, 2 per 11" canister: by colour or **U**pper / **L**ower	E04U

Daisy goblet segments: 11 coloured + central visotube

Black	K	Violet	V
Red	R	Mint (pistachio)	M
Dove grey	D	Blue	B
Pink	P	Brown / rust	N
Orange	O	Green	G
Yellow	Y	White	W

E04U-K

12 locations per goblet

Segments can be further sub-divided using 1 or 2 small round visotubes (12mm or 9mm): up to 23 locations per goblet

CBS goblets, 2 per 11" canister: by colour or **U**pper / **L**ower E04L

Visotubes within each goblet by:

Shape: **H**exagonal, **P**olygonal, **R**ound

Colour:			
Red	R	Violet	V
Orange	O	Brown ('rust')	N
Yellow	Y	Turquoise	T
Green	G	Dove grey	D
Blue	B	Black	K
Pink	P	Clear	C

E04L-PV

up to 25 locations per goblet

Hexagonal visotubes can be further sub-divided using 6 × 7.1mm round visotubes of different colours. E04L-YR *49 locations per goblet*

Can also add 6 7.1mm round visotubes peripherally (name as '**X**' and colour); use 1 or 2 × 9.2mm visotubes to secure everything within the goblet. E04L-XO *55 locations per goblet*

<u>Note</u>: CBS goblets are 65mm Ø to fit in 67mm canisters

Figure 10.6 Explanation of common cryotank inventory systems. For more information on canes and cassettes see www .nordiccell.com; for goblet-based systems see www.cryobiosystem.com. Within the images the asterisks identify the location specified in the Example column.

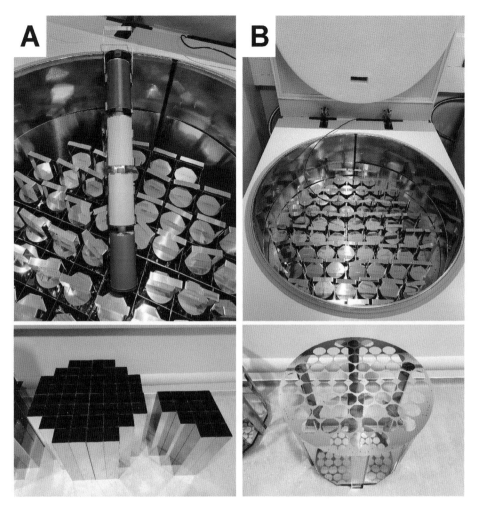

Figure 10.7 Illustration of two types of inventory systems for large capacity cryostorage tanks (shown in Thermo Scientific™ CryoPlus™ 3 vessels), intended for liquid storage of High Security straws and vitrification devices. (A) = a system with each four-level carrier located in a square grid frame made of four symmetrical components (52 carriers = 208 daisy goblets); (B) = a higher density system where the carriers are located in spaces defined simply by a frame (66 carriers = 264 daisy goblets). Goblets are held securely in the carrier sections and can be easily removed and replaced while wearing cryo gauntlets. The base of each section acts as a cover for the one below to prevent specimens floating out when immersed in LN2, with an extra cover above the topmost level. While system B requires more practice to remove and replace the carriers (which must be done absolutely vertically), system A is more forgiving and can be used with a motorized Cryo-Lift® (see www.cryo-lift.com). The upper panels show the systems installed, the lower panels show the structural units outside the cryotank for clarity. These custom inventory systems are from Lifestart Solutions Ltd (Ashford, UK; see www.lifestartsolutions.com).

(Table 10.1) whose semen are going to be frozen should be screened for major viral markers in advance to minimize the risk of potentially infective material (see 'Donor Screening', below). Semen should not be stored in the same cryotanks as embryos or oocytes.

Donor Tanks

Tanks for specimens from all types of sperm donors

Pre-Screening Patient Tanks

Autoconservation for patients who have time for screening, e.g. pre-vasectomy, or patients with repeat screenings.

Unscreened Patient Tanks

Autoconservation for patients without time for screening, for example cancer patients.

Infectious Disease Patient Tanks

Autoconservation for patients with an infectious disease. In theory there should be more than seven tanks for the various combinations of infectious disease patients, notwithstanding the consideration that different clades of a virus might be isolated in separate cryotanks. This number is excessive, but when CBS *High Security Straws* are used, all specimens can be stored in the same tank since these straws achieve effective biocontainment of their contents.

Quarantine Tank

According to some authorities or regulations, reproductive material (semen, oocytes or embryos) from patients with positive serology for HIV, HBV or HCV are initially stored in tanks reserved exclusively for these patients. If a viral load determination is made on semen or washed spermatozoa before cryopreservation, the specimens are stored in quarantine tanks while awaiting the result. Then, after obtaining a negative result, the specimens are transferred into the dedicated tanks for patients with positive serology until being used in ART.

In some banks, the quarantine tank is used to store semen from donors for six months in order to wait for all donor samples in a quarantine tank to be 'cleared' before allowing any samples to be transferred to a 'definitive' donor storage tank – but if even one sample tests positive for a pathogen then the entire tank contents should be discarded and the tank emptied and sterilized (which, from experience, is rarely actually done). An adequate cost-benefit analysis of this tank should be made in each bank [51]. However, such quarantine tanks are not necessary when using CBS straws, since they achieve effective biocontainment of all specimens. This should also meet, in principle and effect, the requirement for 'separate storage' under Directive 2006/17/EC, e.g. as in Annex III, ¶2.3.

Emergency Tanks or Cleaning of Other Tanks

These are used in the case of an accident with one of the other tanks or when other tanks are to be cleaned. A periodic cleaning of the storage tanks should be carried out by allowing the cryotank to warm, wiping with a disinfectant solution and rinsing with distilled water. Allow to dry before re-filling [56]. If CBS *High Security Straws* are not used, cleaning should be carried out annually. However, if these secure straws are used, the major source of the material that forms the white 'slurry' at the bottom of cryotanks is the fog composed of frozen moisture from room air or the exhaled breath of operators when a cryotank is opened. Consequently, cleaning should only be carried out perhaps every five years.

Reserved Samples

A protocol to reserve spermatozoa from a donor for further pregnancies by a patient should exist.

Storage Systems

When a frozen sample stored below −132°C warms above this temperature, a recrystallization of frozen water molecules takes place. This recrystallization can induce incipient damage to the cryopreserved cells, damage that will not become evident until months or years later when the sample is finally thawed. Moreover, this damage is cumulative; each incident of warming above −132°C will contribute to decreasing the functional survival possibilities of the cryopreserved cells. However, spermatozoa that have been vitrified with non-permeating CPAs have much less residual intracellular water, making it possible to consider storage at higher temperatures [69].

There are four types of storage systems for cryogenically frozen samples: liquid phase nitrogen, vapour phase nitrogen, super cold air and mechanical freezers. The factors to keep in mind to decide what type of storage to utilize are: storage temperature, temperature fluctuation during audit, theoretical cross-contamination risks, staff safety, equipment cost, packaging systems, and the size and space of the cryobank [31,47,51,52]. Clearly, the lower the storage temperature, the greater the margin of safety when a specimen is removed briefly to check its identity. The lowest storage temperature is reached with storage in liquid phase nitrogen; the slightly higher theoretical cross-contamination risk in such cryotanks can be essentially eliminated using CBS *High Security Straws* [31].

Inventory Control Systems

Each sample to be processed by a sperm bank is immediately identified in accordance with the bank's sample identification protocol (i.e. at least two identifiers: the subject's name and an ID number). This identification system should be mechanized, whenever possible, for greater clarity of references. The final identification of the straws can be carried out using a double system of barcodes and alphanumeric characters on labels.

Straws are generally located by a local inventory code (straw, visotube and flag colour, canister, tank). Inventory details must be recorded in a dedicated inventory logbook and in a password-protected electronic inventory database, with varying levels of access to users.

Straw codes should be linked so that key individuals with appropriate access rights can interrogate other relevant datasets, e.g. clinical data, follow-up data. The local inventory code and straw-code can be used in conjunction with a national or international code [70] to ensure straw traceability, and straws issued for use should be accompanied by all relevant documentation. According to the EU Tissues & Cells Directive [71], a Single European (identifying) Code ('SEC code') must be assigned to all donated semen specimens distributed for human application. Semen cryopreserved for autologous use, or when the donated semen is used only in patients treated in a clinic/hospital having the same location as the ART establishment that is authorized for non-partner donation activities, do not require a SEC code. This SEC code incorporates information on both the donation identification (identification of the tissue establishment and unique donation identification number) and the product identification (product code and split number). Due to the length of the code (40 characters), where the label size precludes the application of the SEC, the code shall be unambiguously linked to the packaging device with such a label through the accompanying documentation.

Traceability

A system to ensure the traceability of frozen sperm samples must be established, and this would also make it possible to verify compliance with quality and safety standards. Traceability should operate both from the donor to the recipient and *vice versa*, and include all products and materials that come into contact with the semen that could have an effect on specimen quality and safety. Traceability should also include the chain of custody: who received a semen sample, who performed the cryopreservation, who audited the frozen straw, etc. [70].

Legal Considerations

Sperm banking includes a variety of ethical concerns pertaining to such values as dignity, bodily integrity, autonomy, ownership and privacy. These ethical concerns have been translated into a complex and incoherent apparatus of private, public, national and international standards and provisions. All these norms not only differ with respect to whether they are legally binding, but also reveal that there is no clear national or international consensus on pivotal issues in sperm banking. The framework of norms relating to sperm banking is under permanent reconstruction. The main factors considered in this regard are: commercialization, confidentiality, informed consent, and regulatory safeguards. Information registries concerning donation must be kept for at least 30 years in order to enable the traceability of the donors and to fulfil the possible need for information about the donor [70]. Other regulatory aspects of sperm cryobanking (e.g. air quality) have been discussed previously [72].

Posthumous Reproduction

Since one category of people who cryopreserve their gametes or reproductive tissues are patients affected by serious diseases, there is a real chance that some people will die with their reproductive material in storage. Such a possibility must be raised and talked through in counselling sessions prior to banking material. Posthumous use is regulated in some countries, so a specific procedure is necessary for proper management of these samples [73].

Storage Period

While the longest period of cryopreservation that has resulted in a human birth is 40 years [74] in most countries there is a legal limitation on semen storage. Reproductive tissues and gametes should only be stored until the age at which it is considered acceptable for them to be used for the achievement of a pregnancy [71].

Maximum Number of Children Born from a Donor

The regulation of live births per donor varies greatly between countries. However, it is generally accepted that the limit on the maximum number of children per donor should be by families created and not by patients treated [64,75].

Transportation

Dry Shippers

To ensure the maximum performance of a shipping tank, its integrity has to be tested periodically. Weigh the shipping tank empty and then after filling (allow it to cool slowly with repeated additions of liquid nitrogen over a period of several hours to ensure maximum performance), monitor its static evaporative loss over a few days to verify its integrity [19]. A thermal camera can be used for dewar failure detection.

Transport

To achieve safe transportation of biological material, international recommendations for transportation of biological material must be observed. International and national regulatory agencies require that anyone involved in the shipping and packaging of dangerous goods must receive training and certification in the proper regulations that govern the transport, packaging, and labelling of those materials. Consequently, patients should not transport frozen sperm samples themselves.

Returning Sperm Samples

As a general rule, if returning semen to the provider cryobank (e.g. cancelled insemination cycle), a cryobank can only accept the return of samples when the following three conditions are met: (1) the samples have not been thawed; (2) the integrity of the package can be demonstrated (the seals are intact); and (3) proper storage temperature for the sample has been maintained throughout the transport (and can be demonstrated). Because of the difficulty in adequately proving the last item, many cryobanks will not accept any returned samples.

Donor Screening

The recruitment of sperm donors is an increasingly difficult process. At most, one out of ten men initially evaluated is accepted as a donor [21,22]. The three principal reasons for this acceptance rate are lack of interest after the initial phone interview or after completing the intake questionnaire, issues arising from the serology testing or medical history, and on the basis of semen quality or post-thaw sperm survival.

In many jurisdictions the recruitment, selection and management of sperm donors is not just covered by recommendations from professional societies but also highly regulated. Examples include the Tissues and Cells Directives in the European Union [76], FDA regulations and guidelines from the American Society for Reproductive Medicine in the USA [77,78], and Health Canada's regulations and guidance [79,80]

Especially where there are regulations, it is required that a lab follow them, often under significant penalty. Consequently, any recommendations made in this chapter are intended only as general guidelines and will be superseded by local regulations. However, it must be recognized that there is no way to totally preclude all risks of genetic or infectious disease transmission to offspring resulting from donor sperm treatment.

Clinical History and Physical Screening

A complete personal and sexual history should be obtained and an abbreviated version of the donor's personal history should be obtained before each donation, thus highlighting changes that might require a donor to be excluded from the donation programme [78]. Semen from donors older than 45 years should not be admitted, and in many jurisdictions an upper age limit is established by legislation. Psychological screening is an expected part of medical screening, and needs to focus on looking at motivation, looking at pattern of personal stability, discussing the psychological ramifications of being a gamete donor, giving psychological guidance in the preparations for becoming a gamete donor, and ruling out pathology or coercion. Psychological screening that exceeds these objectives should not be done. Sperm donor candidates should undergo a complete physical examination, including tests for urethral discharge, warts and scattered ulcers, disseminated lymphadeno-pathies, anal injures and venous punctures [78,81]. These physical examinations should be repeated every six months, as long as the donor is participating in the donation programme.

Routine biochemical and haematological laboratory screening, including tests for blood group and Rh factor, are also typically recommended.

Genetic Screening

A karyotype study should be carried out for donations of gametes [81,82], and a donor's family history up to three generations should be compiled. Donor candidates are rejected if their antecedents present a significant risk, for example with respect to certain specific polygenic diseases, that is deemed to be greater than that of the general population. When genetic diseases with family associations, for which there are no genetic screening tests, because they are polygenic or multifactorial (e.g. congenital myopia, multiple sclerosis, autism, etc.), occur in first degree relatives, these donor candidates should not be accepted. If the antecedents are of dominant or recessive diseases, screening is easier because diagnostic tests are available.

Extended genetic carrier screening studies aim to identify whether or not a recipient of donor semen is a carrier of pathogenic or probable pathogenic variants related to serious genetic diseases which respond to a recessive autosomal inheritance or are linked to the X chromosome. With this information, a recipient can be advised of genetic risk to her future offspring and be made aware of the different strategies available to mitigate possible hereditary diseases. However, it must be assumed that, given the sensitive and unique nature of genetic information (it allows individual characterization, it is permanent, predictive and may affect biological relatives), and the cost of this testing, all patients might not agree to carrying out genetic studies. In addition, due to the large number of possible diseases and genetic alterations, and the complexity of studying and interpreting the results, not all centres and gamete banks will process donors' genetic information in the same way.

Hence it is not advisable to define a single genetic screening strategy for gamete donors. Recipients who need to use ART should be informed about possible existing strategies, as well as the limitations of genetic tests. This would allow them to reduce the risk of having offspring affected by a serious hereditary recessive disease or an X-linked genetic disease which, in the event of not taking any preventative measures has an estimated general population prevalence of about 0.5% without other risk factors.

First Strategy

Faced with recipients of donor spermatozoa who have decided not to carry out any genetic screening tests for carriers of recessive diseases, centres which use donor gametes should carry on candidates at least karyotype and ethnicity and population-based genetic screening for carriers of recessive diseases.

Due to prevalence, penetrance, genotype-phenotype correlation and seriousness, this basic genetic screening should include at least:

- Cystic fibrosis in Caucasian populations (analysis of pathogenic variants of the CFTR gene with high demographic frequency and which show clear association with the development of a severe phenotype of cystic fibrosis, testing should reduce by at least 75% the baseline risk of being a carrier of this disease)
- Glucose-6-phosphate dehydrogenase deficiency
- α or ß-Thalassaemia in Mediterranean populations
- Sickle cell disease in African and Afro-Caribbean populations
- Tay-Sachs disease in Jews of Eastern European descent
- Spinal muscular atrophy (SMN1) in all donors

Semen donors with X-chromosome-linked diseases will be ruled out by anamnesis and medical history.

Second Strategy

Where a recipient agrees to carry out a genetic carrier screening study of recessive diseases (as well as having the donor karyotype), the recommended strategy aimed at reducing the risk of having offspring affected by a serious hereditary recessive disease consists of selecting donors who do not share pathogenic variants on the same gene as the recipient (genetic matching). Nonetheless, it will be necessary to warn recipients of the very small but real risk of the appearance of unknown mutations, or technical limitations of testing, which mean that there is always a residual risk of offspring being affected by the diseases studied in the genetic matching. With this strategy, the reduction in the risk of having a child affected by a recessive genetic disease only applies to the diseases where the recipient has been studied.

Serological and Microbiological Tests

Screening for infectious diseases (HIV-1 and HIV-2, HCV, HBV and syphilis) is essential before the cryopreservation of donated semen, although no method exists to ensure total effectiveness regarding the non-transmission of infectious agents [31]. Laboratory tests used in the screening of semen donors should be approved by the FDA [78], or by the EU [82], or other regulatory bodies as appropriate. Serological tests of semen donors should be performed seven days before the first freezing for treatment purposes, and every six months while they are making donations [82]. Quarantine can be reduced to three months if serology and PCR are carried out after this time has passed [81]. There is no need to perform repeat screening for transmissible infectious diseases if every donation is screened using PCR [70].

Tests for anti HTLV-I and II antibodies should be performed for all donors who reside in or who come from zones of high incidence of specific diseases, or whose spouse/partner or family come from these zones [70,81] – or where required by regulation. A donor with a non-specific positive test for syphilis should not be rejected if a specific test produces a negative result [70]. Reject donors with active cytomegalovirus (CMV) infections (positive CMV IgM antibodies or a recently positive IgG seroconversion). Matching according to the anti-CMV serological status, and using donor semen with negative CMV IgM antibodies and positive CMV IgG (indicative of past infection, and low probability of virus-containing semen) for recipients with the same serological status, is a practise recommended in some countries [e.g. 78,81], but not in others [e.g. 80,82].

NAT testing for *Neisseria gonorrhoeae* and *Chlamydia trachomatis* on urine or a swab obtained from the urethral meatus must be negative at the initial screening, and again after three [81] or six months [78].

Collaboration with the local Sexually Transmitted Disease (Genito-Urinary Medicine) Clinic concerning the type of screening tests, testing intervals, etc., is extremely valuable.

Screening for the West Nile virus (WNV) is recommended (using PCR) if the donation is made during the time of year when WNV is potentially transmissible to humans in the donor's country of residence (e.g. from 1 June through to 31 October in the USA and Canada) [78,80], or if in the preceding 56 days a donor has lived in or travelled to an area where WNV is endemic [80]. Although there is currently no definitive evidence linking WNV transmission with reproductive cells, it is recommended that practitioners defer gamete donors who have confirmed or suspected WNV infections in the preceding 120 days [78].

Regarding the Zika virus, temporary exclusion as sperm donors of those who have visited countries and areas affected by indigenous transmission of the Zika virus is recommended for six months following their return, and for six months following cessation of symptoms in those diagnosed with Zika virus infection. The list of affected areas and countries can be consulted in the epidemiological updates published by the European Centre for Disease Prevention and Control (www.ecdc.europa.eu/en/zika-virus-disease).

The risk of transmission of SARS-CoV-2 via semen remains unclear at this time, but the precautionary principle would support the opinion that sperm donors with a positive triage for SARS-CoV-2 infection, and perhaps even only with significant symptoms if the local risk of infection is high, should postpone donating semen for at least 21 days or be studied with laboratory tests.

Semen Analysis

A classical semen examination must be done on all sperm donor candidates according to the guidelines described in this handbook (see Chapter 3). To avoid unnecessary freezing of donor specimens, a baseline of acceptable pre-freeze sperm characteristics should be established in order to guarantee a minimum acceptable motile sperm count after thawing (e.g. sperm concentration $>50 \times 10^6$/ml, $\geq 40\%$ progressively motile, and other seminal parameter within reference values). However, no agreement exists with respect to these parameters between the different authors [19,22,23] due to the high inter-individual variability of sperm cryopreservation [20–22]. In consideration of the aforementioned factors, we can only expect to be able to estimate the post-thaw survival rate from the pre-freeze sperm characteristics, recognizing the sensitivity of such predictions to measurement error [58]. But, nonetheless, cryopreserved donor semen with low post-thaw characteristics (notably the number of progressively motile spermatozoa per unit or 'dose') would not seem to be fit for purpose, especially if being provided as a commercial product.

References

1. Arav A, Natan Y. The near future of vitrification of oocytes and embryos: looking into past experience and planning into the future. *Transfus Med Hemother* 2019; **46**: 182–7.

2. Öztürk AE, Bucak MN, Bodu M, et al. Cryobiology and cryopreservation of sperm. In: Quain M ed., *Cryopreservation. Current Advances and Evaluations.* London: InTechOpen, 2020. www.intechopen.com/books/cryopreservation-current-advances-and-evaluations/cryobiology-and-cryopreservation-of-sperm

3. Fahy GM, Wowk B. Principles of cryopreservation by vitrification. *Methods Mol Biol* 2015; **1257**: 21–82.

4. Yeste M, Morató R, Rodríguez-Gil JE, et al. Aquaporins in the male reproductive tract and sperm: functional implications and cryobiology. *Reprod Domest Anim* 2017; **52**: 12–27.

5. Morris GJ, Acton E, Murray BJ, Fonseca F. Freezing injury: the special case of the sperm cell. *Cryobiology* 2012; **64**: 71–80.

6. Fuller B, Paynter S. Fundamentals of cryobiology in reproductive medicine. *Reprod Biomed Online* 2004; **9**: 680–91.

7. Mazur P, Leibo SP, Farrant J, et al. Interactions of cooling rate, warming rate and protective additive on the survival of frozen mammalian cells. In: Wolstenholme GE, O'Connor M, eds., *The Frozen Cell.* London: Churchill Press, 1970, 69–88.

8. Nei T. Mechanism of haemolysis of erythrocytes by freezing, with special reference to freezing at near-zero temperatures. In: Wolstenholme GE, O'Connor M, eds., *The Frozen Cell.* London: Churchill Press, 1970, 131–47.

9. Merryman HT. The exceeding of a minimum tolerable cell volume in hypertonic suspension as a cause of freezing injury. In: Wolstenholme GE, O'Connor M, eds., *The Frozen Cell.* London: Churchill Press, 1970, 565–9.

10. Nijs M, Ombelet W. Cryopreservation of human sperm. *Hum Fertil* 2001; **4**: 158–63.

11. Thomson LK, Fleming SD, Aitken RJ, De Iuliis GN, Zieschang JA, Clark AM. Cryopreservation-induced human sperm DNA damage is predominantly mediated by oxidative stress rather than apoptosis. *Hum Reprod* 2009; **24**: 2061–70.

12. Schulz M, Risopatrón J, Uribe P, et al. Human sperm vitrification: a scientific report. *Andrology* 2020; **8**: 1642–50.

13. Gao D, Liu J, Liu C, et al. Prevention of osmotic injury to human spermatozoa during addition and removal of glycerol. *Hum Reprod* 1995; **10**: 1109–22.

14. Isachenko E, Isachenko V, Sanchez R, et al. Cryopreservation of spermatozoa: old routine and new perspectives. In: Donnez J, Kim SS, eds., *Principles and Practice of Fertility Preservation.* Cambridge: Cambridge University Press, 2011, 176–98.

15. Tao Y, Sanger E, Saewu A, Leveille MC. Human sperm vitrification: the state of the art. *Reprod Biol Endocrinol* 2020; **18**: 17.

16. Isachenko V, Maettner R, Petrunkina AM, et al. Cryoprotectant-free vitrification of human spermatozoa in large (up to 0.5 ml) volume: a novel technology. *Clin Lab* 2011; **57**: 643–50.

17. Mansilla MA, Merino O, Risopatrón J, et al. High temperature is essential for preserved human sperm function during the devitrification process. *Andrologia* 2016; **48**: 111–13.

18. Gilmore JA, Liu J, Gao DY, et al. Determination of optimal cryoprotectants and procedures for their addition and removal from human spermatozoa. *Hum Reprod* 1997; **12**: 112–18.

19. Mortimer D. *Practical Laboratory Andrology.* Oxford: Oxford University Press, 1994, 301–23.

20. Centola GM, Raubertas RF, Mattox JH. Cryopreservation of human semen. Comparison of cryopreservatives, sources of variability, and prediction of post-thaw survival. *J Androl* 1992; **13**: 283–8.

21. Keel BA, Webster BW. Semen cryopreservation methodology and results. In: Barratt CLR, Cooke ID, eds., *Donor Insemination.* Cambridge: Cambridge University Press, 1993, 71–96.

22. Barratt CL, Clements S, Kessopoulou E. Semen characteristics and fertility tests required for storage of spermatozoa. *Hum Reprod* 1998; **13 Suppl 2**: 1–7.

23. Yogev L, Kleiman S, Shabtai E, et al. Seasonal variations in pre- and post-thaw donor sperm quality. *Hum Reprod* 2004; **19**: 880–5.

24. Holt WV. Basic aspects of frozen storage of semen. *Anim Reprod Sci* 2000; **62**: 3–22.

25. Amidi F, Pazhohan A, Shabani Nashtaei M, et al. The role of antioxidants in sperm freezing: a review. *Cell Tissue Bank* 2016; **17**: 745–56.

26. Len JS, Koh WSD, Tan SX. The roles of reactive oxygen species and antioxidants in cryopreservation. *Biosci Rep* 2019; **39**: BSR20191601.

27. Jannatifar R, Piroozmanesh H, Naserpoor L. Supplementation of freezing media with cyclic adenosine monophosphate analog and isobutylmethylxanthine on sperm quality. *Res Mol Med* 2020; **8**: 201–8.

28. Stacey G. Validation of cell culture media components. *Hum Fertil* 2004; **7**: 113–18.

29. Nallella KP, Sharma KK, Allamaneni SS, et al. Cryopreservation of human spermatozoa: comparison of two cryopreservation methods and three cryoprotectants. *Fertil Steril* 2004; **82**: 913–18.

30. Banihani SA, Alawneh RF. Human semen samples with high antioxidant reservoir may exhibit lower post-cryopreservation recovery of sperm motility. *Biomolecules* 2019; **9**: 111.

31. Mortimer D. Current and future concepts and practices in human sperm cryobanking. *Reprod Biomed Online* 2004; **9**: 134–51.

32. Stanic P, Tandara M, Sonicki Z, et al. Comparison of protective media and freezing techniques for cryopreservation of human semen. *Eur J Obstet Gynecol Reprod Biol* 2000; **91**: 65–70.

33. Morris J. *Asymptote Cool Guide to Cryopreservation*. Cambridge: Asymptote Ltd 2002. https://docplayer.net/64129364-Asymptote-guide-to-cryopreservation.html [last accessed 25 August 2021].

34. Henry MA, Noiles EE, Gao D, et al. Cryopreservation of human spermatozoa. IV. The effects of cooling rate and warming rate on the maintenance of motility, plasma membrane integrity, and mitochondrial function. *Fertil Steril* 1993; **60**: 911–18.

35. Isachenko V, Isachenko E, Katkov II, et al. Cryoprotectant-free cryopreservation of human spermatozoa by vitrification and freezing in vapor: effect on motility, DNA integrity, and fertilization ability. *Biol Reprod* 2004; **71**: 1167–73.

36. Calamera JC, Buffone MG, Doncel GF, et al. Effect of thawing temperature on the motility recovery of cryopreserved human spermatozoa. *Fertil Steril* 2010; **93**: 789–94.

37. Wang M, Isachenko E, Todorov P, et al. Aseptic technology for cryoprotectant-free vitrification of human spermatozoa by direct dropping into clean liquid air: apoptosis, necrosis, motility, and viability. *Biomed Res Int* 2020; 2934315.

38. Shah D, Rasappan, Shila, Gunasekaran K. A simple method of human sperm vitrification. *MethodsX* 2019; **6**: 2198–204.

39. Berkovitz A, Miller N, Silberman M, et al. A novel solution for freezing small numbers of spermatozoa using a sperm vitrification device. *Hum Reprod* 2018; **33**: 1975–83.

40. Le MT, Nguyen TTT, Nguyen TT, et al. Cryopreservation of human spermatozoa by vitrification versus conventional rapid freezing: effects on motility, viability, morphology and cellular defects. *Eur J Obstet Gynecol Reprod Biol* 2019; **234**: 14–20.

41. Cassou R. La méthode des paillettes en plastique adaptée a la généralisation de la congélation. *5th Int Cong Anim Reprod Artif Insem Trento* 1964; **4**: 540–6.

42. Cryo Bio System. CBS™ High Security Cryobanking Systems Product Monograph. L'Aigle. CryoBioSystem 2021. www.cryobiosystem.com/cbs-high-security-cryobanking-systems-product-monograph/ [last accessed 25 August 2021].

43. Russell PH, Lyaruu VH, Millar JD, et al. The potential transmission of infectious agents by semen packaging during storage for artificial insemination. *Anim Reprod Sci* 1997; **47**: 337–42.

44. Liu S, Li F. Cryopreservation of single sperm: where are we today? *Reprod Biol Endocrinol* 2020; **18**: 41–52.

45. Tyler JP, Kime L, Cooke S, et al. Temperature change in cryo-containers during short exposure to ambient temperatures. *Hum Reprod* 1996; **11**: 1510–12.

46. Byers KB. Risks associated with liquid nitrogen cryogenic storage systems. *J Am Biol Safety Assoc* 1998; **3**: 143–6.

47. Clarke GN. Sperm cryopreservation: is there a significant risk of cross-contamination? *Hum Reprod* 1999; **14**: 2941–3.

48. Nalge Nunc International. *Cryopreservation Manual*. Rochester: Nalge Nunc International Corporation (now part of Thermo Fisher), 1998.

49. Wood MJ. The problems of storing gametes and embryos. *Cryo-Letters* 1999; **20**: 155–8.

50. Tedder RS, Zuckerman MA, Goldstone AH, et al. Hepatitis B transmission from contaminated cryopreservation tank. *Lancet* 1995; **346**: 137–40.

51. Tomlinson M, Sakkas D. Is a review of standard procedures for cryopreservation needed? Safe and effective cryopreservation – should sperm banks and fertility centres move towards storage in nitrogen vapour? *Hum Reprod* 2000; **15**: 2460–3.

52. Mortimer D. Setting up risk management systems in IVF laboratories. *Clinical Risk* 2004; **10**: 128–37.

53. Mortimer ST, Mortimer D. *Quality and Risk Management in the IVF Laboratory*, 2nd edn. Cambridge: Cambridge University Press, 2015.

54. Parmegiani L, Accorsi A, Cognigni GE, et al. Sterilization of liquid nitrogen with ultraviolet irradiation for safe vitrification of human oocytes or embryos. *Fertil Steril* 2010; **94**: 1525–8.

55. Isachenko V, Rahimi G, Mallmann P, et al. Technologies of cryoprotectant-free vitrification of human spermatozoa: asepticity as criterion of effectiveness. *Andrology* 2017; **5**: 1055–63.

56. Elder K, Baker D, Ribes J. *Infections, Infertility and Assisted Reproduction*. Cambridge: Cambridge University Press, 2005.

57. Carrell DT, Cartmill D, Jones KP, et al. Prospective randomized, blinded evaluation of donor semen quality provided by seven commercial sperm banks. *Fertil Steril* 2002; **78**: 16–21.

58. Castilla JA, Sánchez-León M, Garrido A, et al. Procedure control and acceptance sampling for donor sperm banks: a theoretical study. *Cell Tissue Bank* 2007; **8**: 257–65.

59. Chan CC, Chen IC, Liu JY, et al. Comparison of nitric oxide production motion characteristics of sperm after cryopreserved in three different preparations. *Arch Androl* 2004; **50**: 1–3.

60. Grizard G, Chevalier V, Griveau JF, et al. Influence of seminal plasma on cryopreservation of human spermatozoa in a biological material-free medium: study of normal low-quality semen. *Int J Androl* 1999; **22**: 190–6.

61. Palomar Rios A, Gascón A, Martínez JV, et al. Sperm preparation after freezing improves motile sperm count, motility, and viability in frozen-thawed sperm compared with sperm preparation before freezing-thawing process. *J Assist Reprod Genet* 2018; **35**: 237–45.

62. Cohen J, Garrisi GJ, Congedo-Ferrara TA, et al. Cryopreservation of single human spermatozoa. *Hum Reprod* 1997; **12**: 994–1001.

63. David G, Czyglik F, Mayaux MJ, et al. Artificial insemination with frozen sperm: protocol, method of analysis and results for 1188 women. *Br J Obstet Gynaecol* 1980; **87**: 1022–8.

64. Le Lannou D, Thepot F, Jouannet P. Multicentre approaches to donor insemination in the French CECOS Federation: nationwide evaluation donor matching, screening for genetic diseases and consanguinity. *Hum Reprod* 1998; **13 Suppl 2**: 35–54.

65. Ofeim O, Brown TA, Gilbert BR. Effects of serial thaw-refreeze cycles on human sperm motility and viability. *Fertil Steril* 2001; **75**: 1242–3.

66. Isachenko E, Mallmann P, Rahimi G, et al. Vitrification technique: new possibilities for male gamete low-temperature storage. In: Katkov I ed., *Current Frontiers in Cryobiology*. London: InTechOpen, 2012, 41–76. Available at www .intechopen.com/books/current-frontiers-in-cryobiology/vitrification-of-fish-and-dog-spermatozoa [last accessed 25 August 2021].

67. Bennet J, Grout B. *Operating a Successful Cryopreservation Facility*. Sunbury (UK): Planer plc, 2018. See www.planer.com.

68. Igbokwe N, Tomlinson M. The use of radio frequency identification (RFID) and track and trace technology in reducing the risks and cost of sperm cryopreservation. *Ann Clin Lab Res* 2020; **8**: 308.

69. Sanchez R, Risopatrón J, Schulz M, et al. Vitrified sperm banks: the new aseptic technique for human spermatozoa allows cryopreservation at -86°C. *Andrologia* 2012; **44**: 433–5.

70. European Union 2004. Directive 2004/23/EC of the European Parliament and of the Council of 31 March 2004 on setting standards of quality and safety for the donation, procurement, testing, processing, preservation, storage, and distribution of human tissues and cells. https://eur-lex.europa .eu/legal-content/EN/TXT/?uri=celex:32004 L0023 [last accessed 25 August 2021].

71. European Union Commission. Commission Directive (EU) 2015/565 of 8 April 2015 amending Directive 2006/86/EC as regards certain technical requirements for the coding of human tissues and cells. Official Journal of the European Union L 93/43. http://eur-lex.europa.eu/legal-content/EN/TXT/PDF/?uri=CELEX:32015L0565&from=EN [last accessed 25 August 2021].

72. Mortimer D. A critical assessment of the impact of the European Union Tissues and Cells Directive (2004) on laboratory practices in assisted conception. *Reprod Biomed Online* 2005; **11**: 162–76.

73. The ESHRE Task Force on Ethics and Law. Taskforce 7: Ethical considerations for the cryopreservation of gametes and reproductive tissues for self use. *Hum Reprod* 2004; **19**: 460–2.

74. Szell AZ, Bierbaum RC, Hazelrigg WB, Chetkowski RJ. Live births from frozen human semen stored for 40 years. *J Assist Reprod Genet* 2013; **30**: 743–4.

75. Janssens PM, Thorn P, Castilla JA, et al. Evolving minimum standards in responsible international sperm donor offspring quota. *Reprod Biomed Online* 2015; **30**: 568–80.

76. European Union Commission. Commission Directive 2006/17/EC of 8 February 2006 implementing Directive 2004/23/EC of the European Parliament and of the Council as regards certain technical requirements for the donation, procurement and testing of human tissues and cells. https://eur-lex.europa.eu/legal-content/EN/TXT/?uri=CELEX:32006L0017 [last accessed 25 August 2021].

77. US Food & Drug Administration. Tissue & Tissue Products. www.fda.gov/vaccines-blood-biologics/tissue-tissue-products [last accessed 25 August 2021].

78. Practice Committee of the American Society for Reproductive Medicine and the Practice Committee of the Society for Assisted Reproductive Technology. Guidance regarding gamete and embryo donation. *Fertil Steril* 2021; **115**: 1395–410. https://doi.org/10.1016/j .fertnstert.2021.01.045

79. Government of Canada. Safety of Sperm and Ova Regulations (SOR/2019–192). https://laws-lois.justice.gc.ca/eng/regulations/SOR-2019-192/index.html

80. Health Canada Directive. Technical requirements for conducting the suitability assessment of sperm and ova donors. Ottawa (Canada): Health Canada 2019. Available at: www.canada.ca/content/dam/hc-sc/documents/services/publications/drugs-

health-products/technical-directive-sperm-ova-donors/technical-directive-sperm-ova-donors-en.pdf [last accessed 25 August 2021].

81. Clarke H, Harrison S, Perez MJ, Kirkman-Brown J on behalf of the Association of Clinical Embryologists, the Association of Biomedical Andrologists, the British Fertility Society, and the British Andrology Society. UK guidelines for the medical and laboratory procurement and use of sperm, oocyte and embryo donors (2019). *Hum Fertil* 2019; 1–13. https://doi.org/10.1080/14647273.2019.1622040

82. EDQM (European Directorate for the Quality of Medicines & HealthCare of the Council of Europe). *Guide to the quality and safety of tissues and cells for human application*. Strasbourg: 4° ed Council of Europe, 2019. https://register.edqm.eu/freepub [last accessed 25 August 2021].

83. Katkov I, Bolyukh V, Chernetsov OA, et al. Kinetic vitrification of spermatozoa of vertebrates: what can we learn from nature? In: Katkov I ed., *Current Frontiers in Cryobiology*. London: InTechOpen, 2012, 1–40. Available at: www.intechopen.com/books/current-frontiers-in-cryobiology/kinetic-vitrfiication-of-sperm-of-vertebrates-what-can-we-learn-from-nature- [last accessed 25 August 2021].

Preparation of Surgically Retrieved Spermatozoa

Background

For many men with azoospermia, of both excretory and secretory types, spermatozoa for use in ART (nowadays almost always using ICSI, and ideally after their cryopreservation) can be recovered directly from the epididymis or testis. Since this is a laboratory handbook, clinical procedures for surgically recovering spermatozoa from the male reproductive tract are not included, but are reviewed elsewhere [1,2]. Prior screening of azoospermic subjects for microdeletions in the AZF region of the Y chromosome can be clinically useful in excluding some cases with extremely poor prognosis; this testing should be a part of the clinical work-up prior to attempting surgical retrieval of spermatozoa [3].

Strategies for processing and selection of surgically retrieved spermatozoa have been reviewed recently [4,5], but in simple terms, in cases with obstructive azoospermia or bilateral absence of vas deferens, the first approach is typically percutaneous sperm aspiration (PESA) or micro-epididymal sperm aspiration (MESA). If no spermatozoa can be recovered from the epididymis, then testicular sperm recovery can be attempted.

In non-obstructive azoospermia (NOA) the cause is at the level of the seminiferous epithelium, with severe impairment of spermatogenesis. Testicular biopsy can provide tissue in which foci of spermatogenic activity can be found and spermatozoa recovered by testicular sperm aspiration (TESA) or testicular sperm extraction (TESE). In conventional TESE (cTESE), one or multiple biopsies are taken randomly, whereas in microdissection TESE (micro-TESE), a large incision is made through the tunica albuginea, and the seminiferous tubules are examined at 20–25× magnification using an operating microscope. Tubules showing distension might contain usable spermatozoa.

Systematic reviews of studies comparing the outcome of various methods for retrieving spermatozoa in cases with NOA indicate greater success with micro-TESE compared with cTESE [6,7], and better with cTESE than with TESA [7]. However, the populations and procedures vary across the studies, and good randomized clinical studies are lacking.

Preparation of Epididymal Spermatozoa

Principle

Fluid is aspirated from the epididymis through a fine needle (PESA) or obtained by making a small cut into the epididymis (MESA). The spermatozoa are ideally isolated from the epididymal fluid by density gradient centrifugation, although in cases when there are very few spermatozoa, simple centrifugal washing might have to be used. This can, however, increase the risk of ROS-induced damage to the spermatozoa, especially their DNA.

Specimen

- Aspirated epididymal fluid

Equipment

See also Appendix 2.

- Microscope configured for andrology with phase contrast optics (10×, 20× and 40× objectives)

- Centrifuge
- Tally counter
- Air-displacement pipetter, 500-µl volume
- Rubber bulb to control Pasteur pipettes

Disposable Materials

- Centrifuge tubes
- Glass Pasteur pipettes (sterile), 5.75"
- Microscope slides
- Coverslips, 22 × 22 mm #1½ or #2 thickness
- Pipette tips

Reagents

Sperm Buffer: Any HEPES- or MOPS-buffered ART culture medium known to support human spermatozoa that is supplemented with at least 5 mg/ml (ideally 10 mg/ml) of HSA. The medium must be at 37°C prior to use.

Calibration

The incubator used to warm the media must be set at 37°C and its operation verified using an independent temperature measuring device.

Quality Control

No special QC procedures are required for this technique.

Procedure

1. Upon receiving a specimen of aspirated fluid, empty the syringe into a sterile Falcon tube, pumping the plunger several times to expel all the fluid.
2. Prepare a wet preparation using 10 µl of the diluted aspirate on a clean slide with a 22 × 22 mm coverslip. Examine under the microscope at 200× magnification.
3. Check for the presence of spermatozoa, and assess their approximate concentration (e.g. as 'high', 'average' or 'low') and motility (e.g. <1%, 1%, 5%, 20%, etc.); 5–10 motile spermatozoa per 20× objective field constitutes an average quality specimen.
4. Report the findings immediately to the surgeon and record the % motility on the Falcon tube from which the sample was taken. Also note on the tube anything that might affect the freezing process, e.g. a lot of blood, or low sperm concentration, compared to the other samples.
5. Once the sample has been evaluated, store it in a 37°C air (non-CO_2) incubator.
6. Repeat steps #1 through #5 for each aspirated specimen.
   Note. If cases are done in or adjacent to the surgical procedure room, the urologist will likely ask when there is 'enough specimen to freeze'. Individual judgement is required here and, while not going too far, estimates should be on the cautious side.
7. Combine all aspirates which contain motile spermatozoa into one tube using sterile Pasteur pipettes and measure the total volume for cryopreservation.
8. Determine the concentration and motility of the total sample using a Makler chamber and evaluate the amount of debris at the same time. Fixed-depth chambers that fill by capillary action are not recommended due to inconsistent loading and errors consequent to the Segré-Silberberg effect (see Chapter 6).
9. If the concentration of the sample is so low as likely to provide insufficient motile spermatozoa per straw post-thaw to perform ICSI, the sample can be concentrated by centrifuging at 500 *g* for 10 min and

257

resuspending the pellet in sperm buffer. Re-assess the sperm concentration of the concentrated specimen using a Makler chamber.

10. If possible, perform a semen analysis on the final specimen.

11. a) If the specimen has to be held for some time before performing ICSI, this should be done at ambient temperature rather than 37°C, to protect the spermatozoa from ROS-induced damage.

b) Ideally, specimens should always be cryopreserved for later use, i.e. the procedure should have been performed before the ART treatment cycle. Even if the procedure is performed on the day of oocyte retrieval, some of the specimen should be cryopreserved, if possible, for use in a subsequent cycle.

Calculations and Results

Ensure that all laboratory forms and reports are completed.

Notes

1. Samples showing extremely poor sperm motility (even 0%) can be treated with pentoxifylline to try and stimulate sperm motility immediately prior to use. Spermatozoa to be used for ICSI are treated post-thaw, but any likely effect should be established by an earlier trial if there is sufficient material. Spermatozoa must be washed free of any pentoxifylline before being used to inseminate oocytes [4,5].

Preparation of Testicular Spermatozoa

Principle

Seminiferous tubule tissue is aspirated from the testis into a needle (TESA) or excised as one or more open testis biopsies (TESE). In micro-TESE, dilated tubules identified under magnification are sampled. The spermatozoa must be recovered from the seminiferous tubules and washed using techniques that will not cause harm to them, in particular to their DNA. This is achieved by simple mincing of the tissue. Enzymatic digestion and/or physical homogenization (e.g. using a micro-tissue grinder) seriously compromise the quality of the spermatozoa and can result in substantial levels of ROS-induced damage to the sperm DNA; the sample also often ends up as a gelatinous mass that is hard to handle.

Incubation of the retrieved testicular spermatozoa can lead to the acquisition of sperm motility. While this can sometimes be seen after just 3–4 h, many workers culture specimens overnight and even for up to three days.

This protocol was generously provided by Carole Lawrence (Laboratory Director, Pacific Centre for Reproductive Medicine, Edmonton, AB, Canada; see www.pacificfertility.ca).

Specimen

Testicular tissue specimens containing seminiferous tubules. Specimens should be placed in a HEPES- or MOPS-buffered culture medium as quickly as possible (this will allow the specimen to be kept under an air atmosphere without compromising the pH of the medium), and must be kept within a temperature range of 20–38°C.

Equipment

See also Appendix 2.

- Microscope configured for andrology with phase contrast optics (10×, 20× and 40× objectives)
- Air incubator
- CO_2 incubator
- Centrifuge
- Tally counter

- Air-displacement pipetter, 500-μl volume
- Sterile fine dissecting scissors
- Rubber bulb to control Pasteur pipettes

Disposable Materials

- Scalpels with disposable blades
- Sterile fine (e.g. 25G) hypodermic needles, use 1-ml syringes as handles
- Culture dishes, e.g. Falcon #1007
- Centrifuge tubes
- Glass Pasteur pipettes (sterile)
- Microscope slides
- Coverslips, 22 × 22 mm #1½ or #2 thickness

Reagents

Sperm Buffer: Any HEPES- or MOPS-buffered ART culture medium known to support human spermatozoa that is supplemented with at least 5 mg/ml (ideally 10 mg/ml) of HSA.

Sperm Medium: Any bicarbonate-buffered ART culture medium known to support human spermatozoa that is supplemented with 10 mg/ml of HSA.

All culture media must be at 37°C prior to use.

Calibration

1. Incubators must be set at 37°C and their operation verified using an independent temperature-measuring device.
2. The CO_2 incubator must be set at the appropriate pCO_2 for the proper equilibration of the Sperm Medium and the %CO_2 verified by an independent CO_2 analyser.

Quality Control

No special QC procedures are required for this technique.

Procedure

Processing the Tissue

1. Place the testicular biopsy tissue in a small Falcon Petri dish in a small volume of Sperm Buffer. Tease the tissue apart into very small pieces using small dissecting scissors, fine scalpel blades and small-gauge hypodermic needles. (Do not try disrupting the tissue by aspirating it in and out of the needles.)
   Hint: Bend an additional small-gauge needle in the middle at 90° and use this to press on the small pieces in the dish in order to extrude material from the tubules by compression.
2. Examine the cell suspension using the inverted (ICSI) microscope by phase contrast or Hoffman optics. If there are large numbers of spermatozoa showing significant motility it is possible to proceed directly to step #8, but even such samples would show increased yield if incubated for 24 h.
3. Add some more Sperm Medium and place the dish at 37°C in a CO_2 incubator overnight. This will increase the motility and result in more motile spermatozoa per straw later.
4. Wash the spermatozoa:

a) Following overnight incubation, rinse the contents out of the dish, and transfer them into a Falcon #2095 conical centrifuge tube.

b) Centrifuge at 200–300 g for 10 min.

c) Remove the supernatant and resuspend the pellet with Sperm Buffer to 1.0–2.0 ml according to its size.

d) Make a standard wet preparation (10 µl under a 22 × 22 mm coverslip) and assess the specimen for motile spermatozoa under phase contrast optics.

e) If there are sufficient motile spermatozoa, go to step #8.

f) If there are no motile spermatozoa, advise the patients and the urologist. Proceed to step #5.

Note: All further washing and preparation of the spermatozoa will be done after thawing (see step #11), not before cryopreservation.

5. Transfer the specimen into a small Falcon dish containing fresh medium and return it to culture at 37°C in the CO_2 incubator overnight.

6. The following morning repeat step #4 unless the specimen has already been cultured for 72 h, in which case proceed to step #7.

Note: At step #4d, if there are sufficient motile spermatozoa, go to step #8; if not, then the specimen can be incubated for a third night (maximum).

7. If there are still no motile spermatozoa after 72 h in culture, advise the patients and the urologist.

Freezing the Spermatozoa

8. Process the specimen for cryopreservation (see Chapter 10). If there is a high concentration of motile spermatozoa, extend the specimen using Sperm Buffer before slowly adding the cryoprotectant medium dropwise so as to be able to freeze more straws. Ensure that the subject has signed a sperm cryopreservation consent form.

9. Perform a test-thaw. See Note #3.

10. Complete the laboratory report form and transcribe the relevant information onto the necessary clinical report form(s). Make sure the nurse or clinician managing the partner's stimulation cycle is advised of the results as soon as possible.

Thawing the Spermatozoa for Use in ICSI

11. Thaw one or more straws of the specimen as necessary (see Chapter 10). The dilution step should use at least a 5× volume of Sperm Buffer, and ideally a 10× volume, added slowly dropwise.

12. Make a standard wet preparation (10 µl under a 22 × 22 mm coverslip) and assess the specimen for motile spermatozoa under phase contrast optics.

13. Depending on the number of motile spermatozoa seen, either:

a) If there are very few motile spermatozoa, wash the sample by centrifugation (500 g × 10 min), and resuspend in the pellet in about 100 µl Sperm Buffer, regardless of the amount of debris present.

b) For specimens containing many sticky cells, wash the spermatozoa using a single layer (2.0–4.0 ml) of 40% gradient colloid only (i.e. do not use a two-layer gradient) by centrifuging at 500 g × 10 min. Discard the entire supernatant, and resuspend the pellet in about 100 µl Sperm Buffer, regardless of the amount of debris present.

c) For most specimens the spermatozoa can be readily identified and picked out directly.

14. Make a standard wet preparation (10 µl under a 22 × 22 mm coverslip) and assess the specimen for motile spermatozoa under phase contrast optics. Record the observations on the lab form.

15. Proceed to preparing the sperm dish for ICSI.

Calculations and Results

Ensure that all laboratory forms and reports are completed.

Notes

1. Processing testicular tissue on the day of an ICSI procedure is not recommended due to the risk of not having any spermatozoa after the woman has undergone stimulation.
2. Extensive experience (Carole Lawrence, personal communication) using this protocol over many years, including sperm cryopreservation using Nidacon's *Sperm CryoProtec* cryoprotectant medium and a CryoLogic programmable freezer (i.e. not cooling in a static vapour phase), has shown that:
   a) If there are motile spermatozoa pre-freeze (even <1%) then there should always be some motility post-thaw.
   b) Sperm motility post-thaw often improves during the period between processing and commencing ICSI injections; there should be no need to resort to using any 'motility enhancing' chemicals such as pentoxifylline.
   c) Clinical pregnancy rates of >70% per oocyte retrieval can be achieved after ICSI in women <40 years of age.
3. While some workers advocate lysing the red blood cells (RBCs) present, there seems to be little real need for this, and it not only results in the release of large amounts of potassium from the lysed RBCs, but all the cell 'ghosts' remain in the specimen. Experienced ICSI operators have little trouble picking up spermatozoa from around intact RBCs.

References

1. Shin DH, Turek PJ. Sperm retrieval techniques. *Nat Rev Urol* 2013; **10**: 723–30.
2. Tournaye H, Krausz C, Oates RD. Concepts in diagnosis and therapy for male reproductive impairment. *Lancet Diabetes Endocrinol* 2017; **5**: 554–64.
3. Verheyen G, Popovic-Todorovic B, Tournaye H. Processing and selection of surgically retrieved sperm for ICSI: a review. *Basic Clin Androl* 2017; **27**: 6.
4. Flannigan RK, Schlegel PN. Microdissection testicular sperm extraction: preoperative patient optimization, surgical technique, and tissue processing. *Fertil Steril* 2019; **111**: 420–6.
5. Rowe PJ, Comhaire FH, Hargreave TB, Mahmoud AMA. *WHO Manual for the Standardized Investigation, Diagnosis and Management of the Infertile Male.* Cambridge: Cambridge University Press, 2000.
6. Deruyver Y, Vanderschueren D, Van der Aa F. Outcome of microdissection TESE compared with conventional TESE in non-obstructive azoospermia: a systematic review. *Andrology* 2014; **2**: 20–4.
7. Bernie AM, Mata DA, Ramasamy R, Schlegel PN. Comparison of microdissection testicular sperm extraction, conventional testicular sperm extraction, and testicular sperm aspiration for nonobstructive azoospermia: a systematic review and meta-analysis. *Fertil Steril* 2015; **104**: 1099–103.

Chapter 12

Quality Management and Accreditation

Overview of Quality Management

Quality Concepts

Quality is the degree to which a product or service conforms to accepted standards and/or to the requirements of internal and external customers, thus quality is definitely in the eye of the beholder. Obviously, the main customers are the patients, but others include the referring doctors who use the facilities of the andrology lab, the management team, external providers, employees, regulatory authorities and certification agencies. Before beginning the discussion of quality, we must consider which dimensions or perceptions of quality the customer/consumer may have. The following is a quick overview of the possibilities:

1. Administration and management focus on continuous quality improvement in an effort to improve the level of performance across the entire organization and achieve higher levels of customer satisfaction = culture of quality.
2. Clinical and laboratory personnel, i.e. physicians, nurses and scientists, focus on the delivery of medical care while consistently incorporating current professional knowledge = clinical quality.
3. Employers, healthcare purchasers, patients and families may assess the quality of their healthcare delivery based on personal treatment, courtesy, environment, access to care and medical outcomes, i.e. 'do they get better' = quality of service/healthcare quality.

The quality of a product or service is not random, but rather can be programmed, measured, and improved: quality is part of everyday management. The approach to quality issues is not a science – hence there is not, and can never be, a single 'ideal solution'. It is the job of management to assess and choose from the many possible solutions or approaches the one they think will be appropriate for their particular needs. Quality can be managed using various systems. For example, Total Quality Management (TQM) is an integrated management philosophy and set of practices that emphasizes, among other things, quality control (QC), quality assurance (QA) and quality improvement (QI).

QC is an activity designed to ensure that a specific element within the laboratory is functioning correctly by means of the monitoring of indicators [1]. QC is about making sure that each task is done correctly. QC also includes corrective measures to ensure that procedures are up to standard. QC is a component of QA and should include all the phases of the total testing process: pre-analytical, including the phase before the test is even ordered where the clinician decides which test to order, analytical and post-analytical phase, including how the clinician responds to the laboratory results [2].

QA is a comprehensive programme designed to look at a laboratory procedure as a whole and to identify risks and act in a proactive rather than reactive way so as to prevent or reduce undesired effects. 'Risk' is defined as 'the effect of uncertainty'. QA is the overall scheme to ensure that deviations from the expected result do not occur, e.g. the spermatozoa provided by a cryobank are suitable for use in artificial insemination. QA relates to the way in which work is done, and to this end it will be fundamental to use tools which help us to know the starting point (e.g. SWOT analysis, flowcharts, etc.) [3,4], where we want to be (objectives, mission) and the risks we should prevent ('risk-based thinking'). Risk-based thinking ensures that risks are identified, considered and controlled throughout the design and use of the quality management system [5,6].

QI is a comprehensive, perpetually reiterative, monitoring process designed not only to detect and eliminate problems, but also to enhance a laboratory's performance by exploring innovation and developing flexibility and effectiveness in all processes. This process refers to the Plan-Do-Check-Act (PDCA) circle, also known as the 'Deming wheel' [7]. It is a very simple concept which helps coordinate an organization's quality improvement efforts: just as a circle has no end, the PDCA cycle repeatedly executes in pursuit of continual improvement. The PDCA cycle provides general guidance for quality management, enabling any organization to meet the requirements of interested parties, taking the organizational context into account. The four stages are leadership-dependent and embrace the risk-based thinking aspects of a quality management system. The PDCA cycle emphasizes and demonstrates that improvement programmes must start with careful planning by top management to achieve specified targets, which should be based on intended use. The planning should include and guarantee support to the activities in the process (human resources, infrastructure and environment for the operation of processes). The total testing process begins when a specimen and request form are received in the laboratory and finishes by creating a report as well as appropriate interpretation and use. All the phases of the total testing process should be controlled and periodically monitored by appropriate quality indicators, as well as by regular internal audits, control of non-conforming results, implementation of corrective and preventive actions and verification of the achievement of the intended quality of results and services. Customer satisfaction must also be measured. Reviewing all these performance evaluation activities must result in effective action, and must move on again to careful planning in a continuous cycle (Figure 12.1) [8].

Hence, when a clinical laboratory such as an andrology laboratory is considering adopting systematic quality management such as TQM, it must take into account the six dimensions of healthcare quality: effectiveness, safety, efficiency, timeliness, equity and patient centeredness. The management system should monitor that these six dimensions are taken into account in the andrology laboratory. With this change, the challenge shifts from a simple question such as 'was the test done correctly?' to 'was the right test carried out on the right specimen and was the right result and right interpretation delivered to the

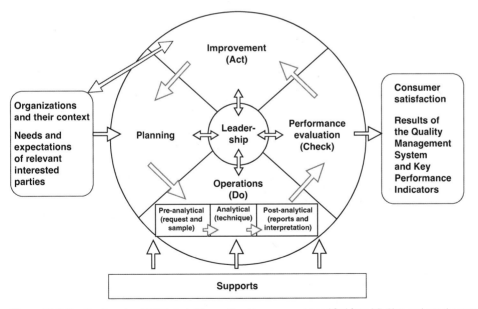

Figure 12.1 The Deming wheel ('PDCA Cycle') for continual improvement (modified from [8]). Plan: evaluate the current situation and define a plan about how and which activities need improvement; Do: conduct a small-scale implementation of the plan; Check: monitor and evaluate the plan; adopt and adjust the plan where necessary; Act: implement the definitive plan. The process is iterative, new cycles are started to continually improve the system and assure quality.

right patient at the right time, and all at the lowest cost possible and adapting to the specific needs of the patient (social, health and educational level)?'

A Quality Management System

A quality management system (QMS) is the entire system developed by an organization that involves the establishment of a quality policy and quality objectives, and the processes to achieve those goals. In order for a QMS to be effective, the objectives must be measurable, reflect the laboratory's overall goals, and be clearly defined. It must also be practical, reviewed regularly, measured for effectiveness, and be accessible to all employees. A QMS consists of documented policies and procedures for the establishment and effective implementation of the system itself, as well as records to provide evidence that the system is in compliance. The documents include: Quality Manual (philosophy of the laboratory); procedures (principles and strategy); test methods (Standard Operating Procedures or SOPs); and records (results, evidence, proof). There are software packages that facilitate the implementation of a QMS.

With the objective of increasing the likelihood of quality positive health outcomes, seven principles are considered in a QMS:

Customer-Focused

As previously mentioned, this is one of the dimensions of healthcare quality as described by various authors. The Picker Institute presented the most complete model of patient-centeredness for general healthcare services [9]. In patient-centred care, eight dimensions are described:
1. Access to care (availability of health services with toilets adapted to disabled patients)
2. Information, communication, and education (to facilitate autonomy and health promotion)
3. Involvement of family and friends (to recognize the patients' needs and role)
4. Respect for patient preferences (to encourage patients' decision-making and dignity)
5. Co-ordination of care (support services and front-line patient care)
6. Continuity and transition (to inform self-care after discharge)
7. Physical comfort (a clean and comfortable waiting room and toilet)
8. Emotional support (to alleviate the fear and anxiety produced when a semen sample has to be collected)

Similarly, andrology laboratories should know the referring doctor's current and future requirements and should periodically evaluate andrology laboratory customer satisfaction. There are several specific experiences to measure patients' perception of medicine laboratories [10] or infertility health services which can be very well adapted to the activity of the andrology laboratory [11,12]. Other studies have evaluated the satisfaction of the referring doctor [10,13].

Leadership

This means the directors of the andrology lab must be actively involved in the operation of their QMS, and that quality should become embedded in routine business operations and not a separate and discrete activity – leadership is at all levels: 'everything' and 'everywhere'.

People Engagement

To manage an organization effectively and efficiently it is important to involve all people at all levels and to respect them as individuals. Recognition, empowerment and enhancement of competence facilitate people's engagement in achieving the organization's quality objectives.

Process Approach

A series of continuous actions or tasks, or a method by which something is done, is termed a process. The group of techniques used to understand all factors involved in a process is called Process Mapping, with examples being flowcharts, top-down process maps, swim-lane analysis, and the IDEF0 modelling method

[3]. However, a QMS is not only a description of isolated processes, but also the management of inter-related processes.

The necessary information must be available to operate and improve the processes and to monitor, analyse and evaluate the performance of the overall system and SOPs are a key tool for this. An *SOP* is a document which describes the regularly recurring operations relevant to the performance and quality of an investigation. The purpose of an SOP is to carry out the operations correctly and always in the same manner. An SOP should be available at the place where the work is done and is a compulsory instruction. If deviations from this instruction are allowed, the conditions for these should be documented, including who can give permission for this and what exactly the complete procedure will be. The original SOP should be kept in a secure place while working copies should be authenticated with stamps and/or signatures of authorized persons [3].

In addition to SOPs, nowadays an overall QMS is needed to manage risks that can affect the outputs of the processes and overall outcomes (see Chapter 13 'Risk Management').

Improvement

The key is to monitor the performance of a process over time. Monitoring requires the definition and use of Key Performance Indicators (KPIs). KPIs can measure how well an organization meets user needs and requirements, as well as the quality of all operational processes [3,14,15]. A KPI should measure quality in a valid and reliable manner, with little inter- and intra-observer variability so that it is suitable for comparison between professionals, practices and institutions. Indicators are selected from research data with consideration for optimal patient care (preferably an evidence-based guideline), supplemented by expert opinion. Within the selection procedure, feasibility (such as measurability and improvability), is important alongside validity and reliability [16,17]. Nevertheless, problems can appear when it comes to interpreting the results [18].

Key Performance Indicators should be defined and monitored for each of the six dimensions of healthcare quality (see Tables 12.1 and 12.2) [19,20]. A KPI must be expressed in numerical terms and most of the time must be expressed relative to a value relating to the incidence for proper performance interpretation, only rarely as relative to measuring desirable events. There are three types of KPI [21].

- Structural: Relative to production or support processes.
- Key processes indicator: Relative to three phases of the overall testing process: pre-analysis; analytical; and post-analysis.
- Outcome measures.

Some indicators are more suitable for internal quality improvement (clinical indicators) and others are especially appropriate for external appraisal (outcome indicators). The two techniques most frequently used for evaluating KPIs are control charts and rolling averages.

Moreover, as the choice to order a laboratory test is the first step of the total testing process, the 'Choosing Wisely' initiative can be viewed as an international effort to improve the earliest part of the pre-analytical phase. This campaign seeks to improve medical decision-making by physicians and patients through the creation of a list of procedures or treatments that are often used excessively or inappropriately. In the field of andrology labs, the American Society of Reproductive Medicine has made recommendations such as: 'Do not perform advanced sperm function testing, such as sperm penetration or hemizona assays, in the initial evaluation of the infertile couple' and 'Do not perform a post-coital test (PCT) for the evaluation of infertility' [22]. Andrology labs should monitor compliance with these recommendations.

Evidence-Based Decision Making

This principle impacts both clinical decisions and Health Technology Assessment (HTA).

Clinical practice guidelines are fundamental for making sound clinical decisions. These are documents containing systematically developed recommendations, algorithms, and other information to assist healthcare decision-making for specific clinical circumstances. The Appraisal of Guidelines Research and Evaluation (AGREE) Instruments provide a framework for assessing the quality of clinical

Table 12.1 Examples of structural and outcome Key Performance Indicators for the andrology laboratory

Type	Activity	KPI	Healthcare quality dimensions
STRUCTURAL			
Support processes	Employee competence	Number of training events organized for all staff, per time period	Effectiveness, safety
	Laboratory information system	Number of laboratory information system unplanned downtime episodes, per time period	Efficiency, timeliness
	Laboratory equipment	Time laboratory equipment is unable to properly process samples	Efficiency
	Documents	Guidelines revised, per time period	Effectiveness, safety
		Guidelines in accordance with healthcare recommendations concerning equity, ethical or legal limitations (e.g. no sperm freezing for surrogacy in another country)	Equity
Production processes	Resource utilization	Number of semen analyses per microscope or technician	Efficiency
		Number of samples stored per cryotank	Efficiency
		Reagent and culture medium wastage	Efficiency
		Consumption of liquid nitrogen per cryopreservation procedure	Efficiency
		Number of broken transport containers per month	Efficiency, safety
	Throughput	Number of processed samples per time period	Efficiency
OUTCOME			
Clinical	Health status	Pregnancy rate following AIH cycle	Effectiveness
		Fertilization rate when using cryopreserved semen for IVF	Effectiveness
		Pregnancy rate following IUI with cryopreserved semen donor	Effectiveness
Client	Client satisfaction	Percentage of: (sum of points given in the enquiry to the question of overall patient satisfaction) / (maximum point defined in the enquiries × the number of enquiries)	Patient-centredness
		Percentage of: (sum of points given in the enquiry to the question of overall satisfaction with the referring doctor) / (maximum point defined in the enquiries × the number of enquiries)	Effectiveness, timeliness
		Numbers of patients who commented that they are not respected by laboratory staff / total number of patients interrogated	Equity

practice guidelines: see www.agreetrust.org. The SEMQUA Guide, which was specifically developed to evaluate the studies carried out on semen quality, evaluates the reporting quality of the reports considered in a clinical practice guideline on this subject [23].

Health Technology Assessment also depends on evidence-based decisions, and HTA may be defined as a form of research which systematically analyses the health, social, economic, ethical, and legal consequences derived from the use of technology, produced in both the short- and long-term, with such analyses including both desirable and undesirable effects. The International Network of Agencies for Health Technology Assessment (INAHTA) is sub-grouped into national agencies of Health Technology Assessment (www.inahta.org). International guidelines exist for reporting HTA (see CHEERS (Consolidated Health Economic Evaluation Reporting Standards)) [24].

Relationship Management

Andrology laboratories must establish relationships with interested parties to enhance their ability to create value. The laboratory must define and inform suppliers about their purchase requirements for products or services, and the providers should understand the laboratory's requirements.

Table 12.2 Examples of Key Performance Indicators concerning the total testing process

Phase	Activity	KPI	Healthcare quality dimensions
Pre-analytical	Inappropriate test ordering	% of inappropriate orders of semen cryopreservation (not meeting minimum sperm parameters according to semen cryopreservation SOP)	Effectiveness, efficiency, timeliness
		% of misidentified or unintelligible requests	Safety
		% of ART patients without appropriate serological testing	Safety
		% of patient specimens accepted for cryopreservation without informed consent	Safety
		Patient or donor waiting time for an appointment	Patient-centredness, timeliness
	Sample collection, identification, transport	% of misidentified or unintelligible samples	Safety
		% of inadequate or inappropriate transportation conditions	Efficiency, safety
		Patient waiting time at the lab	Efficiency, safety
		% of incomplete semen samples collected	Effectiveness, efficiency, safety,
		% of patients unable to collect sample (blocked)	Efficiency, safety
Analytical	Unacceptable performance in IQC	% of prepared samples (for IUI and IVF) with post-preparation sperm motility below competence level (<90%)	Effectiveness, safety
		% of internal quality control results outside defined limit	Effectiveness, safety
		Incubator temperature outside defined limit (control chart)	Safety
		% cooling rate outside defined limit	Safety
		% of cryopreserved normozoospermic samples with sperm cryosurvival rate below competence level	Safety
	Unacceptable performance in EQA	% of unacceptable performances in external quality assessment programme	Effectiveness, safety
	Data transcription error	% of incorrect results for erroneous manual transcription	Efficiency, safety
Post-analytical	Inappropriate turnaround times	% of reports delivered outside the specified time	Timeliness
		% of prepared sperm specimens delivered outside the specified time	Timeliness
		Average time to communicate cryopreservation results to patients	Timeliness
	Result interpretation	% of patients with an abnormal semen analysis result without at least one extra semen analysis	Efficiency, safety
		In case of normozoospermia, patients who repeat semen analysis before three months have passed	Efficiency, timeliness

Accreditation

Within quality assurance, accreditation is an effective tool for implementing internationally recognized quality systems in medical service and healthcare. Accreditation of management systems is internationally accepted for conformity assessment. Accreditation is defined as a collegial process based on self- and peer-assessment, whereby an authoritative body (usually a non-government organization) gives formal recognition that an organization is in voluntary compliance with one or more standards set by the authoritative body. Accreditation 'Standards' are published documents that contain technical specifications or criteria to be used consistently as rules, guidelines, or definitions of characteristics to ensure that materials, products, processes and services are fit for their purpose.

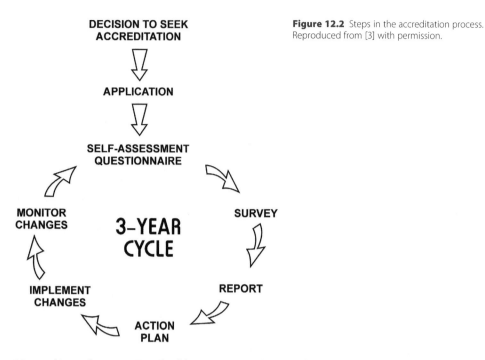

Figure 12.2 Steps in the accreditation process. Reproduced from [3] with permission.

Note: 'Accreditation Standards' must not be confused with 'performance standards' or 'minimum standards' (also called 'quality specifications' or 'performance specifications') since these define the minimum technical requirements for a process to be performed or undertaken, and do not usually consider anything beyond basic quality control.

Nevertheless, certain semantic confusions exist between the terms 'accreditation' and 'certification' and 'registration'. The ISO Council Committee on Conformity Assessment has attempted to resolve the semantics problem by standardizing the following definitions.

Accreditation: A procedure by which an authoritative body gives formal recognition that a body or person is competent to carry out specific tasks. A planning for typical steps in the accreditation process is in Figure 12.2.

Certification: A procedure by which a third party gives written assurance (certificate of conformity) that a product, process or service conforms to specified requirements.

Registration: A procedure by which a body indicates relevant characteristics of a product, process or service, or particulars of a body or person, in an appropriate, publicly available list.

Put simply, certification assesses that an entity does what it says and accreditation assesses that it does what it says and also does it well.

Note: Internationally, certification has become the dominant term. But common terminology in the USA is not always in harmony with this international guidance, nor with European practice. The European approach is to identify both quality system registrars and product certifiers as certification bodies. There is very little use of the term registration in Europe.

In general terms, 'accreditation' is a formal recognition that a body is competent to carry out specific tasks; while 'certification' is a formal evaluation by a third-party that a product conforms to a standard, and 'registration' commonly refers to certification of quality systems. Hence, laboratory accreditation is defined as a formal recognition that a laboratory is competent to carry out specific tests or specific types of tests (i.e. ISO 15189:2012; note a new, revised standard is expected in 2022) [14,15]; and quality system registration or certification is a formal attestation that a supplier's quality system is in conformance with an appropriate quality system model such as 9001:2015 [6].

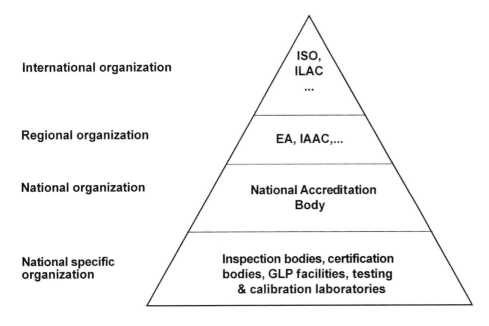

Figure 12.3 Worldwide accreditation infrastructure.

Worldwide Accreditation Infrastructure

The standards of accreditation most often followed were established by the International and Regional Standards and Conformance Bodies. The international organization responsible for 'Documentary Standards Development' is the International Organization for Standardization (ISO: www.iso.org), while at the regional level, for instance, the European Committee for Standardization (Comité Européen de Normalisation, CEN, www.cen.eu) collaborate with the ISO and national organizations for standardization (e.g. DIN, AFNOT, BSI, SIS). A body specifically designated for laboratories is the International Laboratory Accreditation Cooperation (ILAC). At a regional level accrediting bodies have been established (e.g. the European Cooperation for Accreditation or ECA, and the Inter-American Accreditation Co-operation, or IACC). In each country, accreditation is performed by qualified government agencies or private sector professionals or trade organizations operating in accordance with appropriate international requirements such as ISO/IEC 17011. A listing of international accreditation bodies that are signatories to the 'ILAC mutual recognition arrangements' may be found on the ILAC website, www.ilac.org. (Figure 12.3).

Most national accreditation bodies follow an international guideline developed by the International Organization for Standardization (ISO) for testing laboratories in general (ISO/IEC 17025:2015, entitled *General Requirements for the Competence of Testing and Calibration Laboratories*, with a particular version adapted for medical laboratories: *ISO 15189:2012, Medical Laboratories – Particular Requirements for Quality and Competence*; note that a new, revised version of this Standard is expected in 2022) [15,25]. Some countries prefer a local guideline such as CCLK (Coördinatie Commissie ter bevordering van de Kwaliteitsbeheersing op het gebied van Laboratoriumonderzoek in de Gezondheidszorg) in The Netherlands, CPA (Clinical Pathology Accreditation) in the UK, or UNE179007:2013 Systems of quality management for assisted reproductive laboratories (AENOR) in Spain.

Most national accreditation bodies follow developed international, regional or national guidelines. The standard entitled *General Requirements for the Competence of Testing and Calibration Laboratories* (ISO/IEC 17025:2015) applies to laboratories in general, and for medical laboratories specifically there is the *Medical*

Laboratories – Particular Requirements for Quality and Competence standard (ISO 15189:2012, under revision, with a new version expected to be published 2022) [15,25].

Globally, most clinical andrology laboratories follow the methodology guidelines/recommendations of either the World Health Organization or ESHRE SIG Andrology [26–31], although not always very well [32]. Hopefully, the recent publication of a specific ISO Standard on semen analysis (*ISO 23162:2021 Basic Semen Examination – Specification and Test Methods*) will improve standardization in the future [33].

Training

Standardization of semen analysis requires clear, detailed and robust methods. However, these alone are not enough. There must also be an effective training system for staff, and this must be followed-up by ongoing QC and QA. Reading even the most detailed manual or handbook can never replace proper, basic technical training; practical hands-on training is essential. Many technicians, through no fault of their own, are performing semen analysis using inappropriate methods with inadequate training [32]. Importantly, this can easily be addressed using proven training methods [26,29]. Everyone involved in andrology laboratory work is encouraged to determine/assess if their current systems comply with current best practice.

Training of new personnel to perform techniques in an andrology laboratory constitutes the corner stone of the quality assurance. The 'learning curve' is the effort required to acquire a new skill over a specific period of time. The type of curve (steep or gradual) depends on the inherent technical difficulty as well as the heterogeneity of the caseload. Thus, sperm preparation is technically easy, but one must individualize the techniques employed for each step to ensure optimum results; hence the learning curve will be a gradual progression. Meanwhile, sperm cryopreservation is technically complicated, but generally the same protocol is employed for all semen samples.

A standardized training system is essential to avoid future problems. Training progress has to be closely followed, documented, and be approved by the laboratory director. Therefore, it is important to establish training criteria and performance thresholds that should be met in order to attain the experience necessary to perform procedures independently. Equally, it is desirable that appropriate quality control measures be implemented in order to ensure that such performance thresholds, once achieved, are maintained. Different levels of ability have been described for the andrology laboratory [34]:
1. Basic understanding established
2. Able to work under supervision
3. Allowed to work without supervision
4. Able to train other people

Step-by-Step (Slow and Steady)

The first requirement should be that the trainee is fully conversant with the setting-up and operation of the andrology laboratory equipment. This may seem like an obvious statement, but an eagerness to perform semen analysis sometimes enables trainees to convince themselves, and others, that they know how to use the equipment properly when in fact they do not. Once the trainee has become familiar with the equipment and material, and after observing an experienced staff member perform the technique, the trainee can practise with 'left-over' semen not required for analysis. Familiarity with the material and reagents allows the trainee to progress using them concurrently so that they can manipulate the semen in a way that mimics a 'real' scenario. Only once these techniques have been perfected should the trainee proceed to attempt to prepare or cryopreserve a 'real' semen specimen, under supervision.

Criteria for Competence

- For cryopreservation, an expected survival rate for donor semen of ≥25% (ideally >30%).
- For sperm preparation by direct swim-up from semen, a recovery rate ±10% of the progressively motile spermatozoa with a ≥20% increase in progressive motility.

- For sperm preparation by density gradient centrifugation, a minimum of 90% progressive motility in the final preparations from normal semen samples, with a benchmark of ≥95% [34,35].
- Semen analysis should be based on an expectation of meeting generally accepted analytical quality specifications [36].

Once a trainee has demonstrated an ability to achieve this goal, they can be considered ready to progress to dealing with half of the semen specimens in a given case, under supervision. When a trainee has demonstrated an ability to achieve the goal on three consecutive occasions, they can progress to handling an entire case independently, under supervision. A trainee will be allowed to work independently after 10 cases of sperm cryopreservation or 50 cases of ejaculated semen preparation with optimum results. Only after completing training and after gaining experience from a certain number of cases, can someone instruct beginners. Annual reports on the percentage of recovery rate or cryosurvival rate provide a good form of quality assurance. Naturally, pregnancies resulting from sperm preparation or cryopreservation provide further quality assurance, but they are also subject to variables other than andrology laboratory techniques.

In addition to the processes already described, for proper training in semen analysis, it is advisable that trainees attend a technique standardization course. The effectiveness of these courses to diminish the variability between observers has been demonstrated with the completion of a single course [29] or refresher courses [37]. After an introductory course, future training is mandatory until the individual is fully trained [38]. This can only be done with serious commitment. To support continued training 'at home', control material from an EQA scheme can be used, or a specific programme for continuous training can be employed [39]. When proper training has been completed, IQC should be implemented as a tool to decrease both inter- and intra-technician variability, and to ensure that semen analysis technical skills are maintained at a high standard.

Comparing the Results of an Expert and a Trainee

Discrete variables: Comparing a discrete variable with two categories requires use of the Kappa statistic (K). With more categories, use the weighted Kappa [40]. It must also be taken into account that the K value represents a proportion of accuracy greater than that expected by chance. However, this coefficient assumes a generally equal distribution of prevalence for the attribute under study (e.g. 60% progressive motility *vs* 40% non-progressive motility). If this prevalence is not equally distributed (e.g. only 3% of spermatozoa with post-acrosomal vacuoles) then the K value is distorted and becomes less meaningful (lower), a problem known as the Kappa Paradox. To avoid the Kappa Paradox, the Gwet coefficient may be used [41] and to optimize the interpretation of the Gwet coefficient and the Kappa value it is recommended to take into consideration the concepts of positive readings (those where at least one of the observers detected the presence of the characteristic) and negative readings (those where at least one of the observers did not detect the presence of the characteristic), and to calculate the proportions of positive agreement (the number of positive readings agreed upon both by the expert and trainee, divided by all of the positive readings for the observers), and of negative agreement (the number of negative readings agreed upon both by the expert and trainee, divided by all of the negative readings for the observers) [42].

Continuous variables can be compared using paired *t*-tests or Wilcoxon matched pairs tests, interclass correlation coefficients, or Bland & Altman charts (Figure 12.4; also see the section on 'Selecting Methods' later in this chapter) using the mean of the differences between observers and ±2SD control limits, or using the combined inherent CV of each observer as control limit [43].

A training scheme based on goal-orientated targets using libraries of reference materials has also been described [26].

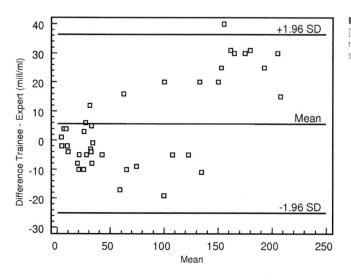

Figure 12.4 A Bland & Altman chart (see [61]) revealing a trainee's tendency to count more spermatozoa when analysing semen samples with higher sperm concentration.

Training for Sperm Morphology Assessments

Process

For sperm morphology evaluation training, the trainee is first given a lecture on the biology of spermiogenesis and the theoretical aspects of sperm morphology evaluation [44], followed by the practical application of this information taught in a one-on-one situation using a dual-headed microscope or video imaging system attached to a microscope. In these sessions, the basic ideal and abnormal morphological forms are seen and described under the microscope. The trainee is then allowed to evaluate routine morphology samples without the knowledge of the results of the original assessments. The results of the trainee are then compared to the routine laboratory results and then taken back to the one-on-one situation to discuss the trainee's results along with possible reasons for discrepancies e.g. misinterpretation of sperm size where, especially in the case of large-headed spermatozoa, misclassification as ideal can be common. In this situation, the trainee should be encouraged to use a built-in eyepiece micrometer to first routinely measure the size of spermatozoa until the image of a morphological ideal, and especially normal-sized spermatozoa, is imprinted on their mind.

The general tendency will be that the trainee will first over-estimate the percentage of morphologically ideal spermatozoa and then, after the first few training sessions, become over-critical and under-estimate the percentage of morphologically ideal spermatozoa. With proper guidance, the trainee will move closer to the target value so that, after about three weeks of daily training sessions, they will be able to produce acceptable results.

Extreme care must continue to be taken as there will always be a general tendency to be over critical, and thus to under-estimate the percentage of morphologically ideal spermatozoa, especially when working in isolation in a small laboratory. For this reason, it is important to take part in a refresher course within a year after the initial training, as well as to participate in an EQC programme. Access to reference slides is highly beneficial.

Evaluation

Due to the uniqueness of sperm morphology results, a system equivalent to the z-score measurement has been developed [45], using a so-called SD-score, where the results of a trainee can be monitored on a quarterly basis and expressed as marginal, good or excellent (excellent is where the (quarterly) readings are always within –0.2 to +0.2 SD score levels). The SD score is calculated according to the following formula:

$$SD = \frac{\text{Trainee score} - \text{Reference laboratory score}}{\text{SD of reference laboratory}}$$

Where: $SD = \sqrt{p(100-p)}$

p = morphology result (%ideal) as evaluated by the reference laboratory personnel

This system is especially useful for small laboratories which receive slides on a regular (quarterly) basis for EQC purposes. The results can be plotted on a graph and trends, scoring too strictly or too leniently, can be observed.

Quality Control

Control is the action of measuring, examining, testing and calibrating one or several characteristics of a product or of a service, and the comparison with the specified requirements in order to establish their conformity. Control is used for different aspects of quality in laboratory andrology:

- Control of an analytical process: pre-analytical, analytical and post-analytical (e.g. semen analysis).
- Control of any step necessary to guarantee the quality of sperm preparation or cryopreservation: freezer and cryotank temperatures, pipetter calibration, liquid nitrogen level in cryotanks, etc.
- Control of the relations with the patients, clinicians, donors or clinics (e.g. complaints).
- Control of the quality level of the services (outcome or clinical result) associated with the andrology laboratory (e.g. pregnancy rate).

It remains inevitable that errors will be made. Therefore, the control system should have checks to detect them. In this text we will concentrate on the quality control of analysis techniques.

Internal Quality Control

The internal QC involves in-house procedures for continuous monitoring of operations and systematic day-to-day checking of the produced data to decide whether these are reliable enough to be released. Two types of material can be used: control material or patient samples. An internal quality control scheme requires several steps.

Control Materials

1. Selection of materials:
   - Similarity to 'real' patient specimens.
   - Availability in large enough quantities to allow evaluation over a long period of time.
   - Similarity in concentration from aliquot-to-aliquot (precision).
   - Stability over a period of use (note that frozen sperm samples do not meet all these conditions for semen analysis [46–48]).
2. Recommended quality control materials [46,48,49]:
   - Sperm concentration: pools of formalin (1%) fixed semen suspension.
   - Sperm motility: digital recordings on DVD or PC-based, older videotapes are also acceptable, depending on image quality.
   - Sperm morphology: unstained and stained smears.
   - Sperm vitality: eosin-nigrosin smears.
   - Biochemical analysis of semen frozen or lyophilized (freeze dried) seminal fluid.
   - Anti-sperm antibodies: positive frozen serum or seminal fluid (positive and negative control materials are also commercially available from FertiPro, Beernem, Belgium).

No certified reference materials exist at the moment for semen quality control. However, sufficient homogeneity and stability can be established for in-house control material [50,51].

273

3. Selection of levels (decision points): Test material should be available in important medical decision-making levels: low (lower than reference limit), medium (near reference limit) and high (above reference limit). Also see Appendix 1.

4. Definition of the quality requirement: The maximum allowed analytical error can be defined by various strategies [52,53]. Ideally, quality specifications should be derived from clinical need. However, it is not possible to simply measure how much, for example, the pregnancy rate decreases with an increased variability in sperm motility analysis. Other strategies include components of biological variation, analysis of clinicians' opinions, guidelines based on state-of-the-art, or by external quality assessment schemes (EQAS) [34,46,54,55].

   Three levels of KPI performance specifications should be defined: minimum or passable; desirable or competence; and optimal or benchmark. The rationale underlying these three levels affects the expected or required response to failure to meet the performance specifications. 'Optimal or benchmark' indicates no need for further improvement, while 'desirable or competence' indicates satisfactory performance, and 'minimum or passable' indicates considerable room for improvement [56]. If only competence and benchmark performance specification are taken into account, there is a risk that many laboratories might not reach a desirable level of performance. This situation could endanger the survival of many centres, especially if such a recommendation were incorporated into guidelines, codes of practice or government regulations [57]. Finally, these quality specifications can vary according to the intended clinical applications (e.g. toxicological or epidemiological studies) [53].

5. Variation of a method: To assess the variability (imprecision) of a method, the control material is assessed repeatedly over a period of time (e.g. at least 20 days). Independent control checks during this period should verify that the method is under control for the entire assessment time. The mean and standard deviation (SD) of the assessed control values are used to calculate the within-observer analytical CV. If the obtained value is less than the specified requirements, the performance of the method is acceptable. The values obtained should also be plotted into a classic control chart (also called Shewhart chart or Levy-Jennings chart). Note that this assessment only reflects the variability of the method, not the accuracy, which can only be evaluated with External Quality Assessment [58,59].

6. Stability of method: Aliquots of the same control material (e.g. fixed sperm suspension) are analysed on consecutive days and the obtained values are plotted in a Shewhart control chart [60]. As long as the control values recorded on the Shewhart chart vary randomly around the control mean with no more than 5% of the points falling outside the ±2SD control limits, the method is in control. Points falling outside the ±2SD control limits are taken to be warning signals, while a single point falling outside the ±3SD control limits signals rejection of the associated assay and immediate action is required to investigate and rectify any problem that could have caused the error. Note that a stable method is not the same as a clinically useful method, but an unstable method cannot produce clinically useful results.

Patient Material

When patient specimens are used, repeated measurements need to be done in order to establish the same basic parameters as is the case for control material (see above).

Inter-Observer Quality Control

All methodology described previously, including control charts, can be used to assess systematic differences between technicians [r]. Another technique is the classic Bland & Altman chart, using the mean of the differences between observers and ±2SD control limits, or using the combined inherent CV of each observer as control limit [43,61].

Some external quality assessment programmes (EQAPs) include the option to include an unlimited number of individual staff from a specific laboratory. In this way, the quality manager can also review staff performance as an internal quality control process.

Quality Control in Other Areas of the Andrology Laboratory

In addition to the technique control chart, the accumulative histogram or rolling average have been used to control the quality in other fields of the andrology laboratory [62]. These techniques can be used to control any quality indicator (see the 'Overview' and 'Accreditation' sections). A procedure to control the quality of all frozen semen coming out of a sperm bank should exist (see 'Cryopreservation Methods' in Chapter 10) [63].

Coefficient of Variation

Using the coefficient of variation (CV) gives no indication about what the coefficient relates to, e.g. within-observer or total random error, or to the level of the parameter to which the CV applies. Furthermore, a CV of 8 does not mean a 95% error range or ±8, but ±16. The interpretation of the CV is also confused because semen analysis exhibits a non-constant error variance that is proportional to the parameter level: sperm concentration is directly related, while percentages (motility, vitality and normal forms) are inversely related [38,64]. Use the CV if you must, but use it carefully, and appropriately [65].

Selecting Methods

That assessments of sperm concentration, motility and morphology are frequently subject to wide variations due to technical error is well-established and has been known for many years [38,66–71]. This is despite the availability of methods whereby intra- and inter-operator variability can be reduced [e.g. 26,27,36,72–77]. Careful technical design to reduce inherent variability and minimize opportunities for operator errors is key to implementing robust reference methodology, and a checklist for basic semen analysis methods has been published [31], and is at the heart of the new ISO Standard 23162:2021 *Basic Semen Examination – Specification and Test Methods* [32].

The basic requirements for achieving accuracy, precision and reproducibility are simple: (a) use robust methods that reduce technical error as much as possible, and (b) train staff carefully in the correct performance of the methods. This was the philosophy behind the basic semen analysis courses run by the ESHRE (the European Society of Human Reproduction and Embryology) Special Interest Group in Andrology (ESHRE SIG-A), courses that have provided eloquent evidence of the validity of this approach [29], which employed the goal-orientated training approach first promoted by Mortimer [26]. As a fundamental philosophical principle, expending effort on establishing standardization is logically and practically to be preferred to expending effort on demonstrating/confirming that staff have not been properly trained and/or methods have not been correctly standardized against established definitions [e.g. 78].

Consequently, we are left with the inescapable conclusion that the only reason sperm assessments are not performed more reliably in many diagnostic laboratories and IVF centres can only be that those responsible for the medical and scientific direction of those laboratories just do not care. As a result, the often-expressed opinion that sperm counts, etc., do not have any value becomes a self-fulfilling prophesy – how could observations with error components of up to 50% be taken seriously or used intelligently? Yet the basic standards by which all medical laboratories should function are well-established, and clearly expounded in ISO 15189:2012 [3,14,15].

Basic Requirements of a Robust Method

Establishing the criteria to be used for specifying a technical procedure, or for selecting one from several available (and, similarly, for choosing a particular piece of equipment) can be simplified if it is considered as a process [14]. This approach allows the following generic questions to be used as basic principles for establishing the method's specifications and evaluating candidate methods' suitability.

What does it need to do?

Basically, what do you want to measure? If necessary, define the criterion, or its sub-classifications, quantitatively. For example, the following definitions for human sperm motility classification have been accepted by international consensus since the early-/mid-1990s [26,60,74]:

class *a* = rapid progressive motility	definition: ≥25 µm/s progression velocity at 37°C
class b = slow progressive motility	definition: 5–25 µm/s progression at 37°C
class *c* = non-progressive motility	definition: flagellar activity but <5 µm/s 'space gain' at 37°C
class *d* = immotile	definition: no flagellar activity

While WHO5 reduced these assessment to only progressive (PR), non-progressive (NP) and immotile (IM), on the supposed grounds that technicians cannot reliably sub-classify progressive spermatozoa in rapid and slow categories, this 'dumbing down' was rejected by the ESHRE SIG-A [30], and the four-category classification has been adopted in ISO 23162:2021 [33] as well as in WHO6 [27], and also continues to be used in this handbook (see Chapter 3).

How well must it do it?

What precision is necessary for the purpose of the measurement? For example, knowing the proportion of progressively motile spermatozoa to a greater precision than an integer percentage would confer no additional benefit, but would greatly increase the effort required. Also remember that results can only be presented to a degree of precision appropriate to the statistical validity of the measurement. In this regard we must consider all factors that can affect the method's accuracy and precision, including being able to establish – and respect – its 'uncertainty of measurement' (see below).

What are the options?

Review the available methods but exclude those for which no robust or validated methodology or protocols are available. Is the method being used by other respected diagnostic andrology labs? Are there established performance indicators for the method?

How well does a method do it?

Review all possible sources of error and bias within the method. Does the method control them to practical levels commensurate with achieving the necessary uncertainty of measurement? Can the method be improved so that it controls these problems better, or should a better method be designed?

How well can it be controlled?/Can we make it better?

What reference materials and calibrators are available (remember that calibration ≠ quality control)? Is QC for the method practical in the routine setting (remember that QC must be continual)? Is there an EQAP for the method (remember that participating in an EQAP cannot replace QC, and that, for it to be useful, an EQAP must also include both QA and QI capabilities)? This is particularly important with assessments for which no metrological standards exist or can be easily fabricated (e.g. semen viscosity, colour and odour). Purists might say that such assessments are without value and should not be made, but if they can provide information of value to those requesting the tests (clinical andrologists, infertility subspecialist physicians) when observations are abnormal, then there is sufficient reason for them to be 'reported by exception'.

Is it practical?

Evaluate each method's feasibility in terms of the equipment, reagents and time that will be required, as well as the method's complexity and any need for specialized training. Basically, undertake comparative cost/benefit analyses.

Will help be available?

What training courses are available? Will specialized training be required from the originator of a particular technical procedure (e.g. the SCSA™)? For specialized equipment, will support be needed/available from the manufacturer or distributor?

Measurement Uncertainty

Every measurement has an error associated with it and, without a quantitative statement of the error, a measurement lacks worth, even credibility. The parameter that quantifies the boundaries of the error of a measurement is the 'measurement uncertainty' or MU [79,80]. An uncertainty statement must have an associated confidence level, most usually a 95% confidence level, i.e. effectively 2× the combined uncertainty. In practical terms, for diagnostic semen analysis purposes, an uncertainty of ±10% is adequate and readily achievable in practical terms (the methods described in this handbook, if properly implemented, will achieve this).

Sources of Uncertainty

In addition to the earlier ISO Guide [79] there is also ISO/TS 20914:2019 *Medical Laboratories – Practical Guidance for the Estimation of Measurement Uncertainty* [81].

Common sources of MU include:

- Incomplete definition of the measurand
- Incomplete realization of the definition of the measurand
- Non-representative sampling
- Inadequate knowledge of the effects of environmental conditions on the measurand (or imperfect measurement of those conditions)
- Personal bias in reading analogue instruments – or making subjective assessments
- Finite instrument resolution or discrimination threshold
- Inexact values of measurement standards and reference materials
- Inexact values of constants and other parameters obtained from external sources
- Approximations and assumptions incorporated in the measurement method and procedure
- Variations in repeated observations of the measurand under apparently identical conditions ('repeatability')

Determination/Controlling the Uncertainty for a Method

This process is very similar to undertaking a Failure Modes and Effects Analysis or 'FMEA' [3]:

1. Construct a model of the measurement system (process mapping).
2. List all the factors that can contribute errors to the final result (this requires a good understanding of the measurement principles, the equipment and environment), and then categorize each one as either random or systematic.
3. Ensure that each source of error has been controlled, as far as is practical, within the method.
4. Either compute their combined uncertainty [80,81] or derive it by comparing results with known reference values.

Comparing Methods

Discrete variables such as modal progression ratings or subjective rankings of debris or round cells should never be averaged. Instead, frequency distributions should be compared or proportion above/below a particular threshold. When comparing two series of assessments (e.g. novice and expert), individual pairs of values should not differ by more than one rank, and be identical in, say, >90% of cases. For example, in a group of 30 paired assessments, no more than two ratings can be different, and then by no more than +/– 1 rank each. See also 'Discrete variables' in the section 'Comparing the Results of an Expert and a Trainee', above.

Continuous variables such as sperm concentration and the percentages of sperm motility, live spermatozoa, and spermatozoa with ideal morphology can be analysed using paired *t*-tests or, better, the method described by Bland & Altman [61], e.g. using MedCalc software (see www.medcalc.org). This latter method considers the average discrepancy between two sets of values (calculated as the mean of a series of individual difference values) compared to the average of the individual paired measurements. For training situations, the difference values should be calculated as 'trainee – expert', so that an over-estimate by the trainee yields a positive difference and the expert value used instead of the average (since there is no evidence that the trainee is able to generate reliable values, e.g.

277

Figure 12.4) [26]. In subsequent exercises, e.g. post-training proficiency testing or QC, the original method plotting the difference against technician-average values should be employed. Arcsin transformation of percentage values should not be necessary, but because the range of sperm concentration values is extremely wide, each difference value is expressed as a percentage of either the expert's value for training situations, or of the average value for other purposes.

Alternative statistical methods include Passing & Bablok analysis [82] and Deming's regression method, which can also be used to establish concordance between different methods tested in duplicate, including giving the coefficient of variation (both also available in MedCalc).

The aim is to achieve consistency between the methods (or competence of a trainee against an expert). Consequently, the goal is to achieve a zero mean difference and a 95% range of differences that is within a pre-determined level of acceptability, e.g. ±5%. The 95% range of discrepancy is calculated by multiplying the SD by the value of the 't' statistic for that number of observations and the appropriate level of significance. For example, for a 5% significance level with n = 20, $t = 2.086$, for n = 30, $t = 2.042$ (the SD is not multiplied by 2.0 until n = 60).

Making Your Lab Better

For each technical procedure, employ the quality cycle ('plan, do, check, act' or 'PDCA' cycle) [3].

A. *Review Your Methods*
1. Take your current method apart (process mapping).
2. Assess component steps and procedures (process analysis).
3. Identify all possible sources of error/bias.
4. Are they all being 'trapped', avoided or at least minimized?
5. Is there anything else that can be done?
6. Compare your method with others.
7. Should (can) you change anything?

B. *Uncertainty of Measurement*
1. Can you determine what it is?
2. Do you report results appropriately?
3. Do the report recipients understand the implications?

C. *Review Your Quality Control Procedures*
1. Do they relate to reality? (calibration ≠ QC)
2. Do they actually increase reproducibility: between observers? over time?

D. *External Quality Assurance*
1. Is it more than proficiency testing?
2. Does the feedback help you apply corrective action?
3. Does it include ongoing quality improvement?

External Quality Assurance Schemes

External Quality Assurance

Participation in an external quality assurance (EQA) scheme allows an evaluation of the analytical performance of a laboratory by comparison with the results of other laboratories. In addition, these schemes can be a useful source of reference samples which can be put to good use internally by participating laboratories. The main objective in using an EQA programme in laboratory andrology is to compare the results with other laboratories and thereby achieving measurement of how correct the results are (accuracy). There are different types of EQA, some giving approval only to laboratories achieving results with certain limits (proficiency testing), others mainly providing a measure for the participating laboratories as one tool in their own work for improved quality (educational schemes), and other schemes mainly giving the opportunity for participating laboratories to compare the results (peer comparison).

Analytical Performance Evaluation

The usual procedure is that sub-samples of a large sample are distributed to participating laboratories at regular intervals. Furthermore, sub-samples of certain large samples can be sent repeatedly without the participants knowing this [68]. When sub-samples have been analysed by participating laboratories for one or more attributes, the results are sent to the scheme organizer. Here the data are processed and reports of each round are returned to the participants. After a number of distributions, a more extensive report can be made since more data allow more and better statistical conclusions. Participating laboratories are supposed to analyse their results and, when significant or systematic deviations are noticed, they are supposed to take corrective action in the laboratory.

The design of each PT differs according to goals chosen, and schemes for the same seminal parameter can, under the management of different organizers, produce varying information on laboratory performance [83]. These variations depend, in particular, on difference in methods used for the selection of control materials, statistical procedures (identification of assigned value), and the assessment of laboratory performance.

The use of human frozen semen in EQA poses several difficulties and is therefore not recommended.

It is very important to define the analytical performance specifications for an EQAP: 'target' values and acceptable variability. A 'target' value is assigned for each sample and each assessment type. There are two ways to obtain 'target' values for a semen analysis EQAP:

- Value from expert laboratories: average (and variation) of result from at least three expert laboratories. This method is used in the EQAP initiated by the ESHRE Special Interest Group in Andrology.
- Average value from all participating laboratories: The mean or median (and variation by standard deviation or central 50 percentiles, respectively) calculated from the results from all participating laboratories. When the 'target' value is calculated on the basis of all results, it will be influenced by the results from the majority of the laboratories, irrespective if they use the correct methods or not.

There are different strategies for estimating acceptable variability in EQAP [56,84].

External Quality Control/Quality Assurance Schemes

A number of External Quality Control and Quality Assurance schemes now exist around the world (see Table 12.3). However, the QA functionality of some schemes is higher than others and laboratories should investigate whether a particular scheme meets their needs before enrolling (and take out a trial subscription).

External Quality Assessment Programmes can be classified into six categories (category 1 being the most desirable), according to how well they are able to evaluate performance. Evaluation capability depends on three characteristics: sample commutability, the process for target value assignment, and inclusion or non-inclusion of replicate samples. EQAPs for semen analysis belong to category 6 because the commutability of their materials has not been demonstrated, their target values are not established by a reference system and non-replicate samples are included in the programme. This means limiting evaluation to peer group comparisons and failing to provide information on bias between different measurement procedures. The information obtained from inter-laboratory CV is for a measurement procedure only [85].

External Quality Control/Quality Assurance Schemes in Other Areas of the Andrology Laboratory

As mentioned in Chapter 9, 'Sperm Preparation', it is very important that the materials used in sperm preparations for ART do not have any negative effects on sperm viability. In order to identify possible sources of sperm toxicity, the human sperm survival test (hSST) is recommended [86]. The validity of the hSST is crucial to the quality achieved by an andrology laboratory, since inadequate performance of this

Table 12.3 Examples of External Quality Control/Quality Assessment Schemes

Country	Scheme name and website	Contact person
Belgium	Sciensano, National External Quality Assessment Scheme www.wiv-isp.be/QML/activities/external_quality/_fr /sperma.htm	Dr Arnaud Capron, PhD, Head of Service 'Quality of Laboratories' Arnaud.Capron@sciensano.be Dr S Wathlet, PhD, Coordinator EQA Scheme Andrology Sandra.Wathlet@sciensano.be
Denmark	DEKS www.deks.dk	Bente Mortensen bente.mortensen@deks.dk
Europe	ANOVA – Karolinska University Hospital and Karolinska Institutet www.anova.se	Dr Lars Björndahl Lars.Bjorndahl@ki.se
Finland	Labquality www.labquality.fi	Jonna Pelanti jonna.pelanti@labquality.fi
Germany	The German External Quality Control Programme for Semen Analysis (QuaDeGA) www.quadega.de	Barbara Hellenkemper (MTA) info@quadega.de
International	FertAid (Internet-based) www.fertaid.com	office@fertaid.com
Italy (Tuscany)	Verifica Esterna di Qualità (Azienda Ospedaliera Universitaria di Careggi) https://crrveq.aou-careggi.toscana.it	Massimo Quercioli crrveq@aou-careggi.toscana.it
Mexico	Programa de Aseguramiento de la Calidad (PACAL) www.pacal.org/n/home/	Dr Sergio Alva Estrada
Netherlands	Stichting Kwaliteitsbewaking Medische Laboratoriumdiagnostiek www.skml.nl	Alex MM Wetzels office@skml.nl
Spain	Programa Español de Control de Calidad Externo de Análisis de Semen CEIFER Biobank – NextClinics. Banco de semen y ovocitos www.ceifer.com/calidad/	Dr Jose Antonio Castilla info@ceifer.com
UK	UKNEQAS www.ukneqas.org.uk	repscience@ukneqas.org.uk
USA	Fertility Solutions www.fertilitysolutions.com https://fertilitysolutions.com/training/proficiency.htm	businessmgr@fertilitysolutions.com
	College of American Pathologists www.cap.org/laboratory-improvement/international-laboratories/external-quality-assurance-proficiency-testing-for-international-laboratories	cdm@cap.org contactcenter@cap.org
	American Association of Bioanalysts www.aab-pts.org	customerservice@aab-pts.org

See European Organization for External Quality Assurance Providers in Laboratory Medicine (EQALM) www.eqalm.org/site/member.php for more information about EQAP providers in laboratory medicine.

bioassay could lead to spermotoxic materials and/or culture media being used, leading to impaired results, or to the need to discard acceptable materials and/or media, thereby increasing the cost of the process. In any case, a good bioassay system for materials and media would improve the results obtained and reduce costs.

To standardize bioassay systems, various scientific societies (the American Association of Bioanalysts, the Fertility Society of Australia, and the Spanish Association for the Study of the Biology of Reproduction) encourage participation in a cytotoxicity external quality control programme (CT-EQC). In these programmes, participants receive laboratory materials, some of which have been contaminated with toxic substances, and they must determine whether the material in question is toxic or not. The participating laboratories are totally unaware of whether the materials have been altered and of the quantity of materials affected [87].

There is currently no EQAP which helps improve quality in the pre- and post-analytical phases of semen analysis, despite being introduced in other areas of the clinical laboratory and being recommended by scientific societies [88,89].

Continuous Equipment Monitoring

In addition to the expectation that all equipment must be included in a preventative maintenance programme, all 'mission critical' equipment such as cryostorage tanks, incubators, CO_2 supply, and liquid nitrogen supply must be monitored routinely (e.g. by independent manual measurements on a daily basis). In addition, there should be an out-of-hours alarm system that can call or page a list of contact persons, any of whom is capable of resolving the issue, when an alarm condition is detected by the equipment itself. That a piece of equipment remains in control throughout the day is then assumed, and this is why there is growing interest in continuous equipment monitoring systems which make and log measurements of key operating parameters entirely independently of the equipment's own controller, and with zero effort by the lab staff [3].

Although a continuous automated monitoring system does have a significant capital cost, rather than forming a 'knee-jerk' opinion that such a system is 'too expensive', a laboratory should perform a complete cost-benefit analysis against the ongoing costs of human-based monitoring, including the total cost (including test equipment purchasing, servicing and calibration) of monitoring the laboratory equipment – and air quality if appropriate – over at least a three-year period.

A continuous monitoring system monitors a series of temperature (T°C), %CO_2, humidity (%RH) and event or status sensors to monitor the following pieces of critical equipment at frequent intervals:

Specimen (air) incubator	T°C
Culture (CO_2) incubator	T°C, %CO_2 and %RH
Microscope heated stage	T°C
Refrigerators	T°C and door open status
Freezer	T°C and door open status
Cryostorage dewars	T°C and LN2 level
CO_2 gas supply	Low pressure status
Room conditions	T°C and %RH

Key features (e.g. the *DATAssure* system from Planer, Sunbury-on-Thames, UK; see www .planer.com) include:

- Critical out-of-range parameters trigger audible alarms to laboratory staff on a 24/7 basis, and call-out alarms to mobile phones outside laboratory operating hours.
- The Laboratory Manager can access the system for either real-time or historical data, generate graphs from within the system, and export data to Excel.
- Operates on an uninterruptible power supply (as well as being connected to the laboratory's emergency generator power).
- Engineers can access the system via the Internet in case of any issues or for system updates.

As usual, the laboratory has independent devices for measuring temperature (including a certified reference thermometer) and %CO_2 to verify any questionable values, and to provide ongoing confirmation operation of the automated system's sensors.

Other similar systems include Boomerang WiLogical (SparMed, see www.sparmed.dk), Log & Guard (Vitrolife, see www.vitrolife.com), Rees Scientific (see www.reesscientific.com), SmartSense (Digi, see www.smartsense.co), and Xiltrix (see www.xiltrixusa.com), as well as offerings from ThermoFisher and VWR.

Regulatory Aspects

Overview

Increasingly there are clear regulatory guidelines for semen analysis, sperm preparation for assisted conception treatment, and for sperm banking. It is essential that laboratory personnel are aware of both the national and international regulatory/legislative environment they operate within. While each country has (or is likely to have) its own particular system, e.g. CLIA in USA, NATA in Australia, CPA and HFEA in the UK (see below), there are also international systems of regulation. For example, the EU Tissues and Cells Directive (2004/23/EC), which came into operation in 2007, sets standards of quality and safety for the donation, procurement, testing, processing, preservation, storage and distribution of human tissue and cells. While this Directive does not cover basic semen assessment, any processing of the specimen (e.g. sperm preparation for IUI) is subject to the regulations under the directive. As such, any laboratory performing IUI within the EU (and in the EEA, which includes Iceland, Liechtenstein and Norway) will need to be licensed under this Directive. IVF clinics and cryobanks storing either patient or donor spermatozoa also require a licence.

ISO Standards

The ISO Standard 15189:2012 is the current edition of the medical laboratories standard, which was derived from the more general ISO 17025:2017 that specifies requirements for quality and competence in testing laboratories [3,14,15]. ISO 15189 is under revision, with a new version expected to be published in 2022. It is more specific for medical laboratories and assists them in developing their quality management systems and processes for assessing their competence. The overall aim of the standards is to define a management system for quality assurance, including working systems for internal and external audit of all aspects of the laboratory and its administration. ISO 15189 also helps accreditation bodies in confirming or recognizing the competence of medical laboratories.

A specific ISO Standard for diagnostic semen examination has been published recently *(ISO 23162:2021 Basic Semen Examination – Specification and Test Methods)* [33]. This new Standard is applicable to all ISO 15189 accredited laboratories that perform diagnostic semen examination.

Regulatory Environments

The requirement for accreditation or licensing of laboratories varies widely between countries and some examples are given below. Good Laboratory Practice (GLP) refers to a system of management controls for laboratories to ensure the consistency and reliability of results. Various regulatory and non-government bodies have GLP guidelines, rules or regulations. There are great similarities in the expectations of all these schemes, notably in their focus on quality management principles. Consequently, the principles espoused in ISO 15189 can be considered as fundamental for good andrology laboratory management.

European Union (and EEA)

The EU Tissues and Cells Directive (2004/23/EC) is a wide-ranging and comprehensive document covering all handling of human cells and tissues for therapeutic use in humans. In addition to the parent directive there are two technical annexes (Directives 2006/17/EC and 2006/86/EC), which detail the implementation of the primary Directive. Together, these Directives cover a wide range of topics, from administrative organization and quality management to traceability of sample origin and all components, materials and equipment that come into contact with the tissues and cells during their procurement, processing, storage and distribution.

After early concerns regarding some of the draft provisions that would likely have been harmful to gametes and embryos [90–92] the EU member states implemented the directives via national legislation by 1 July 2008. In 2015, two new Commission directives were adopted, one an implementing directive on the procedures for verifying equivalent standards of quality and safety of imported tissues and cells (Directive 2015/566) [93] and a second amending Directive 2006/86/EC, providing detailed requirements on the coding of human tissues and cells (Directive 2015/565) [94]. The EU Coding Platform Reference Compendia for the Application of a Single European Coding System for Tissues and Cells was developed (European Commission EU Coding Platform) pursuant to this latter directive.

The European Commission has supported EU member states in their efforts to implement EU directives on tissues and cells by providing funding for several projects (VISTART, EUROCET, etc.) under the Programme of Community Action in the Field of Health. It is worth highlighting the SoHO V&S (Vigilance and Surveillance of Substances of Human Origin) project, which addressed the harmonization of terminology and documentation relating to adverse events and reactions; and the joint action ARTHIQS (Good Practice on Donation, Collection, Testing, Processing, Storage and Distribution of Gametes for Assisted Reproductive Technologies and Haematopoietic Stem Cells for Transplantation) in building institutional and inspection guidelines for assisted reproductive technologies (Inspection Guidance in Assisted Reproductive Technologies (ART) Curriculum and Vademecum for inspectors) (www.arthiqs.eu). In 2019 the European Commission, through the European Directorate for the Quality of Medicines & HealthCare of the Council of Europe (EDQM), updated their Guide to the quality and safety of tissues and cells for human application [93]. Finally, Directive 95/46/EC on the protection of individuals with regard to the processing of personal data and the free movement of such data must be applied when processing personal data (e.g. data relating to donors and recipients).

Australia

The National Association of Testing Authorities (NATA) accredits all testing facilities including medical laboratories. NATA has assessed all laboratories according to ISO 17025 since January 2000, and medical laboratories according to ISO 15189 since 2004. Any laboratory performing diagnostic testing (e.g. andrology or endocrine) must be NATA accredited to operate. Although IVF labs are not required to have NATA accreditation, an increasing number are seeking it, recognizing that their 'sperm tests' are, in fact, diagnostic tests and must therefore be performed in accordance with proper standards for such tests.

USA

The Clinical Laboratory Improvement Amendment ('CLIA') of 1988 established three levels of laboratory testing: 'waived', moderate complexity, and high complexity, with tests being classified according to the risk of harm to patients, the likelihood of erroneous results, and the simplicity of testing. Almost any test that involves microscopic assessment is rated as high complexity, and only laboratories that meet the regulatory requirements of CLIA 88 can perform moderate or high complexity tests. These laboratories must undergo registration and periodic on-site inspections, and meet a range of other requirements, including: (a) having a QA programme; (b) specific personnel standards; (c) participation in an approved proficiency testing programme; and (d) ensuring that the testing equipment and assays are reliable, including having specified QC measures [95]. A number of organizations have received federal authorization to implement the inspection, licensing, and accreditation of andrology laboratories, including the Joint Commission (previously known as the Joint Commission on Accreditation of Healthcare Organizations or JCAHO), the College of American Pathologists (CAP), the Commission on Laboratory Accreditation (COLA), the American Association of Tissue Banks (AATB), and various state regulatory agencies.

Standards *vs* Guidelines

There are formal differences between different types of publications. The well-known WHO laboratory manual is neither a Standard nor a guideline. The WHO as an organization has specifically defined how its guidelines are developed, and the entire process for evidence-based recommendations for selection of treatment modalities. The WHO laboratory manual on the examination of human semen was not developed according to these principles, it is a manual providing suggestions on how the laboratory should work to obtain reliable results. Suggestions for laboratory techniques should be based on best available laboratory science but it is not a guideline for clinical interpretation of the laboratory results.

A formal guideline should – based on the best available scientific evidence – recommend suitable treatment modalities in specified clinical situations. The principles for such guidelines are well defined as evidence-based medicine and are usually based on specific 'PICO' questions – to define in Principle the clinical problem, the specification of the scientific question (clinically the Intervention), the choice of Comparison (or control), and the desired Outcome which, for a laboratory, needs to include the uncertainty of the results.

A formal Standard describes processes and principles to follow to obtain desired results: ISO 15189 considers the quality of results (appropriate equipment, techniques and trained staff members) as well as procedures to detect and minimize errors including traceability of procedures to detect sources of errors, while ISO 23162 considers the specific essential principles to obtain reliable results from basic semen examination [33].

Framework for Validating New Methods

Expectations of Accuracy and Precision for Medical Laboratory Tests

Standards for medical laboratories are well-established and clearly defined in ISO 15189:2012 [14,15]. Any medical laboratory test quantitative result must be within an acceptable range of the 'right answer', i.e. its measurement uncertainty (MU) must be known relative to established reference standards or methods [31,81,96,97], and this includes semen examination and all related tests of sperm function.

Expert opinion requires that results for semen examination characteristics obtained using CASA in a clinical andrology laboratory setting need to be within ±10% of reference values for an expert andrology laboratory, although ±20% might be adequate for a general diagnostic laboratory [31,97]. The assumption here is that all clinical andrology laboratories conform to current accepted 'Gold Standard' semen examination methodology, with all laboratory staff having been properly trained in all the protocols and quality control systems [31], although low conformity to international guidelines is well known [32,69,98], and seems to be especially low in assisted conception centres (ca. 2%; D Mortimer, unpublished data). The recent publication of the ISO 23162 technical standard for basic semen examination provides true reference methodology for use in accredited laboratories, as well as when validating alternative methods [33].

It must also be emphasized that comparisons between systems cannot be based on average values or on correlations/linear regression between paired values: both techniques conceal the real differences that exist between specific replicate determinations. Instead, Bland & Altman 'limits of agreement' or 'discrepancy' plots must be used [3,26,61], which plot the actual differences between the paired values, and can hence be used to establish whether each 'new method' (or 'trainee') value is within ±10% of the reference method or value. This is a gold standard comparison technique, and reports using other statistical approaches, many of which typically conceal the true extent of the existing discrepancy, must be viewed with caution. Indeed, the outcome of Bland & Altman plot analysis can always be due to chance, a possibility that can be excluded with Passing and Bablok analysis [82] (e.g. MedCalc; see www.medcalc.org). Deming's regression method (also available in MedCalc) can also be used to establish concordance between different methods tested in duplicate, including giving the coefficient of variation.

Finally, internal quality control (IQC) and external quality control or external quality assessment (EQC, EQA) are essential. But for an EQC/EQA scheme to have real value it must include the capability of quality improvement: a lab must know how close its results are to the correct values for it to be able to apply remedial training and improve its accuracy.

Validating a New Semen Examination Method

A framework to validate a method for human semen examination based on the fundamental principles discussed in this chapter will require:

- The study must be performed in an expert andrology laboratory whose staff are all trained (with evidence of competency) in, and employ, reference methodology. The laboratory must function within a proper quality-managed operational environment.
- Sufficient clinical specimens for a robust statistical comparison must be analysed in parallel using reference methodology and by the new method. Ideally, several hundred ejaculates need to be examined, covering the spectrum of ejaculate quality that exists in the population, but 120 should be considered a minimum.
- Each semen characteristic assessment must be performed in at least duplicate, with verification of adequate reproducibility of the replicates before calculating the final result.
- Results need to be expressed to an appropriate degree of precision based on the assessment method (avoid 'false precision').
- The new method's results must have an established measurement uncertainty or error, and need to fall within ±10% of the reference method's result.
- Data must be subjected to appropriate statistical analysis, ideally Bland & Altman or Passing & Bablok analyses, rather than linear regressions. Any linear regression analyses need to include the slope and intercept of the fitted line, as well as a test whether the fitted line is different to 0 or 1, as appropriate.
- Reports need to be published. Ideally in a respected peer-reviewed journal (e.g. impact factor of at least 2.0) using an open access model, but for commercial kits at least initially on the vendor's website.

    Without proper validation, no claims of suitability for purpose should be made.

    See Chapter 6 for specific recommendations related to validating CASA technology.

Validating a New Sperm Preparation Method or Sperm Function Test

A suggested framework to validate a new sperm preparation method or sperm function test, based on the fundamental principles discussed in this chapter, includes:

- The study must be performed in an expert andrology laboratory whose staff are all trained (with evidence of competency) in the relevant predicate and/or analytical methodologies. The laboratory must function within a proper quality-managed operational environment.
- Sufficient clinical specimens covering the spectrum of ejaculate or sperm quality that exists in the population need to be used to support a robust statistical comparison. This could require several hundred ejaculates.
- For a new sperm preparation method, the functional competence of the prepared spermatozoa needs to be verified as being at least comparable to predicate methods using at least *in-vitro* sperm function tests, and clinical ART treatment results if possible.
- For sperm function tests, sensitivity and specificity characteristics, as well as positive and negative predictive values, need to be provided, e.g. using ROC curve analysis.
- Each measurement characteristic must be performed in at least duplicate, with verification of adequate reproducibility of the replicates before calculating the final result.
- Results need to be expressed to an appropriate degree of precision, based on the assessment method (avoid 'false precision').
- The new method's results must have an established measurement uncertainty or error, and if appropriate need to fall within ±10% of a predicate method's result, or be shown to be measuring something different based on biology.
- Data must be subjected to appropriate statistical analysis. Comparisons based on simple linear regressions are generally inappropriate, and any linear regression results need to include the slope and intercept of the fitted line, as well as a test whether the fitted line is different to 0 or 1, as appropriate.

- Reports need to be published. Ideally in a respected peer-reviewed journal (e.g. impact factor of at least 2.0) using an open access model, but for commercial kits at least initially on the vendor's website.

Without proper validation, no claims of suitability for purpose should be made.

References

1. Tomlinson MJ, Barratt CL. Internal and external quality control in the andrology laboratory. In: Keel BA, May JV, De Jonge CJ, eds. *Handbook of the Assisted Reproduction Laboratory*. Boca Raton: CRC Press, 2000, 269–77.

2. Zemlin AE. Errors in the extra-analytical phases of clinical chemistry laboratory testing. *Indian J Clin Biochem* 2018; 33: 154–62.

3. Mortimer ST, Mortimer D. *Quality and Risk Management in the IVF Laboratory*, 2nd edn. Cambridge: Cambridge University Press, 2015.

4. Bento FC, Esteves SC. Establishing a quality management system in a fertility center: experience with ISO 9001. *Medical Express* 2016; 3: M160302.

5. Centola GM. Quality control, quality assurance, and management of the cryopreservation laboratory. In: Keel BA, May JV, De Jonge CJ, eds. *Handbook of the Assisted Reproduction Laboratory*. Boca Raton: CRC Press, 2000, 303–25.

6. International Standard Organization. *ISO 9001:2015 Quality Management Systems – Requirements*. Geneva: International Standards Organization, 2015.

7. Deming, WE. *Out of the Crisis*. Cambridge, MA: MIT Press, 1986.

8. Pereira, P. ISO series update, Part 1 – ISO 9001:2015 applied to medical laboratory scope. Madison: Westgard QC, 2017. www.westgard.com/iso-9001-2015-requirements.htm [last accessed 25 August 2021].

9. Gerteis M, Edgman-Levitan S, Daley J, Delbanco TL (eds.) *Through the Patient's Eyes: Understanding and Promoting Patient-Centered Care*. San Francisco, CA: Jossey-Bass Inc Pub, 1993.

10. Guo S, Duan Y, Liu X, Jiang Y. Three-year customer satisfaction survey in laboratory medicine in a Chinese university hospital. *Clin Chem Lab Med* 201; 56: 755–63.

11. van Empel IW, Aarts JW, Cohlen BJ, et al. Measuring patient-centredness, the neglected outcome in fertility care: a random multicentre validation study. *Hum Reprod* 2010; 25: 2516–26.

12. Boivin J, Takefman J, Braverman A. The fertility quality of life (FertiQoL) tool: development and general psychometric properties. *Hum Reprod* 2011; 26: 2084–91.

13. Koh YR, Kim SY, Kim IS, et al. Customer satisfaction survey with clinical laboratory and phlebotomy services at a tertiary care unit level. *Ann Lab Med* 2014; 34: 380–5.

14. International Organization for Standardization. *ISO 15189:2015 Medical Laboratories – Particular Requirements for Quality and Competence*. Geneva: International Organization for Standardization, 2007.

15. Burnett D. *A Practical Guide to ISO 15189 in Laboratory Medicine*. London: ABC Venture Publications, 2013.

16. Mourad SM, Hermens RP, Nelen WL, et al. Guideline-based development of quality indicators for subfertility care. *Hum Reprod* 2007; 22: 2665–72.

17. Wollersheim H, Hermens R, Hulscher M, et al. Clinical indicators: development and applications. *Neth J Med* 2007; 65: 15–22.

18. Castilla JA, Hernandez J, Cabello Y, et al. Defining poor and optimum performance in an IVF programme. *Hum Reprod* 2008; 23: 85–90.

19. Sciacovelli L, Panteghini M, Lippi G, et al. Defining a roadmap for harmonizing quality indicators in Laboratory Medicine: a consensus statement on behalf of the IFCC Working Group 'Laboratory Error and Patient Safety' and EFLM Task and Finish Group 'Performance specifications for the extra-analytical phases'. *Clin Chem Lab Med* 2017; 55: 1478–88.

20. Tsai ER, Tintu AN, Demirtas D, et al. A critical review of laboratory performance indicators. *Crit Rev Clin Lab Sci* 2019; 56: 458–71.

21. Mainz J. Defining and classifying clinical indicators for quality improvement. *Int J Qual Health Care* 2003; 15: 523–30.

22. American Society for Reproductive Medicine. Ten things physicians and patients should question. Available at: www.choosingwisely.org/wp-content/uploads/2015/02/ASRM-Choosing-Wisely-List.pdf [last accessed 25 August 2021].

23. Sánchez-Pozo MC, Mendiola J, Serrano M, et al. Special Interest Group in Andrology of the European Society of Human Reproduction and

Embryology. Proposal of guidelines for the appraisal of SEMen QUAlity studies (SEMQUA). *Hum Reprod* 2013; **28**: 10–21.

24. Husereau D, Drummond M, Petrou S, et al. CHEERS Task Force. Consolidated Health Economic Evaluation Reporting Standards (CHEERS) statement. *Value Health* 2013; **16**: e1–5.

25. Huysman W, Horvath AR, Burnett D, et al. Accreditation of medical laboratories in the European Union. *Clin Chem Lab Med* 2007; **45**: 268–75.

26. Mortimer D. *Practical Laboratory Andrology.* New York: Oxford University Press, 1994.

27. World Health Organization. *WHO Laboratory Manual for the Examination and Processing of Human Semen*, 5th edn. Geneva: World Health Organization, 2010.

28. World Health Organization. *WHO Laboratory Manual for the Examination and Processing of Human Semen*, 6th edn. Geneva: World Health Organization, 2021.

29. Björndahl L, Barratt CLR, Fraser LR, et al. ESHRE basic semen analysis courses 1995–1999: immediate beneficial effects of standardized training. *Hum Reprod* 2002; **17**: 1299–305.

30. Barratt CLR, Björndahl L, Menkveld R, Mortimer D. The ESHRE Special Interest Group for Andrology Basic Semen Analysis Course: a continued focus on accuracy, quality, efficiency and clinical relevance. *Hum Reprod* 2011; **26**: 3207–12.

31. Björndahl L, Barratt CLR, Mortimer D, Jouannet P. How to count sperm properly: checklist for acceptability of studies based on human semen analysis. *Hum Reprod* 2016; **31**: 227–32.

32. Riddell D, Pacey A, Whittington K. Lack of compliance by UK andrology laboratories with World Health Organization recommendations for sperm morphology assessment. *Hum Reprod* 2005; **12**: 3441–5.

33. International Standards Organization. *ISO 23162:2021 Basic Semen Examination – Specification and Test Methods.* Geneva: International Standards Organization, 2021.

34. Keck C, Fischer R, Baukloh V, et al. Staff management in the in vitro fertilization laboratory. *Fertil Steril* 2005; **84**: 1786–8.

35. ESHRE Special Interest Group of Embryology and Alpha Scientists in Reproductive Medicine. The Vienna consensus: report of an expert meeting on the development of ART laboratory performance indicators. *Reprod Biomed Online* 2017; **35**: 494–510 and *Hum Reprod Open* 2017; hox011. https://doi.org/10.1093/hropen/hox011

36. Aguilar J, Alvarez C, Morancho-Zaragoza J, et al. Quality specifications for seminal parameters based on clinicians' opinions. *Scand J Clin Lab Invest* 2008; **68**: 68–76.

37. Toft G, Rignell-Hydbom A, Tyrkiel E, et al. Quality control workshops in standardization of sperm concentration and motility assessment in multicentre studies. *Int J Androl* 2005; **28**: 144–9.

38. Auger J, Eustache F, Ducot B, et al. Intra- and inter-individuality variability in human sperm concentration, motility and vitality assessment during a workshop involving ten laboratories. *Hum Reprod* 2000; **15**: 2360–8.

39. Björndahl L, Tomlinson M, Barratt CLR. Raising standards in semen analysis: professional and personal responsibility. *J Androl* 2004; **25**: 862–3.

40. Viera AJ, Garrett JM. Understanding interobserver agreement: the Kappa statistic. *Fam Med* 2005; **37**: 360–3.

41. Wongpakaran N, Wongpakaran T, Wedding D, Gwet KL. A comparison of Cohen's Kappa and Gwet's AC1 when calculating inter-rater reliability coefficients: a study conducted with personality disorder samples. *BMC Med Res Methodol* 2013; **13**: 61.

42. Martínez-Granados L, Serrano M, González-Utor A, et al. Special Interest Group in Quality of ASEBIR (Society for the Study of Reproductive Biology). Reliability and agreement on embryo assessment: 5 years of an external quality control programme. *Reprod Biomed Online* 2018; **36**: 259–68.

43. Petersen PH, Stöckl D, Blaabjerg O, et al. Graphical interpretation of analytical data from comparison of a field method with reference method by use of difference plots. *Clin Chem* 1997; **43**: 2039–46.

44. Menkveld R, Stander FSH, Kotze TJvW, Kruger TF, Van Zyl JA. The evaluation of morphological characteristics of human spermatozoa according to stricter criteria. *Human Reprod* 1990; **5**: 586–592.

45. Franken DR, Menkveld R, Kruger TF, Sekadde-Kigondu C, Lombard C. Monitoring technologist reading skills in a sperm morphology quality control program. *Fertil Steril* 2003; **79**: 1637–43.

46. Alvarez C, Castilla JA, Martinez L, et al. Biological variation of seminal parameters in healthy subjects. *Hum Reprod* 2003; **18**: 2082–8.

47. Johnson JE, Blackhurt DW, Boone WR. Can Westgard Quality Control Rules determine the suitability of frozen sperm pellets as a control material for computer-assisted semen analyzers? *J Assist Reprod Genet* 2003; **20**: 38–45.

48. Clements S, Cooke ID, Barratt CL. Implementing comprehensive quality control in the andrology laboratory. *Hum Reprod* 1995; **10**: 2096–106.

49. Lu JC, Xu HR, Chen F, et al. Standardization and quality control for the determination of alpha-glucosidase in seminal plasma. *Arch Androl* 2006; **52**: 447–53.

50. Fearn T, Thompson M. A new test for 'sufficient homogeneity'. *Analyst* 2001; **126**: 1414–17.

51. International Organization for Standardization. *ISO 13528:2015. Statistical Methods for Use in Proficiency Testing by Interlaboratory Comparisons.* Geneva: International Standardization Organization, 2015.

52. Fraser CG, Harris EK. Generation and application of data on biological variation in clinical chemistry. *Crit Rev Clin Lab Sci* 1989; **27**: 409–37.

53. Sandberg S, Fraser CG, Horvath AR, et al. Defining analytical performance specifications: Consensus Statement from the 1st Strategic Conference of the European Federation of Clinical Chemistry and Laboratory Medicine. *Clin Chem Lab Med* 2015; **53**: 833–5.

54. Ricos C, Alvarez V, Cava F, et al. Current databases on biological variation: pros, cons and progress. *Scand J Clin Lab Invest* 1999; **59**: 491–500.

55. Castilla JA, Morancho-Zaragoza J, Aguilar J, et al. Quality specifications for seminal parameters based on the state of the art. *Hum Reprod* 2005; **20**: 2573–8.

56. Jones GR, Albarede S, Kesseler D, et al., for the EFLM Task Finish Group – Analytical Performance Specifications for EQAS (TFG-APSEQA). Analytical performance specifications for external quality assessment – definitions and descriptions. *Clin Chem Lab Med* 2017; **55**: 949–55.

57. Lopez-Regalado ML, Martínez-Granados L, González-Utor A, et al. Special Interest Group in Quality of ASEBIR (Society for the Study of Reproductive Biology). Critical appraisal of the Vienna consensus: performance indicators for assisted reproductive technology laboratories. *Reprod Biomed Online* 2018; **37**: 128–32.

58. Westgard JO. Use and interpretation of common statistical tests in method comparison studies. *Clin Chem* 2008; **54**: 612.

59. Cooper TG, Atkinson AD, Nieschlag E. Experience with external quality control in spermatology. *Hum Reprod* 1999; **14**: 765–9.

60. World Health Organization. *WHO Laboratory Manual for the Examination of Human Semen and Sperm-Cervical Mucus Interactions*, 4th edn.

Cambridge: Cambridge University Press, 1999.

61. Bland JM, Altman DG. Statistical methods for assessing agreement between two methods of clinical measurement. *Lancet* 1986; **I**: 307–10.

62. McCulloh DH. Quality control and quality assurance. Record keeping and impact on ART performance and clinical outcome. In: May JV, Diamond MP, De Cherney AH, eds. *Infertility and Reproductive Medicine: Clinics of North America*, 1998: 285–309.

63. Castilla JA, Sanchez-Leon M, Garrido A, et al. Procedure control and acceptance sampling plans for donor sperm banks: a theoretical study. *Cell Tissue Bank* 2007; **8**: 257–65.

64. Alvarez C, Castilla JA, Ramirez JP, et al. External quality control program for semen analysis: Spanish experience. *J Assist Reprod Genet* 2005; **22**: 379–87.

65. Strike PW. *Statistical Methods in Laboratory Medicine.* Oxford: Butterworth Heinemann, 1991.

66. Jequier AM, Ukombe EB. Errors inherent in the performance of a routine semen analysis. *Br J Urol* 1983; **55**: 434–6.

67. Neuwinger J, Behre HM, Nieschlag E. External quality control in the andrology laboratory: an experimental multicenter trial. *Fertil Steril* 1990; **54**: 308–14.

68. Matson PL. External quality assessment for semen analysis and sperm antibody detection: results of a pilot scheme. *Hum Reprod* 1995; **10**: 620–5.

69. Keel BA, Quinn P, Schmidt CF Jr, et al. Results of the American Association of Bioanalysts national proficiency testing program in andrology. *Hum Reprod* 2000; **15**: 680–6.

70. Filimberti E, Degl'Innocenti S, Borsotti M, et al. High variability in results of semen analysis in andrology laboratories in Tuscany (Italy): the experience of an external quality control (EQC) programme. *Andrology* 2013; **1**: 401–7.

71. Punjabi U, Wyns C, Mahmoud A, et al. Fifteen years of Belgian experience with external quality assessment of semen analysis. *Andrology* 2016; **4**: 1084–93.

72. Eliasson R. Standards for investigation of human semen. *Andrologie* 1971; **3**: 49–64.

73. Eliasson R. Analysis of semen. In: Burger H, de Kretser D, eds. *The Testis.* New York: Raven Press, 1981.

74. Mortimer, D. Laboratory standards in routine clinical andrology. *Reprod Med Rev* 1994; **3**: 97–111.

75. Belsey MA, Eliasson R, Gallegos AJ, et al. *Laboratory Manual for the Examination of Human*

Semen and Semen-Cervical Mucus Interaction. Singapore: Press Concern, 1980.

76. World Health Organization. *WHO Laboratory Manual for the Examination of Human Semen and Semen-Cervical Mucus Interaction*, 2nd edn. Cambridge: Cambridge University Press, 1987.

77. World Health Organization. *WHO Laboratory Manual for the Examination of Human Semen and Sperm-Cervical Mucus Interaction*, 3rd edn. Cambridge: Cambridge University Press, 1992.

78. Yeung CH, Cooper TG, Nieschlag E. A technique for standardization and quality control of subjective sperm motility assessments in semen analysis. *Fertil Steril* 1997; **67**: 1156–8.

79. ISO/IEC Guide 98-1:2009 Uncertainty of measurement - Part 1: Introduction to the expression of uncertainty in measurement. Geneva: International Organization for Standardization, 2009.

80. Cook RR. *Assessment of Uncertainties in Measurement for Calibration and Testing Laboratories.* Sydney: National Association of Testing Authorities, 1999.

81. International Standards Organization. *ISO/TS 20914:2019 Medical Laboratories – Practical Guidance for the Estimation of Measurement Uncertainty.* Geneva: International Standards Organization, 2019.

82. Passing H, Bablok W. A new biometrical procedure for testing the equality of measurements from two different analytical methods. Application of linear regression procedures for method comparison studies in clinical chemistry, Part I. *J Clin Chem Clin Biochem* 1983; **21**: 709–20.

83. Cooper TG, Björndahl L, Vreeburg J, et al. Semen analysis and external quality control schemes for semen analysis need global standardization. *Int J Androl* 2002; **25**: 306–11.

84. Palacios ER, Clavero A, Gonzalvo MC, et al. Acceptable variability in external quality assessment programmes for basic semen analysis. *Hum Reprod* 2012; **27**: 314–22.

85. Miller WG, Jones GR, Horowitz GL, Weykamp C. Proficiency testing/external quality assessment: current challenges and future directions. *Clin Chem* 2011; **57**: 1670–80.

86. Castilla JA, Ruiz de Assin R, Gonzalvo MC, et al. External quality control for the embryology laboratory. *Reprod Biomed Online* 2010; **20**: 68–74.

87. Martínez-Granados L, Gonzalvo MC, Clavero A, et al. Application of a sperm survival test: results from an external quality control programme. *Eur J Obstet Gynecol Reprod Biol* 2018; **230**: 55–9.

88. Lippi G, Banfi G, Church S, et al. European Federation for Clinical Chemistry and Laboratory Medicine Working Group for Preanalytical Phase. Preanalytical quality improvement. In pursuit of harmony, on behalf of European Federation for Clinical Chemistry and Laboratory Medicine (EFLM) Working group for Preanalytical Phase (WG-PRE). *Clin Chem Lab Med* 2015; **53**: 357–70.

89. Vasikaran S, Sikaris K, Kilpatrick E, et al. IFCC WG Harmonization of quality assessment of interpretative comments. Assuring the quality of interpretative comments in clinical chemistry. *Clin Chem Lab Med* 2016; **54**: 1901–11.

90. Mortimer D. A critical assessment of the impact of the European Union Tissues and Cells Directive (2004) on laboratory practices in assisted conception. *Reprod Biomed Online* 2005; **11**: 162–76.

91. Hartshorne GM. Challenges of the EU 'tissues and cells' directive. *Reprod Biomed Online* 2005; **11**: 404–7.

92. Saunders D, Pope A. Response to article – 'A critical assessment of the impact of the European Union Tissues and Cell Directive (2004) on laboratory practices in assisted conception' by David Mortimer. *Reprod Biomed* Online 2005; **11**: 407–8.

93. EDQM (European Directorate for the Quality of Medicines & HealthCare of the Council of Europe). Guide to the quality and safety of tissues and cells for human application, 4° edn. Strasbourg: Council of Europe, 2019. https://register.edqm.eu/freepub [last accessed 25 August 2021].

94. European Commission EU Coding Platform – Reference Compendia for the Application of a single European Coding System for Tissues and Cells. https://webgate.ec.europa.eu/eucoding/reports/te/index.xhtml [last accessed 25 August 2021].

95. Carrell DT, Cartmill D. A brief review of current and proposed federal government regulation of assisted reproduction laboratories in the United States. *J Androl* 2006; **23**: 611–17.

96. Sanders D, Fensome-Rimmer S, Woodward B. Uncertainty of measurement in andrology: UK best practice guideline from the Association of Biomedical Andrologists. *Br J Biomed Sci* 2017; **74**: 157–62.

97. Björndahl L. What is normal semen quality? On the use and abuse of reference limits for the interpretation of semen analysis results. *Hum Fertil* 2011; **14**: 179–86.

98. Bailey E, Fenning N, Chamberlain S, Devlin L, Hopkissen J, et al. Validation of sperm counting methods using limits of agreement. *J Androl* 2007; **28**: 364–73.

Risk Management

Overview

Risk management is a rapidly growing area of concern in modern medicine, with primary areas of focus being on reducing medical errors and enhancing patient and staff safety. Risk management was originally an engineering discipline dealing with the possibility that some future event might cause harm or 'loss', leading to a generic description of 'risk' as being any uncertainty about a future event that might threaten an organization's ability to accomplish its mission. Risk management, therefore, includes strategies and techniques for recognizing and confronting any such threat – ideally before it happens – and provides a disciplined environment for proactive decision-making for the purpose of assessing on a continuous basis what can go wrong, determining which risks need to be dealt with, and implementing strategies to deal with these risks [1–4].

- *Proactive risk management* is concerned with 'What can go wrong?' and 'What will we do to prevent the harm from occurring?'
- *Retrospective risk management* is concerned with 'If something happens, how will we resolve it, put things right (and pay for it) and prevent it from recurring?'

In an effective risk management programme, risks are continuously identified, analysed, and minimized, mitigated or eliminated, and problems are prevented before they occur. In layman's terms, there is a cultural shift from 'fire-fighting' and 'crisis management' to one of proactive decision-making and planning. Conversely, failing to pursue risk management means that catastrophic problems will occur without warning, and that there will likely be no ability to respond rapidly to such 'surprises' – making recovery very difficult and/or costly, requiring resources having to be expended to correct problems that could have been avoided.

In recent years, the Failure Modes and Effects Analysis FMEA approach has been used successfully to identify and resolve risks associated with traceability during various aspects of the ART laboratory (see 'Specimen Identity Verification', below).

Risk Management Tools

There are two main tools used in risk management: a proactive tool called Failure Modes and Effects Analysis or 'FMEA', and a reactive tool called Root Cause Analysis or 'RCA' [1,5]. While FMEAs work towards preventing and minimizing risk, RCAs are used to deal with actual adverse events and with troubleshooting. An FMEA can be seen as a form of 'proactive troubleshooting' [1]. Both tools depend on systems and process analysis, whereby every step or component process in a system is identified (process mapping): each process must be reduced to its fundamental steps, with no lower-level derivative processes, so that the factors acting on every component process can be identified and analysed.

Detailed discussions of risk perception, risk communication and practical risk management tools are available elsewhere [1,5]. For tools such as FMEA and RCA methodology to be effective, they require an enlightened, positive management philosophy and staff committed to quality and risk management. Obviously, an RCA can only be effective if it is accepted throughout the organization that its goal is to aid improvement, and not to assign blame (in keeping with the principles of continuous improvement intrinsic to a 'total quality management' or 'TQM' philosophy). Moreover, it must be understood that most errors result from faulty systems rather than human error: poorly designed processes put people in situations where errors are more likely to occur [1,6–8].

Failure Modes and Effects Analysis

The FMEA is a simple yet powerful tool to identify and counter weak points in the design and execution of processes. Its structured approach (see below) has made it one of the most widely used tools for developing quality designs, systems and services and it can be used to improve processes in any organization. Healthcare applications of FMEA typically identify process steps or components (the 'failure modes') for improvement based upon relative ratings of the anticipated likelihood of them occurring ('likelihood' or 'occurrence') and the 'consequence' or 'severity' of resulting adverse effects or events; nowadays, FMEAs often include a third factor based on the 'detectability' of each failure mode.

Rating schemes for the likelihood, severity and detectability are not standardized beyond the organization employing them (see Tables 13.1 and 13.2). While many organizations employ scales that go up to five, in the examples shown here, we have used scales that go up to 10, on the principle that a wider dynamic range in scales facilitates agreement on assigning ranks, especially since the highest rank should rarely be awarded to anything that might exist in a lab with functional processes. Two-factor Risk Criticality scores can therefore go up to 25 or 100, while three-factor RPN values can go up to 125 or 1000, clearly illustrating the value of wider dynamic range rating schemes for differentiating risks of relatively similar grades.

Table 13.1 Suggested wider dynamic range ratings scheme for performing a Failure Modes and Effects Analysis (modified from [1])

Rating	Occurrence	Consequence or severity	Detectability
0	Impossible – hence it is not a real risk	None – hence it cannot be considered as a real risk	Certain – hence it is not a real risk
1	Very unlikely: well-controlled or minimized risk but cannot be completely eliminated	Trivial: in reality there is no measurable adverse risk	Probable
2	Unlikely: the circumstances for occurrence are all controlled as far as practically possible, but external factors remain which the organization cannot control	Minimal: in reality the risk is more of a nuisance or inconvenience, with no identifiable impact on patient care	Very likely
3	Somewhat possible	Quite minor: e.g. impacts the organization's internal systems only	Likely
4	Possible	Minor: e.g. definite adverse effect on efficiency but without any measurable effect on treatment outcome	Quite likely
5	Very possible	Quite serious: e.g. definite risk of diminished treatment outcome	Very possible
6	Quite likely	Serious: e.g. definite adverse effect on patient management or treatment outcome	Possible
7	Likely	Very serious: e.g. one or more definite adverse impacts upon multiple patients' management or treatment outcomes, or risk of injury to patients or staff	Somewhat possible
8	Very likely	Major: e.g. loss of embryos, OHSS, infection of patients or staff, causes actual injury to patient(s) or staff	Unlikely
9	Probable	Extreme: e.g. loss of life, damage to facility (must be at least of 'very unlikely' occurrence)	Very unlikely
10	Certain: therefore the situation should never exist in the real world	Catastrophic: loss of multiple lives, destruction of facility – in a real-world situation this should apply only to 'acts of God', war or terrorism	Impossible

Table 13.2 Suggested simple (narrow dynamic range) ratings scheme for performing a Failure Modes and Effects Analysis

Rating	Occurrence	Consequence or severity	Detectability
1	Unlikely: circumstances for occurrence are all controlled as far as practically possible	Minimal: more of a nuisance or inconvenience with no identifiable impact on patient care	Probable
2	Possible	Minor: e.g. adverse effect on efficiency but no appreciable effect on patient management treatment outcome	Likely
3	Likely	Serious: e.g. adverse effect on patient management or treatment outcome, or risk of injury to patients or staff	Possible
4	Very likely	Major: e.g. loss of embryos, OHSS, infection of patients or staff, actual injury to patients or staff	Unlikely
5	Probable (but should not be certain)	Extreme: e.g. loss of life, damage to facility (must be at least of 'very unlikely' occurrence)	Very unlikely if not impossible

1. Establish the context of the issue by mapping the process so that its details are readily apparent.
2. Identify possible Failure Modes within the process; each one of these represents a specific risk that is to be considered; classify the likelihood of occurrence of each Failure Mode. Analysing possible contributory factors that explain why something is a possible Failure Mode will likely be needed later in the FMEA process.
3. Determine the Effects of each Failure Mode and rate their severity.
4. Ascertain the likelihood of detecting each Failure Mode under current normal operating conditions.
5. Calculate the Risk Priority Number (RPN) by multiplying the occurrence, severity and detection ratings. If using only occurrence and severity ratings, then their product can be called the Risk Criticality score.
6. Create a Risk Matrix to visualize all the Failure Modes after ranking according to their Criticality or RPN values.
7. Identify any existing or possible future controls for the Failure Mode that might:
   a) Reduce its occurrence
   b) Reduce or mitigate its severity
   c) Identify any means whereby the detection of a Failure Mode might be increased.
8. For each Failure Mode, calculate its revised Criticality or RPN value if the corrective measures were to be successful.
9. Create an Action Plan prioritizing risks based on a combination of the highest current Criticality or RPN values and the largest possible improvements that might be achieved when corrective actions are applied successfully. An Action Plan also needs:
   a) At least one indicator for monitoring the process being improved.
   b) Assignment of someone responsible for its implementation and follow-up.
   c) An expected timeline for its completion.
10. Implement the Action Plan.
11. Review the success of the changes implemented. If unsuccessful, review and repeat the earlier steps as necessary.
12. Record the FMEA and its outcome in the laboratory's Quality Framework.

Risk Management and Regulation

Laboratory accreditation and certification schemes (e.g. ISO 15189:2012 [9,10]) integrate risk management and quality management (especially quality assurance and quality improvement) into an overall operational system. However, laboratory licensing perforce relates to regulations, and typically focuses much more on a perceived need to control risk, most often within the broad-reaching context of 'public safety'. A good example of this, and an illustration of risk analysis and communication, can be seen in the extent to which extreme precautionary measures have been deemed necessary to avoid the theoretical transmission of variant Creutzfeldt-Jakob Disease via sperm donors [11].

What Can Make an Andrology Laboratory 'High Risk'?

As in all areas of laboratory medicine, continual training and proficiency testing are imperative. But these tactics alone will neither ensure quality nor prevent potentially catastrophic errors. The following list covers the most likely areas where risk factors can be found in an andrology laboratory.

Inadequate Physical Resources

Laboratories that are forced to operate with the minimum physical facility or equipment resources will be at greater risk; there must be sufficient capacity in all critical equipment to deal with the busiest of times. All laboratory equipment must be included in a preventative maintenance programme and all 'mission critical' equipment must be monitored on a continual basis, e.g. cryostorage tanks, incubators, CO_2 supply, liquid nitrogen supply. In addition, an out-of-hours alarm system that can call or page a list of contact persons capable of resolving the issue is essential. Real-time monitoring systems are also being installed in more andrology laboratories, especially those with cryobanks. Continuity of electrical power supply to critical equipment must be ensured (e.g. by an in-house generator), while items sensitive to power fluctuations need to be protected by an uninterruptible power supply ('UPS').

As part of the physical resources, the semen collection (masturbation) room and patient care immediately prior to semen collection should not be forgotten. Not paying attention to these two factors results in a high risk of a subject's inability to collect a semen sample (collection block) or collection errors (incomplete sample). The andrology laboratory is responsible for facilitating and managing appropriate conditions in the semen collection room, which should be quiet, private and clean, with optional visual stimuli. In addition, patients should be treated with appropriate empathy by laboratory staff in the moments before semen collection: being provided with information in a place separate from other patients, reassured, and the presence of any accompanying person managed with appropriate sensitivity. For teenagers who want to cryopreserve semen, it is important to exercise caution with the person accompanying them (parent, guardian, or nurse) [12], recognizing rights to privacy and consent rules. For all of the above, it is essential that andrology lab staff are trained in what information to give the patient minutes before entering a room to collect a semen specimen, and how to give this information. Failure to collect the specimen through masturbation could lead to patients having to use more uncomfortable or aggressive methods to obtain spermatozoa (medication, electroejaculation, testicular biopsy), with a corresponding increase in risk.

Inappropriate Methods, Kits, Reagents, Devices or Products

Use of inappropriate methods, e.g. ones with poor accuracy and/or precision, or which cannot provide results with the required uncertainty of measurement, will prevent a laboratory from providing proper service, and can lead to misdiagnosis. All kits and reagents must be 'suitable for purpose', have been stored correctly and not have expired. Similarly, all devices or products used in therapeutic procedures (e.g. sperm preparation for IUI, sperm cryopreservation) must have been approved for medical use by the appropriate regulatory authorities, e.g. The Food and Drug Administration in the USA, CE marking in Europe, etc., wherever possible; non-approved products or veterinary products must not be used.

Inadequate Human Resources

Staffing levels must also reflect the maximum caseload [1,9,10], with some slack in the system so that staff are not constantly working at maximum capacity [1,13] and are able to be alert and not distracted by tiredness – and hence able to perform all aspects of their jobs accurately and reliably, with the lowest possible risk of making mistakes. Any circumstances that contribute to over-tiredness or exhaustion represent serious risk factors. A high prevalence of burnout syndrome in ART laboratory staff has been described [14]. Moreover, even with effective training programmes, a high staff turnover increases the number of people who are less sure of the laboratory's systems, standard operating procedures (SOPs) and usual practices. Laboratories with a higher proportion of relatively inexperienced staff are less equipped to recognize and deal with operational problems as they arise. Comprehensive, formal programmes are essential for training all laboratory staff in new techniques and procedures, and for the orientation, and re-training as necessary, of staff coming from other laboratories. Finally, there is the issue of staff not accepting professional responsibility, e.g. when a member of a team does not take enough care to ensure that they have performed – and completed – all assigned tasks. This can be either intentional or unintentional, but in all cases is unprofessional.

Inadequate Systems

Laboratory 'standard operating procedures' (SOPs) must include sufficient technical/procedural detail for anyone with basic competence to perform the procedure exactly as intended. Methodological variations are thereby excluded, and the incursion of factors that can adversely affect the process prevented. Proper specification of an SOP requires understanding not just how the process in question is regulated by biology, chemistry and physics (and hence engineering), but also how it might be impacted by extrinsic factors, the lab environment, or ergonomics. Incomplete, or poorly written, SOPs create opportunities for laboratory staff to make mistakes, and all staff must follow the laboratory's SOPs exactly. Any changes to documented SOPs must be authorized by the Laboratory Director: the introduction of variations, short-cuts or perceived 'improvements' without authorization must be prevented.

Every time that a specimen is labelled, or moved from one container to another, identity checks must be followed strictly and verified either by a competent witness or some validated process or technological solution [1,15]. Likewise, great care must be taken when completing all documentation to ensure that all records are complete and accurate. Repeated incidents of carelessness or lack of attention to detail (i.e. risk) must be followed-up and remedied; the use of a comprehensive, documented system of notifications and/or task lists to ensure that the laboratory staff know exactly what has to be done each day, will greatly decrease the risk of critical tasks being forgotten.

Unless a comprehensive system of Incident Reports ('nonconformity reports' in ISO 9001:2015 parlance) for all adverse events is in place, enforced, and employed constructively, many mistakes will never be recognized or remedied [10]. In this context, an 'adverse event' can be defined as any event that potentially or actually affects staff safety, patient safety or the provision of testing or treatment according to the patient's care plan or the expected outcome of their treatment [1].

Specimen Provenance

Specimen provenance refers to establishing the origin of a specimen as well as maintaining its chain of custody while being received, analysed, processed, and the pertinent results reported.

Identification of the Person Who Produced a Specimen

It is vital to clearly identify the patient correctly. This might sound obvious, but it is necessary to be certain of the identity of the patient who provides a specimen. In cases where the patient does not speak the local language, there could be particular difficulties. Identification using name, address and date of birth are commonly used. But in some circumstances, particularly if ART treatment is used, more robust methods of identification might be required, such as presenting a driver's licence, passport, or other 'government-issued' identification. In these cases, laboratory personnel can be confident who produced the sample.

In all cases, the patient needs to sign a laboratory form saying that they produced the sample, regardless of whether the specimen was collected on-site or off-site. This is especially important when dealing with situations where the partner delivers to the laboratory a semen specimen produced at home. Here the deliverer must be identified and provide a statement of provenance as to the origin of the specimen, for example saying 'I, Mrs Angelina Smith, have today delivered to the fertility laboratory a semen specimen collected at home by my partner, Mr Brad Smith'. From a risk-management perspective, even if the semen specimen were to have been produced by Mrs Smith's 'friend', she has stated that it was from Mr Smith, so the laboratory would not be at risk for specimen misidentification, the fraud having been committed intentionally by Mrs Smith.

Processing of a Specimen and Reporting the Results

We have stated in this handbook that two unique identifiers must be assigned to each specimen to assist in its correct identification as it is processed through the laboratory. During this process, the individual identifiers are routinely checked when performing specific procedures, e.g. sperm morphology assessments. Additionally, when the final results are collated and the report forms prepared, a final check related to the specimen provenance should be made to verify that the result being prepared does relate to the particular person named on the report.

Specimen Identity Verification

It has already been noted that every time a specimen is labelled or moved from one container to another, identity checks must be followed strictly and verified either by a competent witness or some validated process or technological solution [1,15]. But whether 'double witnessing' – which is merely one tool that can be used to address the problem – can eliminate all risk has been questioned [1,15].

In busy laboratories, manual double witnessing adds additional paperwork to an already busy working environment and can actually have the unintended consequence of increasing risk by creating distractions and interruptions in the process. Identified problems with the procedure include independent redundancy, attentional blindness and ambiguous accountability, and common checking failures include check omission, check incomplete, involuntary automaticity and non-contemporaneous checking. Involuntary automaticity, whereby attention levels decrease when someone performs the same action repeatedly, can reduce the effectiveness of double witnessing [16].

Because one of the main commercial products developed to support this process is called 'Witness', to avoid possible perceptions of favouritism in this handbook the process is termed 'specimen identity verification'.

It is the responsibility of each laboratory to undertake a formal risk assessment of their specimen provenance and identification processes to ensure that the risk of specimen misidentification or confusion is reduced as low as possible (recognizing that risk elimination is rarely possible when a process depends on people actually performing the process).

Several papers have reported FMEA exercises relating to ensuring traceability of gametes and embryos in the ART laboratory [17–22].

Technological Solutions

A great proportion of ART patients are concerned about the possibility of gamete and embryo mix-ups and an electronic specimen identity verification greatly allays those fears [23]. While the situation can be seen as less critical in diagnostic laboratories, many andrology laboratories serve as the specimen reception 'front end' in an ART centre for spermatozoa, and also perform treatment-related processing of spermatozoa directly, e.g. washing for IUI or semen or sperm cryobanking. In these cases, errors in the chain of custody of a specimen would have serious impacts on future paternity, therefore technological solutions for monitoring specimen identity clearly have potential application in andrology laboratories as well.

The two main identification technologies are based on barcodes and RFID tags, and there are several commercial solutions that employ one or other technology, within systems with varied approaches and capabilities. The three main currently available systems, listed alphabetically, are:

- *Gidget®* (Genea BiomedX, Sydney, Australia see www.geneabiomedx.com)
- *Matcher* (IMT Technologies, Chester, UK; see www.imtinternational.com)
- *RI Witness™* (Cooper Surgical Fertility & Genomic Solutions, Måløv, Denmark; see https://fertility.coopersurgical.com/equipment/ri-witness/)

Sperm Cryobanking

The prevalence of adverse events related to staff and sample safety is unknown in a sperm bank, although some evidence suggests that they are frequent [24]. It is important that both patients and physicians are informed of the possibility of failure during storage or accidentally thawing samples. All staff should know the protocols to avoid these risks and how to act should they occur. There is an obsession with analysing the unknown or minuscule risk of cross-contamination between straws, instead of paying attention to other more common risks, such as staff safety or premature warming of specimens during handling (e.g. during audit) [24–26]. Following the revelation of a series of cryotank failures in ART laboratories, a comprehensive assessment of cryogenic storage risk and quality management issues was undertaken in the USA and the resulting publication [27] and a discussion of the legal issues [28] are highly recommended.

For a general guide to operating a cryopreservation facility see [29].

General Measures

Restricted access to the cryobank itself should clearly stipulate that only authorized personnel will be granted entry; patients and donors must not be allowed entry into either the andrology laboratory or the cryobank. There should be a written security procedure and contingency plan for different risks, and registers to record personnel statements that they have read and understood these policies.

Staff Safety

General training in the use of liquid nitrogen and in the use of pressurized nitrogen vessels is a key element in the prevention of risk in the cryobank. Personal protective equipment and suitable equipment for the job must be available. Oxygen monitoring systems must be installed (sensors must currently be replaced annually) and linked to an alarm or some other form of external warning system. There should be an adequate low-level ventilation (forced air change) and the inside of the cryobank should be visible from outside the room (e.g. a reinforced glass door panel).

Liquid Nitrogen Transport

Avoid unnecessary liquid nitrogen transport. Provide easy access for the liquid nitrogen delivery vehicle. Stores should be located on the ground floor. Supply vessels should be checked regularly. There must be a written procedure for the safe handling of liquid nitrogen and a register to record personnel statements that they have read and understood the procedure. Nobody should accompany a vessel being transported in an elevator [30].

Mistaken Identity

Specimen identity verification (a.k.a. 'witnessing') has been proposed to verify all processes involving transfer of gametes, and is mandatory in some countries, e.g. the UK. However, the cost-effectiveness of this measure has not been evaluated. Straws must be identified individually. Automatic labelling systems for straws, or self-adhesive labels, should be used. Labels must be able to withstand immersion in liquid nitrogen. There must be written procedure for dealing with straws with labels that are illegible or missing, and records of samples that are lost.

There is an overall lower risk of confusion between samples when fewer samples are stored. Hence having a protocol to manage unusable samples is key: from deceased patients (once the legal time has passed for post-mortem use), discontinued patients (who do not renew the written informed consent for semen storage), or patients who have requested the destruction of their frozen semen (e.g. due to having become pregnant and having no further reproductive desire). A storage tank inventory should be carried out regularly in order to check that these samples are disposed of, following the established protocols. These inventories should also be carried out when there is a suspected loss of samples or discrepancies between the cryostorage record and the samples in the cryobank [31].

Cryostorage Tank Management

Before starting to use a new storage tank or using one which has not been used for a while, its integrity should be checked. For this, a functional assessment of between one and four weeks should be carried out before starting to use it. Likewise, frequent visual inspections looking for frost, ice, condensation or water pooling, and cracks around the dewar neck should be carried out during its use [27,31]. There should be a renovation plan for the storage tank as its vacuum warranties are limited. Manufacturers' recommendations must be followed.

As general principles, the following areas should be taken into consideration when developing strategies for operating a cryobank safely [27]:

- Administrative and record keeping issues
  - Cryogenic storage tank considerations
  - Liquid and vapour phase
  - Location of storage tanks
  - Static holding time
  - Emergency plan safeguards
- Maintenance and monitoring considerations
  - Tank filling
  - Manual tank monitoring and physical assessments
  - Remote monitoring systems
  - Remote alarm systems
  - Alarm response
  - Sample management and inventory

Many of these aspects have already been discussed elsewhere in regard to quality and risk management, and especially the need for careful monitoring of LN2 levels and for having backup tanks available [1].

Cryostorage Tank Management

Experimental artificial external breaching of an MVE 47/11 liquid storage dewar, created by drilling a 1-mm diameter hole at the shoulder of the tank, showed that it took 20 h for the internal temperature at the level of the stored specimens to rise to −170°C, but then only a further 25–30 min to rise to −100 to −80°C, which is considered to constitute tank failure (the ice transition point of water being *ca.* −132°C) [32; L McNamara, personal communication]. Additional observations on experimental breaches of 10 Taylor-Wharton 35HC and MVE 47/11 tanks that had just been topped-off with LN2 have shown that:

- LN2 vapour was visible within 60 s of all breaches
- With external breaches (holes drilled inside the neck of the tank) vacuum loss was audible for up to 4h
- The tank lid temperature fell below 5°C, due to escaping LN2 vapour, in the first 5 min and stayed there until the tank failed (i.e. specimen level temperature above −150°C)
- Ice 'crowning' of the lid was obvious with external, but not internal, breaches
- There were at least 12 h before tank failure occurred

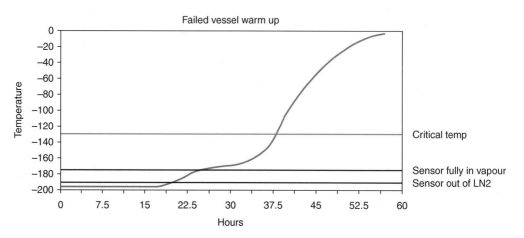

Figure 13.1 Internal temperature in a Statebourne Bio 36 cryostorage tank following artificial breaching (courtesy of J Bennet). See text for detailed explanation.

Monitoring of the ambient temperature at the immediate lid and neck external areas guaranteed immediate notice of a tank failure with *ca.* 14–20 h warning of the tank's failure.

This means that if a lab were to rely only on monitoring temperature rise above –170°C, which is a common practice, then it will only have those few minutes in which to respond, the preceding 14–20 h window of warning while the tank warmed to –170°C, during which samples could have been moved to another cryostorage tank, having not been recognized.

Another tank breaching (induced catastrophic vacuum failure) study performed on a Statebourne Bio 36 cryostorage tank completely full of LN2, with a temperature sensor located at the top of the canisters (i.e. just above the highest samples in the vessel), showed that the temperature remained constant at –196°C while the sensor remained immersed in LN2, until about 18 h after the tank had been breached (Figure 13.1). As the LN2 continued to evaporate, the internal tank temperature increased until a reasonably stable vapour temperature was reached at about 22.5 h; the temperature then slowly increased as more LN2 evaporated until the tank was empty, when the temperature rose quickly (35–37 h) (J Bennet, personal communication; www.lifestartsolutions .com). Clearly, internal tank temperature alone is not an effective way of monitoring compared to the actual LN2 level.

Partially full tanks will obviously warm up sooner, and it must be noted that a vapour storage dewar's internal temperature will fail much faster than that of a liquid storage dewar, perhaps becoming critical within as little as 2 h.

The wireless *TempAlert* system configured to monitor the inside storage temperatures at the canisters as well as the immediate external ambient temperatures at the lid/neck of a cryostorage tank is a relatively simple approach that can provide a warning with sufficient time to respond to imminent tank failure (see www.tempalert.com).

Studies using a continuous weight sensor to monitor similar cryostorage tanks following artificial external and internal breaches showed that a 20% evaporation of LN2 took ~4 h, even though the first temperature alarm at –194°C did not occur until 5.5–6.5 h. Tanks with internal breaches reached –170°C sooner (14–15 h), with 65–75% evaporation, compared to 18–19 h for the externally breached tanks with >95% evaporation; all tanks showed a rapid rise in temperature by 24–25 h [33]. These authors concluded that a WiFi-based weight measurement system, originally intended to monitor the content of LN2 supply tanks, or perhaps high capacity cryostorage tanks, is a robust approach for continuous QC monitoring of cryotanks (TrustGnosis, Brea, CA; see www.trustgnosis.com) [34]. However, this approach would seem impractical for andrology labs with even moderate numbers of cryostorage tanks, unless each tank is permanently located on its own sensor base, making it a very expensive solution. The alternative option of moving each tank onto a weighing base even on a weekly basis would be very time consuming, as well as physically risky, and impractical for labs with larger numbers of cryostorage tanks.

Regardless of the monitoring system, regular physical/visual checks of cryostorage tanks, especially for ice 'crowning' around the lid, should also be performed, and the checks documented.

Dual or Divided Storage

The storage of samples in geographically separate storage facilities or in the same bank but in different containers, and their potential security advantages, should be analysed in a risk management process. If adequate risk management and security measures are in place, then dual or divided storage is not essential for a sperm bank [1].

Transmission of Infection

While there is a risk of cross-contamination during storage in the same cryotank, this risk can be minimized significantly using various strategies such as those described in Chapter 10, 'Sperm Cryopreservation'. Briefly:

1. Following laboratory best practice, *High Security Straws* (Cryo Bio System, L'Aigle, France; see www .cryobiosystem.com) must be used as the specimen packaging system:
    a) Do not allow the outside of the straw to come into contact with either the semen or the sides of the container, this is achieved using the custom filling nozzle.
    b) After sealing, disinfect the outside of each straw using hypochlorite solution, followed by rinsing with sterile water and drying.
    c) Before opening, disinfect the outside of each straw using hypochlorite solution, followed by rinsing with sterile water and drying.
    d) After thawing, use a sterile device (ideally disposable suture scissors) to cut the straw.
2. Use different types of containers according to the serological status of the patient.
3. Keep donor and patient spermatozoa in different vessels.
4. Use emergency (spare) tanks when necessary.

If these measures are followed, vapour phase or supercold containers, previous sample processing, quarantine containers for sperm donor, and high quality air in the sperm bank are not necessary [35,36].

Premature Warming of Cells

Freezing. A contingency plan for malfunction of the controlled-rate freezer during sperm cryopreservation should be in place (e.g. have a spare controlled-rate freezer).

Monitoring system. For secure and effective long-term storage of sperm, it is recommended that a triple-layer alarm system for the storage tanks be employed. Any temperature increase of more than 10% above −196°C must trigger a series of progressive alarms.

- Local alarm (audible and visual), in the room where the containers are located and in a nearby room.
- Distant alarm (audible and visual). If, in a set period of time, the local alarm has not been attended to, an alarm will be activated in a distant room in the same building or complex which is manned by maintenance staff 24 h per day. This alarm will not be effective unless clear and concise written instructions are left, indicating which protocol should be followed.
- In the absence of either local or distant alarms being effective, or if there is no maintenance staff station, a dial-out system should be installed that will contact a series of pre-programmed telephone numbers. It is recommended that a contingency plan be developed and clearly displayed close to the repository, in particular detailing the location of other tanks of similar dimensions and characteristics into which the samples may be transferred in the event of a breakdown or when the tank is being cleaned.

Alarm systems should be able to function in the event of power failure and be tested at least quarterly. However, despite having an alarm system, some guidelines [31] recommend checking tanks three times a week by manual verification, especially when the cryobank space is isolated from the daily laboratory activities.

Packaging system should be related to the type of container. If straws are used, then liquid nitrogen tanks are recommended. Straws have a higher warming rate than cryovials, and the risk of warming when handling specimens outside the cryogenic storage tank for brief periods is higher. Consequently, straws should remain submerged in liquid nitrogen to reduce the risk of premature warming, which is not possible in the vapour phase or supercold tanks.

Supply of liquid nitrogen. Failures can be due to dewar vacuum failure, automated auto-fill system failure, refrigerator over-fills, or failure of the supply company to deliver. Possible solutions include having emergency tanks, establishing a reciprocal cover arrangement with a nearby centre, or maintaining substantial spare capacity [24,25]. It is also possible to have a local liquid nitrogen generator. Modern systems have a relatively small footprint, low power consumption, low noise and vibration levels, and are available from a number of manufacturers around the world.

Interpretation and Diagnosis

As discussed in Chapter 12, 'Quality Management and Accreditation', the post-analytical phase of the total testing process includes how physicians use and respond to laboratory results. Interpretation of results from semen analysis involves more challenges than most other modern laboratory services. Besides the common analytical variability discussed in Chapter 12, there is also considerable variability between men and between semen specimens from one man, variability that does not necessarily imply pathology or reduction of fertility potential. It has not been possible to establish any distinct limits ('cut-offs') between results from fertile and subfertile men – the overlap between populations is considerable, giving a large range of borderline results [37,38]. Therefore, the risk for an incorrect diagnosis is far from negligible if decisions for further investigations or treatment options are based only on a single semen characteristic. Better support for such decisions is of course achieved when several characteristics are evaluated together [2,39].

Furthermore, it is essential for clinicians to be aware of the level of uncertainty for each value reported by the andrology laboratory, so as to be able to determine if, for instance, the difference between two specimens from one patient is more likely to depend on random variation or rather due to physiological or pathological changes in the male reproductive organs. It is therefore important for the laboratory to provide not only guidelines in the form of reference ranges, but also guidance on the analytical variability ('error' or 'uncertainty of measurement') related to each semen characteristic, and what it means when a reported result is close to a decision limit.

A correct diagnosis cannot usually be made based only on laboratory results. The clinical diagnosis, on which decisions for further investigations or treatment choices will be made, should be based on patient history, physical examination and laboratory investigations like semen analysis, as well as other tests such as hormone analyses. Regarding semen analyses results, it is important to again stress the basic principle that correct background information of the patient with each semen analysis should be obtained and presented as part of the semen analysis result to the referring clinician [40].

The risks with incorrect interpretation and diagnosis comprise medical, economical and ethical issues. Among the worst complications includes the possibility when an infertility investigation with sub-optimal results from semen analysis is not followed by an appropriate clinical investigation where an underlying severe, or even fatal if not treated, somatic disease would have been discovered in time for proper medical treatment [41]. Less serious from a medical point of view, but with severe ethical implications, are more chronic disorders with secondary negative influence on semen parameters, where failure of discovery due to lack of proper clinical investigation will result in delayed diagnosis and unnecessarily long suffering. Over-emphasizing 'male factor' infertility in general will cause an exaggerated use of intracytoplasmic sperm injection (ICSI), that will usually mean increased costs for the patient or any other party paying for treatment. On the other hand, poor diagnostic work-up can also mean that a patient with reduced chances for success with ordinary IVF procedures has an increased risk to be given a sub-optimal treatment, also causing economical losses as well as ethical issues [42,43].

In the communication between the laboratory and the clinicians using its service, it is important that the laboratory does not over-interpret the laboratory findings by making assumptions about clinical diagnoses. However, remarks about possible underlying problems that could cause or contribute to discovering abnormalities *should* be communicated to the physician responsible for consideration, together with other information that is usually not available for the laboratory.

Finally, and as with other activities within the total testing process, Key Performance Indicators (KPIs) should be designed and used to monitor the fluency and usefulness of this communication between laboratory and physicians, as well as the correct interpretation of laboratory results by physicians (see Chapter 12).

References

1. Mortimer D, Mortimer ST. *Quality and Risk Management in the IVF Laboratory*, 2nd edn. Cambridge: Cambridge University Press, 2015.

2. Kennedy CR. Risk management in assisted reproduction. *Clin Risk* 2004; **10**: 169–75.

3. Kennedy CR, Mortimer D. Risk management in IVF. *Best Pract Res Clin Obstet Gynaecol* 2007; **21**: 691–712.

4. Mortimer D. Setting up risk management systems in IVF laboratories. *Clin Risk* 2004; **10**: 128–37.

5. Hutchison D. *Total Quality Management in the Clinical Laboratory*. Milwaukee: ASQC Quality Press, 1994.

6. Reason JT. Foreword. In: Bogner MS, ed. *Human Error in Medicine*. Hillsdale: Lawrence Erlbaum Associates Inc, 1994.

7. Bogner MS (ed). *Human Error in Medicine*. Hillsdale: Lawrence Erlbaum Associates Inc, 1994.

8. Leape LL. A systems analysis approach to medical error. *J Eval Clin Prac* 1997; **3**: 213–22.

9. International Standards Organization. *ISO 15189:2012 Medical Laboratories – Particular Requirements for Quality and Competence*. Geneva: International Organization for Standardization, 2012.

10. Burnett D. *A Practical Guide to ISO 15189 in Laboratory Medicine*. London: ACB Venture Publications, 2013.

11. Mortimer D, Barratt CLR. Is there a real risk of transmitting variant Creutzfeldt-Jakob Disease (vCJD) by donor sperm insemination? *Reprod Biomed Online* 2006; **13**: 778–90.

12. Bahadur G, Ling KL, Hart R, et al. Semen production in adolescent cancer patients. *Hum Reprod* 2002; **17**: 2654–6.

13. DeMarco T. *Slack. Getting Past Burnout, Busywork, and the Myth of Total Efficiency*. New York: Broadway Books, 2001.

14. López-Lería B, Jimena P, Clavero A, et al. Embryologists' health: a nationwide online questionnaire. *J Assist Reprod Genet* 2014; **31**: 1587–97.

15. Brison DR, Hooper M, Critchlow JD, et al. Reducing risk in the IVF laboratory: implementation of a double-witnessing system. *Clin Risk* 2004; **10**: 176–80.

16. Toft B, Mascie-Taylor H. Involuntary automaticity: a work-system induced risk to safe health care. *Health Serv Manage Res* 2005; **18**: 211–16.

17. de los Santos MJ, Ruiz A. Protocols for tracking and witnessing samples and patients in assisted reproductive technology. *Fertil Steril* 2013; **100**: 1499–502.

18. Rienzi L, Bariani F, Dalla Zorza M, et al. Failure mode and effects analysis of witnessing protocols for ensuring traceability during IVF. *Reprod Biomed Online* 2015; **31**: 516–22.

19. Intra G, Alteri A, Corti L, et al. Application of failure mode and effect analysis in an assisted reproduction technology laboratory. *Reprod Biomed Online* 2016; **33**: 132–9.

20. Cimadomo D, Ubaldi FM, Capalbo A, et al. Failure mode and effects analysis of witnessing protocols for ensuring traceability during PGD/PGS cycles. *Reprod Biomed Online* 2016; **33**: 360–9.

21. Rienzi L, Bariani F, Dalla Zorza M, et al. Comprehensive protocol of traceability during IVF: the result of a multicentre failure mode and effect analysis. *Hum Reprod* 2017; **32**: 1612–20.

22. Molina I, Gonzalvo MC, Clavero A, et al. Análisis modal de fallos y efectos en la fase pretécnica del Laboratorio de Reproducción. *Medicina Reproductiva y Embriología Clínica* 2017; **4**: 128–35.

23. H. Forte M, Faustini F, Maggiulli R, et al. Electronic witness system in IVF-patients perspective. *J Assist Reprod Genet* 2016; **33**: 1215–22.

24. Tomlinson M, Morroll D. Risks associated with cryopreservation: a survey of assisted conception

units in the UK and Ireland. *Hum Fertil* 2008; **11**: 33–42.

25. Tomlinson M. Managing risk associated with cryopreservation. *Hum Reprod* 2005; **20**: 1751–6.

26. Clarke G. Sperm cryopreservation: is there a significant risk of cross-contamination? *Hum Reprod* 1999; **14**: 2941–3.

27. Schiewe MC, Freeman M, Whitney JB, et al. Comprehensive assessment of cryogenic storage risk and quality management concerns: best practice guidelines for ART labs. *J Assist Reprod Genet* 2019; **36**: 5–14.

28. Rinehart LA. Storage, transport, and disposition of gametes and embryos: legal issues and practical considerations. *Fertil Steril* 2021; **115**: 274–81.

29. Bennet J. *Operating a Successful Cryopreservation Facility*. Sunbury-on-Thames: Planer plc, 2018.

30. British Compressed Gases Association. *Code of Practice 30. The Safe Use of Liquid Nitrogen Dewars. Revision 3: 2019*. Pride Park: British Compressed Gases Association, 2019. www .bcga.co.uk/pages/index.cfm?page_id=111&title= codes_of_practice_[last accessed 25 August 2021].

31. Practice Committees of the American Society for Reproductive Medicine, Society for Reproductive Biologists and Technologists, and Society for Assisted Reproductive Technology. Cryostorage of reproductive tissues in the in vitro fertilization laboratory: a committee opinion. *Fertil Steril* 2020; **114**: 486–91.

32. Graham JR, Applegate CL, Graham SR; Tucker MJ. Cryotank quality control: how to detect a tank that is failing. *Fertil Steril* 2019; **112 Suppl 3**: e268.

33. Schiewe MC, Zozula S, Behnke EJ, et al. The anatomy of liquid nitrogen (LN2) cryo dewar tank failures. *Fertil Steril* 2019; **112 Suppl 3**: e268–9.

34. Schiewe MC, Zozula S, Ochoa T, et al. Usefulness of remote, continuous weight determination for the routine quality management of cryo dewar tanks. *Fertil Steril* 2019; **112 Suppl 3**: e269.

35. Mortimer D. A critical assessment of the impact of the European Union Tissues and Cells Directive (2004) on laboratory practices in assisted conception. *Reprod Biomed Online* 2005; 11: 162–76.

36. Mortimer D. Current and future concepts and practices in human sperm cryobanking. *Reprod Biomed Online* 2004; 9: 134–51.

37. Nallella KP, Sharma RK, Aziz N, Agarwal A. Significance of sperm characteristics in the evaluation of male infertility. *Fertil Steril* 2006; **85**: 629–34.

38. Menkveld R, et al. Semen parameters, including WHO and strict criteria morphology, in a fertile and subfertile population: an effort towards standardization of in-vivo thresholds. *Hum Reprod* 2001; **16**: 1165–71.

39. Jedrzejczak P, Taszarek-Hauke G, Hauke J, et al. Prediction of spontaneous conception based on semen parameters. *Int J Androl* 2008; **31**: 499–507.

40. Menkveld R. The basic semen analysis. In: Oehninger S, Kruger TF, eds. *Male Infertility*. London: Informa Healthcare, 2007, 141–70.

41. Jequier AM. The importance of diagnosis in the clinical management of infertility in the male. *Reprod Biomed Online* 2006; **13**: 331–5.

42. Mortimer, D. Structured management as a basis for cost-effective infertility care. In: Gagnon C, ed. *The Male Gamete: From Basic Knowledge to Clinical Applications*. Vienna, IL: Cache River Press, 1999, 363–70.

43. Mortimer D, Mortimer ST. The case against intracytoplasmic sperm injection for all. In: Aitken J, Mortimer D, Kovacs G, eds. *Male and Sperm Factors 31 that Maximize IVF Success*. Cambridge: Cambridge University Press, 2020.

Reproductive Toxicology

Introduction

Many pharmaceutical, environmental, and occupational compounds may act as male reproductive toxicants [1,2]. Exposure to endocrine-disrupting chemicals during fetal gonadal development has gained considerable attention, but the adult testis may also be vulnerable to chemicals. Reproductive toxicants are associated with disturbances in various processes and sites of the reproductive system, affecting both spermatozoa and the somatic cells of the testis [3,4]. While this field is generally outside the scope of this book, many studies on human reproductive toxicology involve testing the effects of substances or compounds on sperm production or functional competence, methods for which are included here.

Assessment of human male reproductive toxicity represents a great challenge compared to studies with animal models. Data from laboratory animal studies may not be of relevance to human health risk assessment, due to differences between species regarding dose-response relationship, metabolism of the compound and mechanism of action, as well as the high doses of toxicants often used in experimental models.

Reproductive toxicology studies in humans are mostly population-based or use a case-control design. Several studies have revealed regional differences in semen quality, and meta-analyses have indicated a decline in sperm count for decades [5,6]. A growing concern for male reproductive health worldwide has motivated several multicenter studies including comparison of semen parameters at different locations.

Standardization of methods and external quality control are essential for meaningful comparison of data collected at different centres, as well as for monitoring changes over time [7,8].

Studies on Semen Quality

Standardization of Methods

Standardization of semen analysis to improve the reliability of the results is important not only for infertility investigations, but also when assessing male reproductive toxicity at both the individual and population levels. Standardized protocols, training of the technicians, and internal quality control are essential. For multicentre studies, consideration of which type of equipment (e.g. counting chambers, microscopes with phase contrast optics) or methods (e.g. assessment of sperm motility or morphology) give the most useful results should be evaluated as part of the external quality control of the study [9].

Measurement of semen volume should be done by the same method, preferentially by weighing [10], and the same type of counting chamber should be used when determining sperm concentration [8]. It should be noted that in shallow capillary-loaded chambers (e.g. 20 µm) the sample is not uniformly distributed, introducing a significant error that varies according to semen viscosity [11].

For assessment of reproductive toxicity on individuals, or when there are few participants in a study, two ejaculates should be collected for each observation point. In population toxicology studies, however, only one specimen from each individual can be sufficient [12,13], but in all cases, an appropriate power analysis should be undertaken to calculate the number of individuals necessary to detect anticipated differences, if they exist.

When evaluating changes in sperm concentration, either within a population or between populations, abstinence time is an important consideration. Although a specific abstinence time is recommended (e.g.

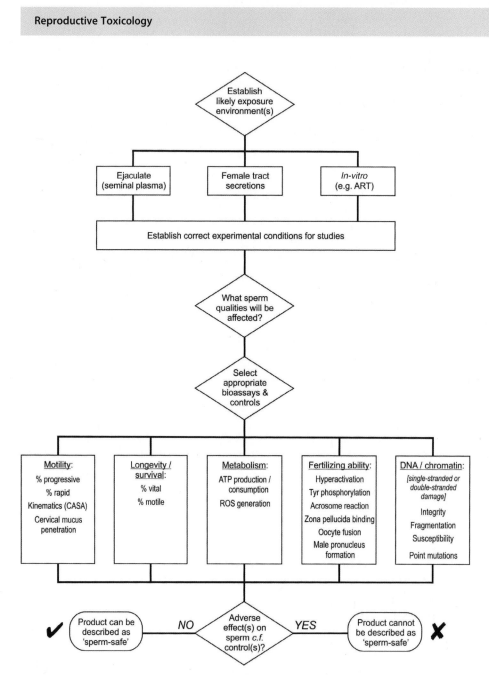

Figure 14.1 Flow chart illustrating a proposed pathway for developing strategies to verify that a product or substance is sperm safe. Reproduced from [3] with permission.

three days, rather than a window such as two to five days), there will be variations which can influence the results and this must be included in the model when performing the statistical analyses. Furthermore, the study populations must be comparable regarding age, ethnicity, and general medical history. In exposure studies, the interval between treatment and sampling should be carefully considered: to detect toxicologic effects on spermatogenesis, the 'follow-up' specimen should be collected after at least one completed spermatogenic cycle (approximately 10–12 weeks, see Chapter 2).

Training of Technicians

Studies have revealed large variation between laboratories, even when the same standardized protocols are used [14,15], and meaningful comparisons depend on strict quality control [8]. Therefore, inter- and intra-technician coefficients of variation should be established for each technique in a pilot study. Furthermore, the mean percentage difference from a chosen standard value should be calculated. Actions to correct errors should be performed when necessary [8]. If possible, technicians from each centre should come together and perform the various assessments side-by-side, in order to minimize differences in method performance.

Detailed discussions of, and techniques for, robust basic semen analysis methods can be found in Chapter 3, extended semen analysis methods in Chapter 4, sperm DNA testing in Chapter 5, and sperm function tests in Chapter 7.

Reproductive Toxicant Testing

In population-based studies, in addition to following standardized methods for assessing reproductive characteristics, the recruitment of participants must be performed to minimize source of bias such as suspected infertility [7]. For compounds or products that are suspected to target the reproductive system, experimental studies are needed that use validated analytical techniques designed to minimize inherent errors, and have carefully defined end-points; detailed recommendations for designing studies have been published (Figure 14.1) [3].

References

1. Pizzol D, Foresta C, Garolla A. Pollutants and sperm quality: a systematic review and meta-analysis. *Environ Sci Pollut Res*. https://doi.org/10.1007/s11356-020-11589-z

2. Semet M, Paci M, Saïas-Magnan J, et al. The impact of drugs on male fertility: a review. *Andrology* 2017; 5: 640–63.

3. Mortimer D, Barratt CL, Björndahl L, et al. What should it take to describe a substance or product as 'sperm-safe'. *Hum Reprod Update* 2013; **19 Suppl 1**: i1–45.

4. Arzuaga X, Smith MT, Catherine F Gibbons CF, et al. Proposed key characteristics of male reproductive toxicants as an approach for organizing and evaluating mechanistic evidence in human health hazard assessments. *Environ Health Perspect* 2019; **127**: 65001.

5. Rahban R, Nef S. Regional difference in semen quality of young men: a review on the implication of environmental and lifestyle factors during fetal life and adulthood. *Basic Clin Androl* 2020; **30**: 16. https://doi.org/10.1186/s12610-020-00114-4

6. Virtanen HE, Jørgensen N, Toppari J. Semen quality in the 21st century. *Nat Rev Urol* 2017; **14**: 120–30.

7. Sánchez Pozo C, Mendiola J, Serrano, M, et al. Proposal of guidelines for the appraisal of SEMen QUAlity studies (SEMQUA). *Hum Reprod* 2013; **28**: 10–21.

8. Björndahl L, Barratt CL, Mortimer D, Jouannet P. 'How to count sperm properly': checklist for acceptability of studies based on human semen analysis. *Hum Reprod* 2016; **31**: 227–32.

9. Brazil C, Shanna SH, Tollner CR, et al. Study for Future Families Research Group. Quality control of laboratory methods for semen evaluation in a multicenter research study. *J Androl* 2004; **25**: 645–56.

10. Cooper TG, Brazil C, Swan SH, Overstreet JW. Ejaculate volume is seriously underestimated when semen is pipetted or decanted into cylinders from the collection vessel. *J Androl* 2007; **28**: 1–4.

11. Douglas-Hamilton DH, Smith NG, Kuster CE, et al. Capillary-loaded particle fluid dynamics: effect on estimation of sperm concentration. *J Androl* 2005; **26**: 115–22.

12. Stokes-Riner A, Thurston SW, Brazil C, et al. One semen sample or 2? Insights from a study of fertile men. *J Androl* 2007; **28**: 38–43.

13. Rylander L, Wetterstrand B, Haugen TB. Single semen analysis as a predictor of semen quality: clinical and epidemiological implications. *Asian J Androl* 2009; **11**: 723–30.

14. Auger J, Eustache F, Ducot B, et al. Intra- and inter-individual variability in human sperm concentration, motility and vitality assessment during a workshop involving ten laboratories. *Hum Reprod* 2000; **15**: 2360–8.

15. Björndahl L, Barratt CL, Fraser LR, et al. ESHRE basic semen analysis courses 1995–1999: immediate beneficial effects of standardized training. *Hum Reprod* 2002; **17**: 1299–305.

Andrology Laboratory Safety

Safety Is the Responsibility of Everyone Working in the Laboratory

Each laboratory is required to work in compliance with the local and national safety guidelines, which vary between countries.

For example, in Canada there is the Workplace Hazardous Material Information Scheme (www.hc-sc.gc.ca/ewh-semt/occup-travail/whmis-simdut/index-eng.php) (WHMIS), which is a hazard communication standard. The key elements of this system are cautionary labelling of containers of WHMIS 'controlled products', the provision of material safety data sheets (MSDSs) and worker education programmes. There is a national standard for the classification of hazardous workplace materials, and all controlled products must be properly labelled and identified using MSDSs. Additionally, workers receive education and training to ensure the safe storage, handling and use of controlled products in the workplace.

In the UK, the Health and Safety Executive (www.hse.gov.uk) is the national body tasked with protecting workers' health and safety by ensuring risks in the workplace are properly controlled. The HSE is responsible for enforcing health and safety at work legislation and plays a major role in producing advice on health and safety issues, and guidance on relevant legislation.

All UK laboratories using chemicals or other hazardous substances are required to perform a detailed assessment covering the following eight points:

- Assess the risks
- Decide what precautions are necessary
- Prevent or adequately control exposure
- Ensure that control measures are used and maintained
- Monitor the exposure
- Carry out appropriate health surveillance
- Prepare plans and procedures to deal with accidents, incidents and emergencies
- Ensure employees are properly informed, trained and supervised.

These themes are common to many regulatory bodies on health and safety and are robust guiding principles. In addition to national guidelines, there are several international resources that provide high quality information related to safety in the laboratory – for example the WHO Laboratory Biosafety Manual [1]. Several excellent web-based safety training programmes are freely available [e.g. 2].

General Recommendations

These recommendations are adapted from those published by the World Health Organization [1,3], ASRM [4] and ESHRE [5].

- All laboratory personnel handling human tissues and body fluids should be vaccinated in accordance with the local recommendations for medical personnel in general.
- *Universal precautions.* Laboratory personnel must handle every specimen of human tissue or body fluid as if it were contaminated with an infectious organism.
- Extraordinary precautions must be taken to avoid accidental wounds from (contaminated) sharp instruments in the laboratory. This includes any sharp edges or corners of microscope slides and coverslips. As far as possible, hypodermic needles should be eliminated from general laboratory use to minimize the risks of 'finger stick' injury. Dispose of all sharp objects in a designated sharps bin.

- Avoid contact between biological materials and open skin lesions. Disposable gloves must be worn at all times when handling fresh or frozen semen, seminal plasma, blood plasma or serum, cervical mucus, follicular fluid and urine, as well as any containers or handling devices (e.g. pipettes) that have come into contact with these materials. Gloves must be removed and discarded as contaminated waste when leaving the laboratory or handling the telephone, etc. Never reuse gloves.
- Either surgical scrubs or a laboratory coat or gown must be worn, fastened, in the laboratory. This protective clothing must be removed on leaving the laboratory. Under no circumstances should such clothing be worn outside the laboratory or assisted reproductive technology (ART) procedures area.
- Suitable footwear is essential; open weave shoes and sandals do not give suitable protection.
- A high standard of personal hygiene must always be maintained. Hands must be washed after removing gowns and gloves. Hands must be washed thoroughly and immediately if they become contaminated with biological material. All hand washing must be with bactericidal soap and hot water. Hand washing sinks must not be used for any other purpose, and hands must not be washed in the general laboratory sink.
- Hands should be kept away from face, nose, eyes and mouth, as must pens, pencils and other objects used in the laboratory.
- Long hair must be tied back.
- Where appropriate, beard covers must be worn.
- If the outside of any sample container is contaminated, it must be disinfected as per the laboratory or institution's approved methods.
- Disposable laboratory supplies should be used whenever and wherever possible. After use they must be collected in special 'CONTAMINATED WASTE BIOLOGICAL HAZARD' containers and properly disposed of as for other infectious material, e.g. by incineration or autoclaving.
- All laboratory equipment that could potentially be contaminated by biological material must be disinfected or sterilized (e.g. by alcohol spray) after a spill or after work activity is completed. This includes equipment handled while wearing protective gloves, e.g. microscopes and pipetting devices.
- Pipetting by mouth is not permitted. Mechanical pipetting devices must be used for the manipulation of all other liquids in the laboratory.
- All procedures and manipulations of biological fluids must be performed so as to minimize the creation of droplets and aerosols. Such procedures include centrifugation or vigorous mixing (especially vortex mixing) of open containers. Only centrifuges fitted with sealed carriers should be used.
- Laboratory work surfaces must be decontaminated with a disinfectant (see above) immediately after any spill occurs, and also on completing work with biological fluids each day.
- Eating (including chewing gum), drinking, smoking, taking of snuff, applying cosmetics, and the wearing of strong perfume or after-shave, etc., are prohibited in the andrology laboratory. Smoking is not permitted in the laboratory. The consumption of food and drink is only permitted in the designated areas e.g. kitchen, staffroom and office areas.
- All working areas must always be kept clean and tidy.
- Faulty equipment must be reported immediately to the laboratory supervisor.
- If you come across a situation that is unsafe, do something about it yourself and report it to your senior.

Accident Prevention

Supervisors' Responsibilities
- Appropriate actions are taken to correct any safety hazards that might exist.
- Proper personal protective clothing and equipment are provided and used.
- Staff are aware of, and abide by, all national, provincial and local government safety regulations.
- Employees receive adequate training in, and information on, safe working procedures.
- An adequate number of workers are trained in first aid procedures.

Employees' Responsibilities

- Report all accidents and injuries to the laboratory supervisor.
- All federal, provincial and local government safety regulations are conformed to.
- Unsafe procedures and conditions are reported immediately to the laboratory supervisor.
- Be aware of hazards in the day-to-day work and that appropriate measures to eliminate any risk of accident are taken.
  - Wear appropriate personal protective clothing and equipment as required and ensure that it is maintained in good condition.
  - Work in accordance with the health and safety training and instruction procedures set by laboratory management, and adhere to the policies, procedures and risk assessments relating to your work activities.

Protective Clothing and Equipment

While performing normal duties, a laboratory worker may be exposed to a variety of hazards. While all steps must be taken to control these hazards at their source(s), personal protective equipment and/or clothing must be used (see discussion of responsibilities, above).

Eye Protection

Eye protection must be worn at any time there is a danger of flying particles, aerosols, irritating substances, liquids or harmful radiation endangering the eyes.

Contact lenses are not a substitute for proper eye protection, and spectacles with plain glass lenses also pose a potential hazard. All workers wearing spectacles who are regularly exposed to this type of hazard should be encouraged to request safety lenses when having prescriptions for new spectacles filled.

Hand Protection

Appropriate gloves must be worn when handling materials or equipment that could be injurious to the skin such as sharp objects, chemicals, biological or extremely hot or cold materials.

Respiratory Protection

Although special equipment such as self-contained breathing apparatus or respirators are not required in an andrology/ART laboratory, suitable surgical face masks should be worn whenever there is a possibility of exposure to aerosols of biological material.

All handling of flammable or noxious substances such as solvents or fixatives should be performed in a fume hood.

Protective Clothing

The general principles governing this issue are that clothing worn in the laboratories or clinical procedure areas must be protected from contamination, and any clothing worn in those areas must not be worn outside them where it might contaminate others.

Fire Safety

While it is the responsibility of the institution to ensure that appropriate fire detection and suppression systems, as required by relevant building and fire safety codes, are installed and serviced – including the provision of portable fire extinguishers – laboratory staff also have specific responsibilities.

Most fires are preventable, see www.hse.gov.uk/toolbox/fire.htm.

General Fire Safety Rules

The following list is not exhaustive:

- Never use naked flames when flammable vapours are present. Smoking is always forbidden in all laboratories.
- Never block fire exit doors, fire/smoke control doors, or access to firefighting equipment.
- Do not store large quantities of flammable solvents in the laboratory. Highly flammable liquids (flash point below 40°C, e.g. ether) must not be stored in ordinary glass containers in quantities of more than 4.5 l. Larger volumes, if essential, must be stored in approved safety containers.
- Never store equipment or materials in hallways or under stairwells.
- Use metal or other approved waste solvent containers. Plastic waste solvent containers are only suitable for small scale use (e.g. under-bench locations).
- Be aware of potential fire or explosion hazards of **any** chemical or material you use.

Dealing with Spills

General Rules

- The primary concern in any spillage incident is the care and safety of all exposed persons, especially those at risk from infection.
- *Always wear gloves and gowns*. Also, wear a face mask and eye protection if appropriate for the particular spill.
- Always read the appropriate safety data sheets for a material before using it and understand risks e.g. Control of Substances Hazardous to Health (COSHH) assessments.

Specific procedures for dealing with spills of biological material and other hazardous substances are described in the following sections.

Biological Materials: Use and Disposal

Modern infection control regulations require that all human tissue samples be considered potentially pathogenic (the principle of **universal precautions**). Therefore, all ART laboratories (including embryology laboratories, andrology laboratories, sperm banks, etc.) must have adequate safety programmes to protect their staff against accidental contamination. This also dictates that laboratory workers recognize the potential dangers of their profession and take every precaution to ensure their own safety. The employers are obligated to provide any necessary safety clothing and equipment to protect its staff from infections or exposure to hazardous materials, and to ensure that all staff know what is required. Failure to follow declared safety procedures may in some circumstances be a disciplinary matter.

The notoriety of HIV has resulted in many individuals being preoccupied with the possibility of AIDS transmission by handling semen or blood. While this is certainly a significant concern, it must not be allowed to overshadow the wide range of other pathogens commonly found in specimens handled by laboratories. AIDS is substantially less infectious through this route than hepatitis, which is the most frequently occurring infection of laboratory workers. Hepatitis B virus has been detected in semen, urine and saliva, as well as blood, and infection can occur from contamination of even a small area of exposed skin if an open lesion such as a scratch or graze is present. Hepatitis C also has similar routes of infection.

In addition, the organisms causing many traditional sexually transmissible diseases (STDs) are found in semen (see Chapter 4). Cases of accidental *Gonorrhoea*, *Chlamydia*, *Mycoplasma* and *Streptococcus* infection of laboratory personnel have been documented. Cytomegalovirus (CMV), *Ureaplasma* and human papillomavirus (HPV) have also been isolated in semen. However, while no documented laboratory-associated infections have been reported for these other pathogens, the possibility of their transmission by exposure to mucous membranes (e.g. ingestion or inhalation of aerosolized material) or accidental inoculation (e.g. finger stick or contamination of an open wound) does exist.

Specific information on dealing with the most commonly encountered biological materials, semen and follicular fluid, follow. There is also a section on other biologically derived materials used in the ART laboratory.

Semen

Collection and Specimen Reception

- Whenever possible, semen specimens should be collected on the premises into the sterile specimen jars provided (see discussion in Chapter 9, 'Sperm Preparation'). The laboratory worker must have the subject verify that their name as printed on the sticky label provided is correct.
- The subject should be instructed to wash their hands before and after collecting the specimen.
- The subject must hand their specimen to one of the laboratory staff and fill in the required documentation (hard copy or electronic).
- Place the specimen in the specimen reception incubator. If the specimen is received on behalf of another section (e.g. by andrology for embryology), then notify a member of staff from the other area that the specimen has been received.
- The laboratory worker handling the specimen must wear gloves from before first contact with the specimen container.

Handling and Processing

This is performed according to the **General Recommendations** listed above. Specifically:

- Ideally all semen specimens should be handled inside a Class II biosafety cabinet. If working in a horizontal laminar air flow cabinet, the fan should be switched off when working with open specimens, to avoid the risk of operator contamination.
- Minimize contamination of the surrounding work area. Do not handle fixtures and fittings that might be touched by others not wearing gloves (e.g. water taps), equipment (e.g. pipetters, microscopes, counters), implements (e.g. pens, calculators), the telephone or paperwork with contaminated gloves.
- Gloves must be removed or a paper tissue used when, for example, turning on a tap.

Disposal

- Contaminated specimen containers, tubes and volumetric pipettes are discarded in designated contaminated-waste bins. Do not over-fill these bins. The lid must be able to be put on the bin without the need for squashing down or breaking long items.
- Used Pasteur pipettes, pipette tips, slides and coverslips are discarded in designated contaminated-sharps boxes. Do not over-fill these boxes.

Spills

- Wear gloves.
- Surround and cover the spillage with paper tissues or towels. Wipe up the spill using paper tissues or towels.
- Sterilize the area of the spill using isopropyl alcohol or ethanol; wipe up excess disinfectant using clean paper tissues or towels.
- Dispose of all paper tissues or towels in a designated contaminated-waste bin.

Other Biologicals

There are a number of other biologically derived materials that might be used in ART laboratories. They arrive either in pure form or as solutions, e.g. in culture medium. Such materials include the following:

Blood products:	Serum albumin (HSA)
Enzymes:	Hyaluronidase, chymotrypsin, trypsin
Others:	Egg yolk, heparin, hyaluronic acid

Since these biological products are obtained as pure, aseptic or sterile preparations they may, in limited quantities, be disposed of down the sink, followed by a significant volume (e.g. 5 l) of cold tap water. However, once they have come into contact with human biological material (i.e. gametes, embryos, semen or follicular fluid) they must be considered potentially infectious and disposed of in the same manner as other contaminated waste.

Contaminated Waste Disposal

All contaminated waste is placed in the appropriate designated CONTAMINATED WASTE bins or boxes which should be sealed for collection by an authorized person or disposal company.

Do not over-fill the bins; no-one should ever have to force long items into the bin or have to try and break them in order to put the lids onto the bins.

Chemical Materials: Receiving, Storing and Disposal

Upon receiving a chemical in the laboratory, locate local data safety sheets e.g. COSHH assessments and store the chemical according to the safety information that is provided. Give all expired, unused or unwanted chemicals to the local Safety Officer for disposal.

Compressed Gases

Safe handling of compressed gasses includes not only the cylinders themselves but also the regulators used to control the flow and/or pressure of the gas at delivery. Gas cylinders must only be transported using special dollies with safety straps around them. In the gas room or during use in the laboratory, cylinders must be stood upright and attached by safety straps to mounting brackets fixed securely to the bench or wall. Cylinders must be protected from mechanical shock and extremes of heat or cold.

Safe, proper use of regulators:

- Regulators must be attached and removed using the correct wrench, spanner or key.
- Ensure that the main (inlet) valve is tightly closed before attaching a regulator to a gas cylinder or removing a regulator from a cylinder.
- Take great care not to damage the screw threads when attaching or removing a regulator.
- When gas is not flowing, close the inlet valve from the cylinder to the regulator and open the outlet valve. Maintaining pressure inside the regulator when not in use will greatly shorten its life.
- Always use appropriate tubing or piping for the gas being used and its purpose. For flammable gases, use butyl rubber tubing; for high pressure gases, use a tubing with a suitable pressure rating as well as any necessary security fittings (e.g. terry clips or worm-drive clamps where the tubing is attached to the regulator outlet).

Note that when using special gases (e.g. CO_2-in-air), suitable tubing must be used. Many materials are permeable to CO_2 and hence the carefully mixed gas could change greatly between leaving the cylinder and reaching its point-of-use.

Cryogenics

Because of its extremely cold temperature (–196°C), the handling and use of liquid nitrogen (LN2) requires extreme care and attention. *Always wear appropriate protective clothing and equipment*, including long sleeves, suitable gloves and a whole-face visor or face shield. Whenever possible, LN2 should be transferred from its supply dewar vessel by transfer hose or other delivery device; open pouring should be discouraged.

Touching the inside of dewar vessels containing LN2, or any object that has been in recent contact with LN2, using bare fingers can cause severe cold burns. If frostbite does occur, warm the affected skin slowly against a warm part of your body (e.g. armpit). ***Do not rub!*** Keep the affected area immobile and cover with a sterile dressing.

Dewar vessels must be protected from mechanical insult. Glass dewar vessels must be treated with extreme caution and it is worth considering the use of styrofoam boxes or stainless steel dewars for short-term uses involving small volumes of LN2. Plastic-cased dewar vessels are perfectly suitable, except that spilling LN2 over the plastic casing, especially at the vessel's open neck, often causes it to split. Remember, even steel or aluminium storage dewar tanks can be punctured, and the loss of vacuum between the outer and inner walls will result in rapid evaporative loss of the LN2, and hence of the cryopreserved material.

Never seal or enclose a dewar vessel containing LN2, as evaporation of the LN2 will cause a substantial build-up of internal pressure that will certainly explode glass dewar vessels (e.g. thermos flasks or jugs). All lids or caps for LN2 dewars must be loose fitting or include an emergency pressure release valve.

Be very careful when handling straws or vials that have been immersed in liquid nitrogen, as there is a genuine risk of explosion. If a cryovial is not completely sealed, LN2 will enter it during its period of immersion. This liquid will rapidly turn to gas when returned to ambient temperature and the sudden huge increase in its volume can cause the vial to explode. This is an extremely serious concern with glass ampoules. With traditional straws, evaporation of the liquid that permeates the cotton plug at the top of the straw often causes violent expulsion of this plug the first time the straw is transferred, even for a few seconds, from the liquid phase to ambient temperature (e.g. while searching for a particular straw or batch of straws). This is not a risk if using *High Security Straws*. Protective goggles or visor must be worn when thawing straws or cryovials. Note that this expulsion of the outer cotton wadding plug does not equate to loss of the seal, which is internal to the outer cotton plug.

Although intended for an animal breeding audience, the double DVD *The Guide to Handling Frozen Semen and Embryos* (www.chipsbooks.com/gdsemen.htm) is an excellent resource on safe handling of specimens in cryogenic storage.

There are several excellent sources of information regarding background, safety, protocols and procedures about the use of compressed gases. For example, that of the British Compressed Gases Association (BCGA) (www.bcga.co.uk/assets/BCGA%20CP30%20-%20Rev%203%20-%2023-07-2019.pdf). ASRM have provided a recent committee opinion on cryostorage of reproductive tissue in IVF laboratories encompassing guidance on the use of liquid nitrogen [6]. Further information is provided in the 'Cryobanking' section in the 'Risk Management' chapter (Chapter 13).

Other Hazards

All hazardous materials, whether in transit, storage or use, must be clearly labelled so as to alert handlers or users of the hazards and safe handling procedures of such materials. Material Safety Data Sheets and information must be kept on file for each chemical used in the laboratory.

Fire or Explosion Hazard

Relevant information includes the substance's conditions of flammability, including its flashpoint, and means of extinction. Sensitivity to mechanical impact and static discharge in relation to explosion hazards must also be identified. Information on any hazardous combustion products should also be available.

Reactivity Data

This information includes description of any conditions under which the substance is chemically unstable or any other substance (or class of substances) with which the substance is incompatible. Information on conditions of reactivity and any hazardous decomposition products is also relevant.

Toxicological Properties

Information on possible routes of entry into the body, including skin contact, skin absorption, eye contact, inhalation and ingestion, as well as the effects of both acute and chronic exposure to the substance, should be available. Other relevant information includes the substance's irritant nature and the likelihood of sensitization to it. Specific information on general toxicity, carcinogenicity, teratogenicity, mutagenicity and reproductive toxicological properties should be clearly identified.

Mercury

- Laboratories should have a policy not to use mercury thermometers. However, in the event of breakage of a mercury thermometer, the spilt mercury must be dealt with as a hazardous material.
- Wear gloves and avoid any skin contact with the mercury.
- Clean up the spill using a specific cleaning kit e.g. *SPILFYTER* Mercury Spill Kit.
- Discard everything in the disposal box that is part of the kit.

Epidemic/Pandemic Responsiveness

Within their quality management systems, each andrology or ART laboratory should develop risk-based safety planning (see Chapter 13, 'Risk management' and [7]) to be prepared for epidemics or a pandemic such as the recent SARS-CoV-2/COVID-19 pandemic.

Studies of semen samples from infected patients have shown conflicting results regarding the presence of SARS-CoV-2, which could be due to the phases and severity of the disease [8]. Nevertheless, every biological specimen must be treated as potentially infected, in accordance with the general recommendations. All staff members must practice precautions to minimize the risk of person-to-person infection and surface contamination according to local, regional and national health authorities' regulations or guidelines.

Incident Reports

An Incident Report form *must* be completed in any situation where an incident occurs that either:

- Impacts the treatment of a patient; or
- Results in injury to a staff member; or
- Creates a safety risk; or
- Creates a security risk; or
- Compromises or actually causes a failure of laboratory QC or QA.

This is a standard requirement of laboratory accreditation schemes, e.g. ISO 15189:2012 [9], as well as a common regulatory requirement [10]. In a number of countries, it is also a legal responsibility of the employer and/or manager.

References

1. World Health Organization. *Laboratory Biosafety Manual*, 4th edn. Geneva: World Health Organization, 2020. Available at: www.who.int/publications/i/item/9789240011311 [last accessed 26 August 2021].

2. www.free-training.com; https://ehs.okstate.edu/online-training.html

3. World Health Organization. *WHO Laboratory Manual for the Examination and Processing of Human Semen*, 6th edn. Geneva: World Health Organization, 2021.

4. Practice Committee of the American Society for Reproductive Medicine; Practice Committee of the Society for Assisted Reproductive Technology. Revised guidelines for human embryology and andrology laboratories. *Fertil Steril* 2008; **90 (5 Suppl)**: S45–59.

5. ESHRE. Revised Guidelines for good practice in IVF laboratories (2015). Available at: www.eshre.eu/Guidelines-and-Legal/Guidelines/Revised-guidelines-for-good-practice-in-IVF-laboratories-(2015) [last accessed 26 August 2021].

6. Practice Committees of the American Society for Reproductive Medicine, Society for Reproductive

Biologists and Technologists, and Society for Assisted Reproductive Technology. Cryostorage of reproductive tissues in the in vitro fertilization laboratory: a committee opinion. *Fertil Steril* 2020; **114**: 486–91.

7. Mortimer D, Mortimer ST. *Quality and Risk Management in the IVF Laboratory*, 2nd edn. Cambridge: Cambridge University Press, 2015.

8. Borges E Jr, Setti AS, Iaconelli A Jr, Braga DPAF. Current status of the COVID-19 and male reproduction: a review of the literature. *Andrology* 2021; **9**: 1066–75. https://doi.org/10.1111/ANDR .13037

9. *International Standard ISO 15189:2012 Medical Laboratories – Particular Requirements for Quality and Competence.* Geneva: International Organization for Standardization, 2012. Available at: www.iso.org/obp/ui/#iso:std:iso: 15189:ed-2:v1:en [last accessed 26 August 2021].

10. European Union Commission Directive 2006/ 86/EC implementing Directive 2004/23/EC of the European Parliament and of the Council as regards traceability requirements, notification of serious adverse reactions and events and certain technical requirements for the coding, processing, preservation, storage and distribution of human tissues and cells. Official Journal of the European Union, L294/32, 24.10.2006.

Appendix 1 Interpreting Andrology Laboratory Results

Understanding Reference Limits and Decision Limits

While most readers might expect a simple table of reference limits in this Appendix, to do so would only support the many current misconceptions and misunderstandings about such 'normal ranges' or 'reference values'. Since the goal of this handbook has been to improve the standardization and quality of semen assessments and other andrology lab procedures, improving the understanding and clinical application of the results from semen examination and other sperm assessments is an essential consequence.

To begin with, the terminology must be clear:

Reference population: A well-defined population, usually without the disorder of interest

Reference values: Results obtained from the reference population

Reference range: The entire range of reference values

Reference interval: A statistically calculated interval, traditionally comprising 95% of the reference values

Reference limits: The values defining the lower and upper ends of the reference interval; when only lower values are considered to be of clinical interest, the reference limit is often equal to the lower fifth percentile of the reference range.

There are a number of major issues that must be borne in mind when developing, or using, reference limits:

1. There is a big difference between a 'normal range' and a 'reference interval' in laboratory medicine, and this has been discussed at length elsewhere [1]. However, in brief, using reference intervals is an important step toward establishing a scientific basis for clinical interpretation of laboratory results, and eliminates the confusion arising from three very different meanings of the word 'normal': relating to the Gaussian statistical distribution; 'normal' *vs* 'abnormal' in the epidemiological sense; and the clinical sense, where normal equates to healthy, or non-pathological. Understanding and applying these concepts is of vital importance to andrology because there is no specific disease 'infertility'; and subfertility is a problem of a couple wishing to have a child, where either – or neither – partner might be 'normal' (i.e. unaffected by a relevant disorder). Moreover, fertility is age-related and also affected by many environmental factors. Consequently, a normal population cannot be either readily defined or studied, but 'reference intervals' can be defined that relate more to the likelihood that a given characteristic is likely to be a contributory factor in determining an endpoint of interest.

2. There are fundamental differences in the endpoints of interest, for which semen examination and other sperm assessments are made. Clearly there is a great difference between attempting to diagnose the etiology of a couple's infertility and attempting to provide a prognosis for any given outcome. As pointed out in the sixth edition of the WHO lab manual [2], semen examination can provide important information about the functional state of the male reproductive organs, which is essential both for the investigation and treatment of the individual man, and for the development of new insights into male reproductive disorders. But there are also great differences between outcomes such as spontaneous pregnancy without treatment (which must also be considered in regard to the time required to achieve such

316

pregnancies, perhaps integrated as an expression of the fecundity rate), and the likelihood of a successful outcome of a particular treatment modality (which, again, needs to include a consideration of time). There are, of course, also substantial differences between treatments, which bypass different levels of the normal process of conception *in vivo* – and hence compensate for different underlying abnormalities in the man's (and/or woman's) physiology, e.g. timed intercourse, cervical insemination, IUI, IVF, or ICSI.

3. A reference limit derived for a particular purpose, or in a particular way, e.g. based on the risk of poor, or no fertilization at IVF ('*in-vitro* subfertility'), cannot be used to diagnose *in-vivo* subfertility (i.e. whether a couple will achieve a pregnancy without treatment, or with some systemic therapy) – or *vice versa*. Moreover, the high intra- and inter-individual variability of semen characteristics can result in someone providing a semen specimen that shows one or more characteristics that are very unusual for them, but the values are well within the reference interval for the population [3,4]. As a result, semen examination reference limits are unsuitable for following longitudinal monitoring and detecting whether change has occurred in an individual.

4. Any reference limit will be dependent upon the technical method by which it was determined, and this also includes the presumption of proper training (achievement of 'competency'), and adequate internal and external quality control. If a value is derived according to a specific protocol, then it cannot be used with the same confidence – or perhaps even the same relevance – when derived using another technique. An obvious example of this is the generally accepted use of 'strict criteria' for evaluating human sperm morphology [5–8], necessitating entirely different reference limits to those used for assessments made using other sperm morphology classification schemes (e.g. [9,10]). Further examples of this problem are given in the following section of this Appendix.

5. Semen examination characteristics are also affected, to varying degrees, by the duration of prior ejaculatory abstinence (and also ejaculatory frequency), as well as post-ejaculatory specimen-holding conditions and pre-examination delay (e.g. [11]).

6. When considering endpoints of interest, there will be further confounding factors related to the clinical management of the couple (e.g. the use of ovarian stimulation, handling of follicular aspirates during oocyte retrieval, and handling of embryos during embryo transfer). Similarly, we must recognize that aspects of laboratory quality will affect the likelihood of achieving success: not just the sperm handling and processing techniques, but also the handling of oocytes and embryos during IVF and ICSI, and the general physico-chemical quality of the culture environment for achieving fertilization *in vitro*, and for supporting embryo development *in vitro* through to transfer.

7. Reference limits should be based on data obtained from well-defined populations and derived using statistical techniques. Consequently, they are subject to a certain degree of uncertainty, and not therefore necessarily as robust when applied to individual cases. They are not 'cut-offs', and there are no absolute values that allow the definition of binary states, e.g. 'normal' *vs* 'abnormal', or 'fertile' *vs* 'subfertile'. While this has been known for many years, far too many workers still seem to believe in such false interpretations. Even what might seem an 'absolute' cut-off of azoospermia cannot necessarily be used in the modern day to define a man as 'sterile': many men who presented with azoospermia have become fathers following surgical sperm retrieval from their testes and ICSI.

8. Issues of ethnicity and geography should also be taken into account. Several studies have revealed ethnic differences concerning the so-called testicular dysgenesis syndrome (a.k.a. the 'falling sperm count' theory). Furthermore, geographical differences in various semen parameters have also been reported between countries or regions that are comparable with respect to ethnicity (e.g. the Nordic countries). But since there are, as yet, no indications of differences in fertility between these regions/ countries, it might be wrong to use common reference ranges. Finally, genetic variations between different ethnic groups could also be of relevance to at least some of the semen parameters. Almost all expert publications on semen analysis have recommended that each laboratory should derive its own reference values (e.g. [12–14]) – yet this has very rarely, if ever occurred. Even using a population of

men who have recently become fathers to define 'normal ranges' for semen analysis remains fraught with confounding factors:

a) Was the age range of the female partners controlled? This is a significant factor affecting a couple's fecundity.

b) How many ovulatory cycles of trying did it take for the couple to achieve a pregnancy?

c) Were either or both partners affected by external factors, e.g. tobacco smoking, recreational drug use, or environmental or workplace reproductive toxins?

d) Is the man actually the biological father? Without paternity testing this cannot be assumed – and there is a generally accepted non-trivial prevalence of non-paternity in many western societies at least.

e) Was any treatment employed but not admitted to? With the growth in 'reproductive tourism' in recent years, especially with the increasing scarcity of gamete donors in many countries, more and more couples go overseas for treatment, and then conceal that fact from at least the regulatory authorities, if not family and friends as well.

Even if these matters have been carefully considered, a further cause for concern is that the probability for normal fertilization and birth of a healthy child is a continuum rather than a dichotomous situation, although the outcome – child or no child – is dichotomous. This means that among couples conceiving within 12 months of trying, some are lucky in spite of poor semen. Furthermore, among couples without success within a year, some men have no semen characteristics indicating male factor infertility. Thus, the selection of men based on couple Time-To-Pregnancy still introduces a largely unknown level of variability due to insufficient definition of the reference population.

Probably the most insightful approach for simple guidelines for interpreting semen analysis results was that promoted by Eliasson in the late 1970s, in which semen analysis evaluation guidelines were provided using three categories: normal, doubtful, and pathological (or not normal), derived from frequency distribution studies on populations of men whose wives were pregnant in the first trimester, and men in a barren union [9,10]. Equivalent values can also be derived from the analysis of the clinical fertility of men attending a fertility clinic after a 20-year follow-up period [15]. This three-category approach was adopted and promoted by Mortimer [16,17], although not by the WHO [12–14], and adopted in the first edition of this handbook [18]. As a final comment in this regard, it must be biologically obvious that no single semen characteristic can be expected to confirm a man's diagnosis of subfertility, nor adequately classify a couple's fertility potential. Indeed, Guzick et al. concluded that while threshold values for sperm concentration, motility, and morphology can be used to classify men as subfertile, of indeterminate fertility, or fertile (see Figure App1.1), none of the measures were diagnostic of infertility [19].

Table A1.1 provides an example of this approach, derived by consensus, and updated for the use of 'strict criteria' sperm morphology assessments. It is well-known that, on a population basis, the quantitative aspects (i.e. sperm concentration and total sperm count), and qualitative aspects of sperm production (i.e. sperm morphology, motility, and vitality) are generally positively inter-correlated [20], although with

Semen characteristic	Fertility status	
	Subfertile ⋯ Indeterminate fertility ⋯ Fertile	
Sperm concentration (10^6/ml)	13.5	48.0
% motile spermatozoa	32	63
% morphologically normal	9	12

Figure App1.1 Figure illustrating the threshold values defined by Guzick et al. (2001) [19].

Table A1.1 General (consensus-based) guidelines for the evaluation of human semen in relation to a general classification of *in-vivo* fertility potential only (may be considered comparable to a diagnosis of subfertility) Values are provided relative to the usual precision of reporting and assume that semen analysis is carried out as per the technical methods, training and QC standards described in this handbook only (given this, all values should be considered to have an uncertainty of measurement of 10%)

Characteristic	Units	Normal	Borderline	Pathological	Notes
Ejaculate volume	ml	2.0–6.0	1.5–1.9	< 1.5	a
Sperm concentration	10^6/ml	20–250	10–20	< 10	a,b
Total sperm count	10^6/ejaculate	> 80	20–79	< 20	a,b
Sperm motility	% motile	> 60	40–59	< 40	c,d
	% progressive	> 50	35–49	< 35	c,d
	% rapid	> 25			c,d,e
	progression grade	3 or 4	2	1 or 0	c,d,f
Sperm morphology	% ideal forms	> 4	4	< 4	g
	TZI	< 1.60	1.61–1.80	> 1.80	g,h
Sperm vitality	% live (vital)	> 60	40–59	< 40	i
Leukocytes	10^6/ml			> 1.0	j
Anti-sperm antibodies	% binding	< 50	50–79	> 80	k

[a] Evaluated after 2–4 days of abstinence.

[b] For ejaculates with 2.0–6.0 ml volume.

[c] Evaluated at 30 min post-ejaculation.

[d] Evaluated at 37°C.

[e] Cut-off for rapid is 25 μm/s 'space gain'; only a normal threshold value is available.

[f] Based on a scale of 0–4: 0 = no progression; 1 = poor; 2 = medium; 3 = good; 4 = very good/excellent.

[g] Evaluated using Tygerberg Strict Criteria (see Chapter 3).

[h] Evaluated as per [12,16] from Papanicolaou-stained smears.

[i] Evaluated by eosin dye exclusion at 30 min post-ejaculation.

[j] Evaluated by cytochemical staining for peroxidase. This value has been carried over several editions of the WHO lab manual and is a consensus opinion for a pathological threshold (see text for more details).

[k] Evaluated using the MAR test method for IgG and/or IgA.

the advent of a narrow dynamic range of 'normal forms', as a result of using stricter criteria, such correlations are less apparent for sperm morphology. From the above discussion, it is evident that a simple table of reference values, no matter how well defined the source population, how rigorous the lab methodology and staff training and QC, or how much statistical analysis or manipulation the data were subjected to, cannot be expected to provide answers for more than one endpoint of interest. Consequently, in the following paragraphs, the applicability of the various reference values, and guidelines for their interpretation, will be provided when available.

Decision Limits

Due to the simple fact that an ejaculate examination can be requested for different purposes, different decision limits will be required, for example:

1. When is a test for Y chromosome deletion or other genetic disorders indicated? There are international recommendations available [21], although based on sperm concentration rather than total sperm number.
2. When is an endocrine work-up for hypogonadism justified?
3. When might treatment for endocrine disorders be effective?

4. Which semen characteristics might provide unambiguous evidence of a significant risk of low or no fertilization by IVF, and hence provide evidence-based guidance on when ICSI should be used in preference to ordinary IVF [22]?

5. For the clinically highly relevant questions at issue, decision limits must be developed as guidance for appropriate health care of men and infertile couples [23–26].

Although answering such questions is outside the scope of this laboratory handbook, the inescapable and vital issue for everyone working in assisted conception is that all WHO reference ranges, even those in the fifth edition of the WHO lab manual, were derived in relation to *in-vivo* conception [27,28], and despite recent expansion of the dataset [29] have *no* relevance to any assisted conception procedure decision making. This includes the use of a supposed 4% ideal forms cut-off, since it has such measurement uncertainty that even 3% and 5% ideal forms cannot be distinguished with confidence unless at least 1500 spermatozoa are assessed. This issue was clearly identified in the Vienna Consensus on laboratory performance indicators in ART [30].

Semen Examination Values

Note: For all semen characteristics, it is assumed that robust technical methods, careful operator training, and both internal QC and external QC/QA, as described in this handbook, have been implemented.

Ejaculate Volume
Pre-Requisites

A known period of prior ejaculatory abstinence; reference limits in this handbook assume two to four days.

In Vivo Significance

Only if the volume is very low is there a risk of the acidic vaginal milieu adversely affecting the spermatozoa. A high volume (>6.0 ml) can also be regarded as an abnormal value, due to likely loss of semen from the vagina. However, no specific risks amenable to routine diagnostic or therapeutic application have been quantified and validated.

In Vitro Significance

No specific relevance to ART outcomes.

Sperm Concentration
Pre-Requisites

Assumes 3 ± 1 days prior ejaculatory abstinence and a complete collection.

Cautionary Note

On a population basis, sperm quality (i.e. motility and progression, vitality and morphology) are positively correlated with sperm concentration; but higher sperm 'quality' (i.e. functional potential) can mitigate the impact of a simple decrease in sperm concentration.

In Vivo Significance

In general, fecundity is decreased with values below 20×10^6 spermatozoa per ml, but only below 5×10^6 per ml will the man's fecundity likely be substantially reduced [15,31]. However, no specific risks amenable to routine diagnostic or therapeutic application have been quantified and validated.

Notes:
1. Only valid where the entire ejaculate has been collected for analysis (the first fraction contains most of the spermatozoa).
2. In cases of hypothalamic hypogonadism undergoing hormonal initiation of spermatogenesis, these reference values are invalid; conception can occur with as few as 0.5×10^6 spermatozoa per ml.
3. One out of 2000 vasectomized men have been reported to father children in spite of a laboratory finding of no spermatozoa, i.e. azoospermia [32].

In Vitro Significance

No generally applicable thresholds beyond whether sufficient spermatozoa can be obtained post-processing for a potential treatment modality.

Total Sperm Count

Pre-Requisites

Only valid for complete ejaculates with normal volumes (i.e. 2.0–6.0 ml) collected after 3±1 days prior ejaculatory abstinence.

Cautionary Note

On a population basis, sperm quality (i.e. motility and progression, vitality and morphology) are generally positively correlated with the total sperm count; lesser impairment of sperm quality will reduce the impact of lower total sperm count. Total sperm count should be used with caution as there are many factors that can influence it. It can be used as a measure of daily sperm production and an indicator of possible number of retrievable spermatozoa after preparation for ART procedures.

In Vivo Significance

Decreasing fecundity with values below 80×10^6 per ejaculate; fecundity will likely be substantially reduced below 20×10^6 per ejaculate. However, no specific risks amenable to routine diagnostic or therapeutic application have been quantified and validated.

A recent analysis of the total progressive motile sperm count (TMSC) as a prognosticator for natural conception revealed that in the overall cohort of subfertile couples (including pregnancies achieved spontaneously or via ART, a TPMC of 50×10^6 best differentiated men who were more likely to father a child within five years. Partners of men with TPMC $\geq 50 \times 10^6$ had a 45% greater chance of conceiving within five years (hazard ratio = 1.45; 95% CI = 1.34–1.58) and achieved pregnancy earlier compared to those men with TPMC $<50 \times 10^6$ (median 19 months, 95% CI = 18–20 vs 36 months, 95% CI = 32–41). Similar results were observed in the natural conception cohort (TPMC cut-off of 55×10^6), while for the natural conception cohort without major female factor, the TPMC cut-off was 20×10^6 [33]. However, a single TPMC threshold could not be used to differentiate fertile from infertile men. All analyses of conception rates revealed 'plateau points' that were consistently higher than the WHO5 reference values. The authors of that paper attested that all semen examinations were performed in a central reference laboratory on samples obtained after two to seven days of abstinence and were in accordance with the 2016 'How to count sperm properly' checklist published by Björndahl et al. [34].

Notes:
1. Only valid where the entire ejaculate has been collected for analysis (the first fraction contains most of the spermatozoa).
2. In cases of hypothalamic hypogonadism undergoing hormonal initiation of spermatogenesis, these reference values are invalid; many reports have shown that conception can occur with as few as 0.5×10^6 spermatozoa per ml.
3. One out of 2000 vasectomized men have been reported to father children in spite of a laboratory finding of no spermatozoa, i.e. azoospermia [32].

4. The total sperm count can also be useful when deciding on ART treatment regimen, since it indicates the total number of potentially functional spermatozoa that might be available.

In Vitro Significance

No generally applicable thresholds beyond whether sufficient spermatozoa can be obtained post-processing for a potential treatment modality.

Sperm Motility

Since sperm function requires progressive motility, simple assessments of the proportion of motile spermatozoa regardless of progression should be expected to have less biological, and hence, clinical relevance. For this reason, they are not recommended for routine clinical use within the context of either diagnosis or prognostic management.

Sperm Progressive Motility

Pre-Requisites

Must be evaluated soon after completion of semen liquefaction, and assessments must be made at 37°C for physiological relevance.

Cautionary Note

On a population basis, progressive motility is positively correlated with other aspects of sperm quality (i.e. concentration, vitality and morphology). Isolated reductions of sperm motility might have less impact upon fertility or fecundity than when seen in conjunction with other evidence of decreased sperm quality. Simple 'bulk' assessment of progression grade has limited value compared to the determination of the proportions of spermatozoa showing grades of progression.

In Vivo Significance

At least 50% of the spermatozoa are expected to show progressive motility (WHO4/6 grades $a + b$); decreasing values below this will be associated with an increasing likelihood of sperm dysfunction, and hence reduced fecundity. However, no specific risks amenable to routine diagnostic or therapeutic application have been quantified and validated.

In Vitro Significance

Poor progressive motility, seen as a reduced proportion of progressively motile spermatozoa and/or reduced quality of progression (i.e. sperm velocity and other kinematic characteristics), is likely to be associated with other impairments of sperm function and hence there will be increased risks of poor or no fertilization at IVF – and hence a likely greater benefit of using ICSI. However, no specific risks amenable to routine diagnostic or therapeutic application have been quantified and validated.

Sperm Rapid Progressive Motility

Pre-Requisites

Must be evaluated soon after completion of semen liquefaction, and assessments must be made at 37°C using an objective definition for 'rapid' (i.e. space gain of >25 μm/s) for optimum physiological relevance.

Cautionary Note

On a population basis, progressive motility is positively correlated with other aspects of sperm quality (i.e. concentration, vitality and morphology), and is essential for effective penetration into and migration through the cervical mucus *in vivo*. An isolated reduction in the proportion of rapid progressive spermatozoa might have less impact upon fertility or fecundity than when seen in conjunction with other evidence of decreased sperm quality.

In Vivo Significance

A reduced proportion of rapid progressive spermatozoa will decrease the potential of an ejaculate being able to achieve effective colonization of the cervical mucus and establish the sperm reservoir within the female reproductive tract [35–37]. However, no specific risks amenable to routine diagnostic or therapeutic application have been quantified and validated.

In Vitro Significance

Poor penetration of cervical mucus (assessed either *in vivo* or *in vitro*), which is often due to impaired sperm motility, has been associated with an increased risk of impaired fertilization at IVF [38,39]. However, no specific risks amenable to routine diagnostic or therapeutic application have been quantified and validated.

Sperm Progression Grading

Since this is a population-averaged subjective assessment, its routine use is no longer considered appropriate in a specialized andrology laboratory. However, various clinicians believe that it is useful to them, and some laboratories will need to continue providing these evaluations to the maximum practicable level of objectivity and standardization.

Sperm Vitality

Pre-Requisites

Must be evaluated soon after completion of semen liquefaction. Typically only assessed when there are <40% motile spermatozoa.

Cautionary Note

On a population basis, vitality is positively correlated with other aspects of sperm quality (i.e. concentration, motility and progression, and morphology), hence isolated reductions of sperm motility might have less impact upon fertility or fecundity than when seen in conjunction with other evidence of decreased sperm quality. Sperm vitality typically exceeds the proportion of motile spermatozoa by at least a small margin, representing those spermatozoa that are 'live' but not motile.

In Vivo Significance

Sperm vitality assessments can clarify cases of 'necrozoospermia' (e.g. due to the presence of spermotoxic antibodies), and help differentiate such cases from ones of immotile cilia syndrome (where motility is essentially zero but many spermatozoa are live). However, no specific risks amenable to routine diagnostic or therapeutic application have been quantified and validated, and the routine assessment of sperm vitality on all semen samples is not recommended.

In Vitro Significance

No specific relevance beyond that for *in-vivo* endpoints.

Sperm Morphology: Ideal Forms

Pre-Requisites

Should be evaluated soon after completion of semen liquefaction. Properly prepared and appropriately stained smears are essential, as are proper training using the defined Tygerberg Strict Criteria and both IQC and EQC/EQA (see Chapters 3 and 12 of this handbook for further information).

Cautionary Note

Sperm morphology is generally positively correlated with other aspects of sperm quality (i.e. concentration, motility and progression, and vitality) on a population basis, although with the narrow dynamic range of 'normal forms' now seen as a result of using stricter criteria, such correlations are less apparent.

Isolated findings of poor sperm morphology can impact fertility or fecundity, even when seen in conjunction with evidence of otherwise apparently normal semen examination findings. Further insight into the possible clinical significance of sperm morphology can be provided by interpreting % ideal forms in conjunction with an assessment of the TZI (see below).

In Vivo Significance

In general, a proportion of morphologically ideal spermatozoa of >4% indicates that sperm morphology is unlikely to be a contributory factor to a couple's subfertility, or an adverse factor influencing prognosis.

Furthermore, the evaluation and recording of all four sperm morphology defect classes can give valuable information about causes for, e.g., decreased motility resulting from a high prevalence of abnormal tails. Large retained cytoplasmic residues can also reveal epididymal disorders.

In Vitro Significance

A proportion of morphologically ideal spermatozoa of >4% indicates that sperm morphology is unlikely to be a contributory factor to poor or no fertilization at IVF, and with <4% many experts recommend the use of ICSI. However, these interpretations should be made in conjunction with the sperm morphology patterns present (small heads, large heads, etc.), and with an assessment of the Teratozoospermia Index (TZI) (since many abnormal spermatozoa show multiple anomalies) and/or the Acrosome Index, and perhaps also sperm function assessments such as hyperactivation analysis using CASA [22].

This might be of particular significance in situations where there is an apparent 'disagreement' between % ideal forms and the TZI (see below): e.g. ejaculates with 0% ideal forms and a low TZI (<1.60) can often result in normal IVF fertilization rates, and >4% ideal forms with a high TZI (>1.80) are at risk of reduced performance in IVF [22].

Sperm Morphology: Teratozoospermia Index

Pre-Requisites

Properly prepared and appropriately stained (Papanicolaou) smears are essential.

Cautionary Note

The TZI provides an additional dimension of information on the production of competent spermatozoa via the process of spermiogenesis [7,40,41]. An elevated TZI indicates an increased risk of abnormal spermiogenesis, and the concomitant existence of sperm dysfunction, even though spermatozoa appear superficially 'normal' at the level of observation used in the sperm morphology evaluation.

In Vivo Significance

A TZI of >1.80 indicates that sperm morphology is more likely to be a contributory factor to a couple's subfertility or a man's fertility potential; with values <1.60 there is considered to be no increased risk over what can be identified from the proportion of ideal forms. Published population data are limited but show – as in all semen characteristics – an overlap between fertile and infertile groups, although ROC analysis revealed a cut-off value of 1.64 [42].

In Vitro Significance

A TZI of >1.80 indicates that sperm morphology is likely to be a contributory factor to poor or no fertilization at IVF and that ICSI should be employed. With values of 1.60–1.80 there is an increased risk of poor or no fertilization at IVF and ICSI might be a cautious approach. With a TZI <1.60 there is considered to be no increased risk over what can be identified from the proportion of ideal forms [22].

Computer-Aided Sperm Analysis

The conclusions and recommendations of the consensus workshop organized by the ESHRE Special Interest Group in Andrology, held in San Miniato in 1997, must be fully considered in any clinical (or research) application of computer-aided sperm analysis (CASA) of human spermatozoa [43] in conjunction with more recent critical reviews of human sperm CASA [44,45].

Further discussion of these issues can be found in Chapter 6 of this handbook, but key points to be noted are:

- Determination of sperm concentration in semen using CASA is subject to a wide range of error factors, and values must be considered suspect unless validated against determinations made using the methods described in this handbook.
- Determination of the percentages of motile and progressively motile spermatozoa in semen using CASA is subject to a wide range of error factors, and values must be considered suspect unless the technique has been validated against determinations made using the methods described in this handbook.
- Population-averaged kinematic values are of limited value. Median and range or centile values will be statistically more meaningful than mean values, but multiparametric kinematic definitions (allowing the classification of individual spermatozoa into specific sub-populations that are correlated with relevant functional endpoints, e.g. 'good mucus-penetrating' spermatozoa), will have greater biological, and hence clinical, relevance.
- Differences between CASA instruments, in both hardware and software, can preclude using reference values derived using one type of instrument to interpret values obtained using a different type of instrument.
- There are no population-based studies using the current generation of CASA systems, to define either:
  - The limits of normal semen quality in fertile men
  - The relationships between CASA variables and the time to pregnancy
  - The relationships between CASA variables (especially hyperactivation) and IVF outcome.

Anti-Sperm Antibodies

In general, controversy continues regarding the prevalence and clinical significance of anti-sperm antibodies (ASABs) in the diagnosis of subfertility and its treatment, but their evaluation remains an integral part of the basic workup for subfertile couples. In the absence of defined decision limits, consensus recommendations are that sperm surface antibodies as revealed by ≥50% bead binding are abnormal and treatment options such as IUI should be considered [27,41,46]. If the bead binding is located on the sperm head then ICSI should be considered, due to an increased risk of impaired sperm-oocyte interaction and fertilization.

Circulating ASABs, especially when they coat the majority of spermatozoa in a particular semen specimen, and are directed against the sperm head, can be of both IgG and IgA isotypes simultaneously (IgA alone has a worse prognosis than IgG alone), are a definite risk factor for impaired sperm transport *in vivo* (especially IgA ASABs) and fertilization. Serum ASABs in women should also be considered a contraindication for both IUI and GIFT, and obviously preclude using affected serum as a supplement for IVF culture medium. ASABs identified in cervical mucus, either by abnormal sperm-mucus interaction tests or by their detection in solubilized cervical mucus, often cause a failure of sperm transport – although this can be amenable to treatment by IUI.

IgM antibodies (from B-cells) mainly reflect an acute reaction, usually disappearing within a few weeks when the acute infection is over. Hence the detection of IgM ASABs on spermatozoa is rare, but definitely pathological, and can indicate either recent trauma to the male genital tract or perhaps testicular cancer. Any man in whom such ASABs are detected should be referred to a clinical andrologist for a thorough investigation.

In biological terms, it must be remembered that ASABs can have three different biological effects: sperm agglutination, cytotoxicity, or just coating the spermatozoa. While the presence of agglutinating antibodies is usually apparent from examination of a wet preparation during semen analysis, and cytotoxic ASABs will result in severely diminished, or even zero, sperm vitality, there is no indication of sperm coating antibodies within a semen analysis. However, sperm coating antibodies can reduce, or even block, sperm penetration of cervical mucus, and can be readily identified using *in-vitro* tests of sperm-mucus interaction, especially via the 'shaking' phenomenon seen in the SCMC test (see Chapter 8 of this handbook).

Ejaculate Biochemistry

Zinc

Pre-Requisites

A completely collected ejaculate.

Cautionary Note

For clinical interpretation it is essential that the complete ejaculate was collected; low ejaculate volume, few motile spermatozoa and low zinc can be caused by incomplete specimen collection. If an incomplete specimen is provided for analysis, provide information to the patient about the importance of reporting any missed part of the ejaculate before allowing collection of a repeat sample.

In Vivo Significance

Low zinc content can be due to reduced secretory function of the prostate, either because of an ongoing prostatitis or as a concomitant of chronic or iterated inflammatory disease of the prostate. A low contribution of prostatic secretion in the sperm-rich ejaculate fractions reduces sperm motility, survival and chromatin stability.

In Vitro Significance

A normal zinc content indicates that prostatic fluid was contributed to the ejaculate.

Fructose

Pre-Requisites

A completely collected ejaculate.

Cautionary Note

The main source of fructose in semen is from the seminal vesicles. The seminal vesicular fluid typically constitutes the last ⅔ of the ejaculate volume, explaining why incomplete collection of the later fractions of the ejaculate can give false too-low values. Because live spermatozoa kept in seminal plasma for an extended period of time will metabolize fructose, seminal plasma for fructose determination should be centrifuged free from spermatozoa within 60 min after ejaculation.

In Vivo Significance

Absence of spermatozoa and low fructose levels indicate possible agenesis of the Wolffian duct system, including the vasa deferentia and seminal vesicles.

In Vitro Significance

A normal fructose content indicates that seminal vesicular fluid was contributed to the ejaculate.

α-Glucosidase

Pre-Requisites

A completely collected ejaculate.

Cautionary Note

Glucosidase is considered mainly a secretory product of the epididymal epithelium, although significant contributions also come from the prostate. Based on a comparison of sperm-free post-vasectomy ejaculates and ejaculates with $>40 \times 10^6$ spermatozoa, the best cut-off was 23.6 mU/ejaculate [47]. There are also indications that post-vasectomy ejaculates collected after prolonged ejaculatory abstinence can have high values for neutral α-glucosidase, especially in ejaculates with a high content of zinc, indicating a possible interaction by prostate α-glucosidase with the assay [47].

In Vivo Significance

Low glucosidase activity in semen primarily indicates a low contribution of epididymal secretion to the ejaculate. This can be due to a partial blockage (in which case spermatozoa can also be lacking in the ejaculate) or due to reduced function of the epididymal epithelium (where sperm function, especially motility, and the reduction of cytoplasmic residues, could be impaired).

In Vitro Significance

A normal α-glucosidase content indicates that epididymal fluid was contributed to the ejaculate.

Oxidative Stress

Reactive Oxygen Species Measurement

There are no defined reference values available. However, using the luminol-based chemiluminescence assay method described in this handbook, values of ≥ 93 RLU/s/10^6 spermatozoa/ml can be considered abnormal (see Chapter 4 of this handbook).

Semen Redox State by MiOXSYS Test

Based on currently available data, the reference value is <1.36 mV/10^6 spermatozoa/ml with higher values indicating oxidative stress (see Chapter 4 of this handbook).

Sperm Function Tests

In-Vivo Sperm-Mucus Interaction Testing: The Post-Coital Test

Pre-Requisites

Appropriate timing of the procedure during the immediate pre-ovulatory period.

Cautionary Note

A cervical mucus Insler score of <10, and/or pH <7.0 can cause a poor PCT. Reading a PCT after a long post-coital delay can show increased numbers of non-progressive spermatozoa (as distinct from shaking spermatozoa), downgrading the test result.

In Vivo Significance

A satisfactory result can be reported when there are either >2500 progressively motile spermatozoa per mm^3 in the cervical mucus, or >1000 rapid progressive spermatozoa per mm^3.

A result of <500 spermatozoa per mm^3, especially when associated with slow progressive or non-progressive motility, indicates decreased sperm penetration ability of the mucus and/or abnormality of the cervical mucus.

Note: Interpretation of the clinical significance of a PCT must be the responsibility of the physician requesting the test. A negative PCT is not always a true negative clinical finding.

In Vitro Significance
None established from population-based evidence.

In-Vitro Sperm-Mucus Interaction Tests
Pre-Requisites
Appropriate timing of the mucus collection during the immediate pre-ovulatory period and the collection of a complete semen sample after 3±1 days prior ejaculatory abstinence.

Cautionary Note
A cervical mucus Insler score of <10, and/or pH <7.0 can affect sperm-cervical mucus interaction and lead to a poor test result.

In Vivo Significance
See Chapter 6 of this handbook for the specific interpretation criteria for the Kurzrok-Miller slide test, the Kremer capillary tube sperm penetration test, and the sperm-cervical mucus-contact (SCMC) test, as well as the value of crossed-hostility format testing.

Note: Interpretation of the clinical significance of any test of sperm-cervical mucus interaction must be the responsibility of the physician requesting the test.

In Vitro Significance
None established from population-based evidence.

Tests of Sperm Fertilizing Ability
There are no evidence-based, population-derived reference values for any *in-vitro* test of human sperm fertilizing ability. See the report from the consensus workshop organized by the ESHRE Special Interest Group in Andrology, Hamburg 1995 [48], and Chapter 5 in this handbook, for further information.

Sperm DNA Tests

Sperm Chromatin Structure Assay
The sperm chromatin structure assay (SCSA) provides a measure of the stainability of double- and single-stranded DNA in the sperm chromatin by acridine orange following acidic pH-induced denaturation *in vitro*, which has been interpreted as a measure of the susceptibility of the sperm chromatin to fragmentation, the DNA Fragmentation Index ('DFI'), as well as an indication of the proportion of spermatozoa that show nuclear immaturity, the High DNA Stainable ('HDS') fraction. It is the only test of sperm DNA/chromatin for which validated clinical interpretation criteria exist, and these are based on many thousands of tests and hundreds of clinical treatment cycles (although the complete nature of the accessibility and stainability of the sperm DNA has not been fully clarified). While there is some controversy in the field regarding the use and interpretation of the SCSA, rational understanding by some workers seems to be confounded by unreasonable expectations (e.g. that the SCSA can predict fertility – no single sperm test can do this, see above), by inappropriate use of the test (e.g. that it is a first-line screening test for all infertile couples), by the uncertainty derived from a number of factors that directly impinge on the predictive value of DNA fragmentation tests [49,50], including confusing different endpoints, iatrogenic induction of DNA damage due to inappropriate

semen processing for ART, the DNA repair ability of the oocyte or whether the type of sperm DNA damage is repairable or not [51], not taking proper account of the female partner's fertility status, and uncritical consideration of some clinical trials.

Because published 'DFI' and 'HDS' results were defined using the SCSA's highly specific testing protocol and objective analysis of the raw flow cytometer data (SCSAsoft®, SCSA Diagnostics Inc), the results from modified or 'improved' assay can only be considered equivalent to DFI or HDS if a directly equivalent test protocol and data analysis algorithms were employed. Unless these basic scientific criteria are met, then the established and validated clinical interpretation criteria for the SCSA cannot be used with such assays, and independent results and clinical interpretation criteria must be established.

In Vivo Significance

While results of >30% DFI do not preclude a natural full-term successful pregnancy, they are associated with a significant reduction in the prevalence of term pregnancies (up to a 7.5-fold difference) and increase in the time required to achieve a pregnancy, and an approximate doubling of miscarriages (due to damaged paternal genes). Also, if there are >15% HDS spermatozoa, a couple should expect a longer time to natural pregnancy.

When IUI treatment is considered, a DFI >25% has been associated with a substantial reduction in fecundity and fertility (at least an eight-fold difference) and the couple should be recommended to consider IVF or ICSI.

In Vitro Significance

The relationship between DFI and HDS values and fertilization *in vitro*, and with subsequent embryonic development, remain unclear, although there does seem to be some association between elevated DFI and impaired sperm function. With >15% HDS spermatozoa, there is a risk of a reduced fertilization rate with IVF, although ICSI might overcome this factor.

Other Tests of Sperm DNA or Chromatin

Specific risk or interpretation criteria amenable to routine diagnostic or therapeutic application have been quantified and robustly validated for any test of sperm DNA fragmentation or chromatin structure or stability other than the SCSA. As noted above, such assays do not give results that are the same as the SCSA's DFI result, and attempts to apply or adapt the threshold DFI values for use with any of these other tests are scientifically unjustifiable. Large-scale, prospective clinical trials are still required to develop, and then validate, robust interpretation criteria for each of these tests separately.

In Vivo Significance

Undefined.

In Vitro Significance

Undefined.

However, based on test methods described in Chapter 5 of this handbook, the following reference limits can be considered.

TUNEL Assay

A value of ≥20% positive spermatozoa is considered abnormal.

Comet Assay

Alkaline COMET: Values of >45% of spermatozoa with single-strand DNA fragmentation are considered abnormal.

Neutral COMET: Values of >60% of spermatozoa with double-strand DNA fragmentation are considered abnormal.

Sperm Chromatin Dispersion/Halosperm Test

Normal range: <15% of spermatozoa have fragmented DNA
Medium range: 15–30% of spermatozoa have fragmented DNA
Abnormal values: ≥30% of spermatozoa have fragmented DNA

References

1. Solberg HE. Establishment and use of reference values. In: Burtis CA, ed. *Tietz Textboook of Clinical Chemistry*. Philadelphia: WB Saunders Company, 1999, 336–56.

2. World Health Organization. *WHO Laboratory Manual for the Examination and Processing of Human Semen*, 6th edn. Geneva: World Health Organization, 2021.

3. Heuchel V, Schwartz D, Price W. Within-subject variability and the importance of abstinence period for sperm count, semen volume and pre-freeze and post-thaw motility. *Andrologia* 1981; **13**: 479–85.

4. Alvarez C, et al. Biological variation of seminal parameters in healthy subjects. *Hum Reprod* 2003; **18**: 2082–8.

5. Menkveld R, et al. The evaluation of morphological characteristics of human spermatozoa according to stricter criteria. *Hum Reprod* 1990; **5**: 586–92.

6. Mortimer D, Menkveld R. Sperm morphology assessment–historical perspectives and current opinions. *J Androl* 2001; **22**: 192–205.

7. van Zyl JA, Kotze TJ, Menkveld R. Predictive value of spermatozoa morphology in natural fertilization. In: Acosta AA, et al., ed. *Human Spermatozoa in Assisted Reproduction*. Baltimore: William & Wilkins, 1990, 319–24.

8. Menkveld R. *The influence of environment factors on spermatogenesis and semen parameters*. PhD Thesis. Stellenbosch: University of Stellenbosch, 1987.

9. Eliasson R. Semen analysis and laboratory workup. In: Cockett ATK, Urry RL, eds. *Male Infertility. Workup, Treatment and Research*. New York: Grune & Stratton, 1977, 169–88.

10. Eliasson R. Analysis of semen. In: Burger HG, De Kretser DM, eds. *The Testis*. New York: Raven Press, 1981, 381–99.

11. Mortimer D, Templeton AA, Lenton EA, Coleman RA. Influence of abstinence and ejaculation-to-analysis delay on semen analysis parameters of suspected infertile men. *Arch Androl* 1982; **8**: 251–6.

12. World Health Organization. *WHO Laboratory Manual for the Examination of Human Semen and Semen-Cervical Mucus Interactions*, 2nd edn. Cambridge: Cambridge University Press, 1987.

13. World Health Organization. *WHO Laboratory Manual for the Examination of Human Semen and Semen-Cervical Mucus Interactions*, 3rd edn. Cambridge: Cambridge University Press, 1992.

14. World Health Organization. *WHO Laboratory Manual for the Examination of Human Semen and Sperm-Cervical Mucus Interactions*, 4th edn. Cambridge: Cambridge University Press, 1999.

15. Bostofte E, Serup J, Rebbe H. Interrelations among the characteristics of human semen, and a new system for classification of male infertility. *Fertil Steril* 1984; **41**: 95–102.

16. Mortimer D. *The Male Factor in Infertility. Part I: Semen Analysis*. Current Problems in Obstetrics, Gynecology and Fertility VIII. Chicago: Year Book Medical Publishers Inc, 1985.

17. Mortimer D. *Practical Laboratory Andrology*. Oxford: Oxford University Press, 1994.

18. Björndahl L, et al. *A Practical Guide to Basic Laboratory Andrology*. Cambridge: Cambridge University Press, 2010.

19. Guzick DS, et al. Sperm morphology, motility, and concentration in fertile and infertile men. *New England J Med* 2001; **345**: 1388–93.

20. Mortimer D, Templeton AA, Lenton EA, Coleman RA. Semen analysis parameters and their interrelationships in suspected infertile men. *Arch Androl* 1982; **8**: 165–71.

21. Pelzman DL, Hwang K. Genetic testing for men with infertility: techniques and indications. *Transl Androl Urol* 2021; **10**: 1354–64.

22. Mortimer D, Mortimer ST. The case against intracytoplasmic sperm injection for all. In: Aitken RJ, Mortimer D, Kovacs G, eds. *Male and Female Factors that Maximize IVF Success*. Cambridge: Cambridge University Press, 2020.

23. Barratt CLR, De Jonge CJ, Sharpe RM. 'Man Up': the importance and strategy for placing male reproductive health centre stage in the political and research agenda. *Hum Reprod* 2018, **33**: 541–5.

24. Aitken RJ. Not every sperm is sacred: a perspective on male infertility. *Mol Hum Reprod* 2018; **24**: 287–98.

25. Cairo Consensus Workshop Group. The current status and future of andrology: a consensus report from the Cairo workshop group. *Andrology* 2020; **8**: 27–52.

26. Barratt CLR, Björndahl L, De Jonge CJ, et al. The diagnosis of male infertility: an analysis of the evidence to support the development of global WHO guidance – challenges and future research opportunities. *Hum Reprod Update* 2017; **23**: 660–80.

27. World Health Organization. *WHO Laboratory Manual for the Examination and Processing of Human Semen*, 5th edn. Geneva: World Health Organization, 2010.

28. Cooper TG, et al. World Health Organization reference values for human semen characteristics. *Hum Reprod Update* 2010; **16**: 231–45.

29. Campbell MJ, et al. Distribution of semen examination results 2020 – A follow up of data collated for the WHO semen analysis manual 2010. *Andrology* 2021; **9**: 817–22.

30. ESHRE Special Interest Group of Embryology and Alpha Scientists in Reproductive Medicine. The Vienna consensus: report of an expert meeting on the development of ART laboratory performance indicators. *Reprod Biomed Online* 2017; **35**: 494–510; *Hum Reprod Open* 2017; hox011. https://doi.org/10.1093/hropen/hox011

31. Jouannet P, Ducot B, Feneux D, Spira A. Male factors and the likelihood of pregnancy in infertile couples. I. Study of sperm characteristics. *Int J Androl* 1988; **11**: 379–94.

32. Smith JC, et al. Fatherhood without apparent spermatozoa after vasectomy. *Lancet* 1994; **344**: 30.

33. Keihani S, et al. Semen parameter thresholds and time-to-conception in subfertile couples: how high is high enough? *Hum Reprod* 2021; **36**: 2121–33.

34. Björndahl L, Barratt CL, Mortimer D, Jouannet P. 'How to count sperm properly': checklist for acceptability of studies based on human semen analysis. *Hum Reprod* 2016; **31**: 227–32.

35. Mortimer D, Pandya IJ, Sawers RS. Relationship between human sperm motility characteristics and sperm penetration into human cervical mucus in vitro. *J Reprod Fertil* 1986; **78**: 93–102.

36. Aitken RJ, Warner PE, Reid C. Factors influencing the success of sperm-cervical mucus interaction in patients exhibiting unexplained infertility. *J Androl* 1986; **7**: 3–10.

37. Mortimer ST. A critical review of the physiological importance and analysis of sperm movement in mammals. *Hum Reprod Update* 1997; **3**: 403–39.

38. Barratt CLR, Osborn JC, Harrison PE, et al. The hypo-osmotic swelling test and the sperm mucus penetration test in determining fertilization of the human oocyte. *Hum Reprod* 1989; **4**: 430–4.

39. Berberoglugil P, et al. Abnormal sperm-mucus penetration test predicts low in vitro fertilization ability of apparently normal semen. *Fertil Steril* 1993; **59**: 1228–32.

40. Mortimer D. Sperm form and function: beauty is in the eye of the beholder. In: Van der Horst G, et al., eds. *Proceedings of the 9th International Symposium on Spermatology*. Bologna: Monduzzi Editore SpA, 2002, 257–62.

41. Rowe PJ, et al. *WHO Manual for the Standardized Investigation, Diagnosis and Management of the Infertile Male*. Cambridge: Cambridge University Press, 2000.

42. Menkveld R, et al. Semen parameters, including WHO and strict criteria morphology, in a fertile and subfertile population: an effort towards standardization of in-vivo thresholds. *Hum Reprod* 2001; **16**: 1165–71.

43. ESHRE Andrology Special Interest Group. Guidelines on the application of CASA technology in the analysis of spermatozoa. *Hum Reprod* 1998; **13**: 142–5.

44. Mortimer ST, van der Horst G, Mortimer D. The future of computer-aided sperm analysis. *Asian J Androl* 2015; **17**: 545–53.

45. Mortimer D, Mortimer ST. Routine application of CASA in human clinical andrology and ART laboratories. In: Björndahl L, Flanagan J, Holmberg R, Kvist U, eds. *XIIIth International Symposium on Spermatology*. Switzerland: Springer Nature, 2021, 183–97.

46. Menkveld R, et al. Detection of sperm antibodies on unwashed spermatozoa with the immunobead test: a comparison of results with the routine method and seminal plasma TAT titers and SCMC test. *Am J Reprod Immunol* 1991; **25**: 88–91.

47. Björndahl L, et al. When is a vasectomy successful? Laboratory aspects. *Andrology* 2019; **7** (**Sup 1**): 96–7.

48. ESHRE Andrology Special Interest Group. Consensus workshop on advanced diagnostic andrology techniques. *Hum Reprod* 1996; **11**: 1463–79.

49. Evenson DP, Wixon R. Data analysis of two in vivo fertility studies using sperm chromatin structure

assay-derived DNA fragmentation index vs. pregnancy outcome. *Fertil Steril* 2008; **90**: 1229–31.

50. Evenson D. DNA Damage: sperm chromatin structure assay. Sperm chromatin structure assay test on its fortieth anniversary. In: Agarwal A, Henkel R, Majzoub A, eds. *Manual of Sperm Function Testing in Human Assisted Reproduction.* Cambridge: Cambridge University Press, 2021, 192–201.

51. Alvarez JG. The predictive value of sperm chromatin structure assay. *Hum Reprod* 2005; **20**: 2365–7.

Appendix 2 Equipment Required for a Basic Andrology Laboratory

The following equipment is required in order for an andrology laboratory to be capable of performing the basic procedures described in this handbook. Sufficient equipment must be available for the number of staff working in the laboratory and for the laboratory to function efficiently at maximum caseload. Back-up equipment should also be available in order for the laboratory's services not to be compromised by equipment failure. Recommendations reflect one or more of the authors' preferences, but do not indicate that other manufacturers or models are not suitable (unless specifically stated).

The equipment has been listed in three general categories:
- Basic andrology laboratory
- Cryobanking
- Equipment for specialized assays: e.g. CASA system, flow cytometer, fluorescence microscope, luminometer

Basic Andrology Laboratory

This section covers the equipment required by any andrology laboratory wishing to employ the methods described in this handbook and operate to proper levels of technical quality and quality control.

Microscope

An upright compound microscope with good quality phase contrast optics is fundamental to a serious andrology laboratory. General features of a microscope configured for andrology (see Figure App2.1) include:
- 10×, 20×, 40× objectives, all PL (positive low) phase contrast
- 100× oil immersion objective (*not* phase contrast)
- Widefield eyepieces, minimum 10× (12.5× can aid sperm morphology assessments)
- Extra eyepiece with built-in **grid reticle**
- Phase telescope (for proper alignment of the phase rings)
- Intermediate magnification capability (vital for sperm motility assessments using video
- Trinocular head with camera oculars, as necessary, and **camera adapter(s)**, e.g. C-mount for video camera
- Green (45G533: IF550), daylight and diffuser filters
- **Heated stage**, ideally built into the microscope's own stage, not one that sits on top of the stage as these stages will adversely affect proper illumination and phase contrast optics (e.g. the Minitüb system with HT-200 controller which also has a warm plate on top of the controller, see www .minitube.com)

Notes
1. Sufficient microscopes should be available for efficient working at maximum caseload.
2. A dedicated sperm morphology workstation microscope would not require either phase contrast optics or a heated stage, but the highest quality possible bright field optics are strongly recommended, especially for the 100× oil immersion objective.

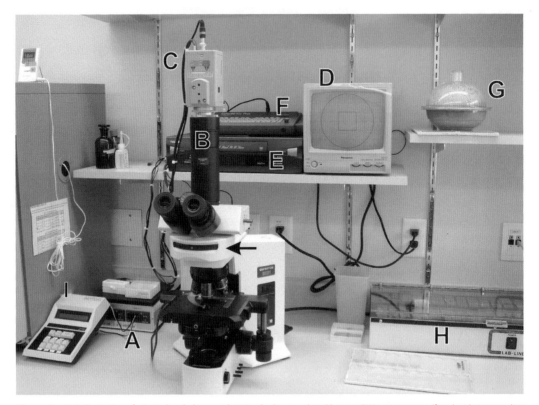

Figure App2.1 Illustration of a typical andrology workstation built around an Olympus BX51 microscope (fitted with intermediate magnification changer module; **arrow**) and attached video display and recording equipment for sperm motility assessments, training and quality control. (A) = Minitüb HT-200 heated stage controller unit; (B) = camera adapter with additional camera ocular; (C) = monochrome video camera; (D) = 9″ monochrome video monitor with acetate overlay showing 25-μm-equivalent ruled grid; E = VHS videocassette recorder; (F) = Video titler device; (G) = Nalgene desiccator used as humid chamber for settling haemocytometers; (H) = large warming plate with hinged clear acrylic cover; and (I) = electronic multichannel counter.

A **videomicrography system** is extremely useful for sperm motility assessments (see Figure App2.1). Ideally a monochrome system, but these old 'surveillance'-type CCTV units are now hard to source and likely to be more expensive than 'low-end' colour systems.

A *digital video camera* (with C-mount, no lens) and *small monitor* are required as a minimum. The monitor should not be too large since it will be viewed close-up (a screen size of about 9″ or 23 cm is ideal), but again these are now hard to find; so select a smaller size display with high resolution so the pixels are small. Ideally, the total magnification on the video screen should be such that 70–100 mm on the screen represents 100 μm in the sample. To facilitate estimating sperm velocity, an acetate sheet with a central circular field and a grid with squares corresponding to 25×25 μm under the microscope can be attached to the video monitor screen.

Video recording is nowadays almost always onto a computer, directly to the hard drive, either via a USB interface or a video 'grabber' (for analogue cameras), and only burnt to disc when necessary for archiving. With older video technology, a *video character generator* or *titler* can be connected between the camera and video recorder to allow identifying text to be added to the video stream before recording.

Note: Although video recording would not be necessary on a dedicated sperm morphology workstation microscope, still video image capture or photography capability is highly recommended.

Other general requirement equipment items are listed alphabetically, below.

Balances

Top-load balance (maximum 100 g, readout to 0.01 g) for weighing semen specimens and their containers.

Note: For retrograde ejaculation urine specimens a larger capacity balance (e.g. 500 g) will be needed.

Analytical balance (maximum 100 g, readout to 0.1 mg) for weighing reagents.

Centrifuge

Needs to have a swing-out rotor and sealed buckets. Ideally this centrifuge should be programmable for ease of use. Adapters should be available for each type of tube to be centrifuged in the laboratory, including the Falcon 15-ml conical tubes for density gradients and the 50-ml Falcon 'Blue Max' tubes for retrograde ejaculation urine specimens. There are many possible models from a wide variety of manufacturers, but the Eppendorf model 5804 performs extremely well and is very quiet with minimal vibration (very important if it has to be located on the same bench as the microscope). There should be sufficient centrifuges for efficient working at maximum caseload.

Counting Chambers

Haemocytometers should be the Improved Neubauer pattern and in sufficient quantity for efficient operation of the laboratory. Remember to buy spare cover glasses.

Note: Disposable haemocytometers are commercially available, see Chapter 3.

Makler chambers for assessing washed sperm preparations. Again, more than one should be available so that the chamber can be warmed back up to 37°C after washing before re-use (total number required will depend on maximum caseload). It is advisable to have at least one spare cover glass.

Dry bath

or warming block with drilled metal blocks for the particular type(s) of tubes to be used.

Freezer

for storing reagents and specimens frozen at a minimum of –18 to –20°C. Can be a combined refrigerator-freezer with separate compartments.

Fume hood

or **fume adsorber** for working with fixatives, stains and solvents, in accordance with local safety and fire regulations.

Heated stirrer

(combination hot plate and magnetic stirrer) for making some reagent solutions and stains.

Hotplate

capable of at least 55°C for running the fructose spot test.

Humid chamber

for allowing haemocytometers to 'settle', e.g. a 15-cm diameter Nalgene desiccator (cat.no. 5315–0150) containing gauze swabs wetted using sterile water. One per workstation is recommended.

Incubators

Air incubator where semen samples can be left at 37°C to liquefy after delivery to the laboratory. A gravity convection type model is adequate. If an orbital mixer can be placed inside the incubator, then the specimens will mix as they liquefy, facilitating their analysis.

CO_2 incubator for sperm function tests. Most bicarbonate-based culture media that support sperm capacitation require 5.8–6.0% CO_2-in-air when used close to sea level (i.e. pCO_2 of 44 mm Hg). If

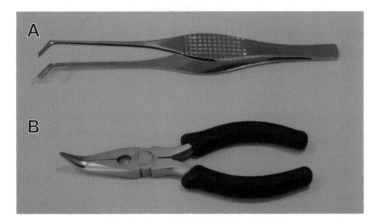

Figure App2.2 (A) Straw handling forceps (NordicCell, Copenhagen, Denmark, see www .nordiccell.com; previously Rocket Medical, Watford, UK; cat.no. R30.722 for 0.5-ml straws and R30.721 for 0.25-ml straws).
(B) Bent-nose radio pliers, ideal for attaching and removing cryovials to/from canes while in cryogenic storage.

a CO_2 incubator is not available, then tubes can be gassed with pre-mixed gas (containing the same amount of CO_2), capped tightly and mixed by inversion to equilibrate with the gas, and then placed in a 37°C incubator with an air atmosphere.

Miscellaneous Minor Items

Calculator for calculating test results (one per workstation).

Forceps of various types and sizes, for handling slides and coverslips during fixing/staining/mounting, small centrifuge tubes, processing surgical sperm retrieval tissue, and also for handling straws and cryovials when frozen (see Figure App2.2).

Glassware:
- Bottles for storing stains and other reagents.
- Coplin jars for fixation and staining of slides.
- Filter funnels for filtering the haemocytometry diluent and stains.
- Measuring cylinders (ideally with stoppers) for preparing fixatives and staining solutions.
- Staining dishes and racks for sperm morphology staining (e.g. the preferred Papanicolaou method).

Iris scissors (stainless steel) for cutting cervical mucus specimens. Several pairs should be available so they can be washed thoroughly and decontaminated after use.

Marker pens for labelling tubes and slides, also special *cryogenic marker pens* for writing on straws.

Pencils for writing on frosted-end microscope slides; *not* to be used for completing laboratory forms or any other permanent record.

Pens for completing laboratory forms and other paperwork; must be indelible (i.e. not water-based gel pens).

Rubber bulbs for using glass Pasteur pipettes. For volumetric work, use either a 3-ml syringe with a short tubing connector or a suitable macro pipetter device.

Safety glasses to protect operators whenever there is a risk of aerosol contamination (as distinct from protection while using liquid nitrogen).

Scissors, general purpose. Not to be used for opening straws as there is a high risk of cross-contamination; even with in-house 'sterilization' (a process that would, of course, require regular validation).

Spatulas of various types and sizes (as per operator preference) for weighing chemicals to prepare diagnostic reagents and stains.

Spotting plates, porcelain for the fructose spot test; can also be used for mixing semen with eosin-nigrosin stain.

Stage micrometer for calibration of microscope fields and magnification.

Pipetters

Air displacement pipetters for dispensing reagents and loading haemocytometers; several models to cover the range from 5–10 µl to 1000 µl, preferably fitted with tip ejectors (e.g. Gilson Pipetman P20, P200 and P1000 units).

Positive displacement pipetter for taking accurate samples of semen. The Gilson M100 unit (1–100 µl) is recommended as it avoids cross-contamination between samples and its tips are available pre-assembled (unlike those for the M50 model).

Macro pipetter to allow volumetric use of glass Pasteur pipettes, for example when preparing density gradients, e.g. the Socorex Acura® Model 835–05 (www.socorex.com). Alternatively, use a 3-ml syringe with a short tubing connector.

Pipette controller for using volumetric pipettes. Ideally a motorized unit or else *Pi-Pump* manual units (the models with an integral release valve are not recommended due to their tendency to leak).

   Note: A set of pipetters is recommended for each workstation.

Refrigerator

For storing culture media and other reagents at *ca.* +4°C. Can be a combined refrigerator-freezer with separate compartments.

Solvent storage cabinet

For safe storage of all flammable solvents and reagents in the laboratory, as per local safety and fire regulations.

Safety cabinets:

Class II biosafety cabinet for working with potentially infectious semen samples, as per local regulations.

Vertical laminar flow cabinet as a 'clean' workstation for handling density gradient preparations and processing spermatozoa for freezing (as per local regulations), and filter-sterilizing diagnostic reagents.

   Note: Sufficient cabinets should be available for efficient, safe working at maximum caseload.

Slide warmer

To keep slides, coverslips, Makler chambers, pipette tips, etc., warm. Should be a large model, ideally with hinged cover. One per workstation is recommended.

Tally counters:

Single channel hand tally counters for counting haemocytometers.

Multi-channel counters, mechanical or electronic, for performing differential counts of sperm motility, vitality and morphology.

   Note: There should be one of each type of counter at each workstation.

Thermometers

For calibrating and checking (operational qualification) all temperature-controlled equipment, including daily-use electronic thermocouple-type devices as well as a calibrated *reference thermometer* for in-house calibration/verification of the daily-use thermometers.

   Note: Electronic thermometers are strongly recommended; spirit-filled thermometers are acceptable but easily broken. Thermometers containing mercury should not be used due to occupational safety concerns.

Vortex mixer

For mixing diluted haemocytometry specimens, *Accu-Beads®*, *SpermMar* beads, biochemistry dilution, etc. One per workstation is recommended. *Warning*: do *not* vortex live spermatozoa!

Waterbath

For heat-inactivating sera and seminal plasma samples for anti-sperm antibody testing, thawing cryopreserved semen and spermatozoa, and in fructose and α-glucosidase assays.

Cryobanking Equipment

Controlled-Rate Freezer

For cryopreserving semen and washed sperm preparations. Ideally it should have built-in programs that allow the specimens to be cooled to at least −160°C before transferring them into storage. Numerous instruments are available from several manufacturers, e.g. *Freeze Control® CL8800i* (CryoLogic, Victoria, Australia), *CTE 2104* (MTG Medical Technology, Altdorf, Germany), *Labotec Cryo Unit* (Labotec, Göttingen, Germany), *Kryo 360–1.7* and *Kryo 360–3.3* (Planer, Sunbury-on-Thames, UK), *Asymptote EF600* (Grant Instruments, Cambridgeshire, UK).

Cryogenic Safety Gear

This is required at *each location* where cryogenic materials will be handled, as per local safety regulations. A set includes **gauntlets** (not 'gardening' gloves), a **full face visor**, and **cryo apron** specifically designed for use with cryogenic materials wherever liquid nitrogen is being handled, and at least gauntlets and safety glasses (but ideally a full face visor) at other locations where only cryogenic specimens are being handled.

Cryogenic Storage Dewars

Vessels for the cryogenic storage of biological specimens in liquid nitrogen. These are available from a number of manufacturers, e.g. Air Liquide, MVE, Taylor-Wharton (later Worthington Industries, now part of Chart Industries). Where they will be moved around within the laboratory or cryobank they must be on **roller bases**. Also, it is highly recommended (and is required in an increasing number of jurisdictions) that each tank used for storing specimens be fitted with at least a low-level alarm sensor, and ideally a combined temperature and level sensor; these are available from a variety of manufacturers including many of those that manufacture the storage vessels, as well as others including Gordinier Electronics, Labotect, and LEC.

> *Note*: While some authorities recommend storage of specimens in the vapour phase, or in super-cold air, this is inherently more risky due to the existence of frequent opportunities for storage temperatures to rise above the transition point of water (i.e. above −132°C) as other specimens are being transferred into/out of storage. Given the biocontainment that is inherent in the use of *High Security Straws* (Cryo Bio System, Paris, France), the use of storage other than immersed in liquid nitrogen is not recommended.

Dry shipper

For transport of cryopreserved samples (e.g. Air Liquide's *Voyageur*, or Taylor-Wharton's *CX100B-11M*).

Label Printer

For secure labelling of straws, e.g. the various models manufactured by Brady that are sold by many distributors, e.g. *TLS 2200* and *LabXpert* models.

Liquid Nitrogen Supply Vessel(s)

These dewars are required for the supply of liquid nitrogen to the laboratory for use with the controlled-rate freezers and for refilling storage and shipper tanks (note that tanks containing patient specimens must never leave the control of laboratory or cryobank personnel and must never be filled directly by the delivery person). The size(s) and number of supply vessels needed will depend on each laboratory's particular requirements, but the following principles must be considered:

- Liquid supply tanks must be on **roller bases** and, ideally, **tipper stands** so that liquid can be poured from the tank without having to lift the tank.
- Large volume users should consider a self-pressuring 'PGS'-type supply vessel, available from major liquid nitrogen suppliers. These vessels require the use of supply hoses fitted with a phase separator.
- Some controlled-rate freezers (e.g. Planer's Kryo-10 models) require the liquid nitrogen to be supplied under pressure, this can be achieved using a **thermal transfer pump** fitted to a standard 25-l supply dewar.

Sealing Device for Straws

The *SYMS* sealer must be used with the *CBS High Security Straws* (the recommended packaging system for cryobanking semen and washed sperm preparations: CryoBioSystem, Paris, France). Automated systems for labelling, filling and sealing straws are available from Cryo Bio System (Paris, France), e.g. the MAPI, PACE and SIDE units, although these are too large-scale for the great majority of human sperm cryobanks.

Note: The Minitube *Ultraseal 21*™ ultrasonic sealing device is not validated for use with CBS *High Security Straws*.

Equipment for Specialized Assays

Computer-Aided Sperm Analysis Instrument

The Boolean sort criteria provided in Chapter 6 have been validated for the Hamilton Thorne IVOS and CEROS computer-aided sperm analysers. These instruments need to operate at a 60 Hz image capture rate and have the 'HDATA', 'Edit Tracks' and 'Sort' function software options installed. The more recent second-generation models running the CASA-II software also include the ability to perform analyses with replicates.

The Microptic Sperm Class Analyzer (SCA) systems are also good CASA instruments, but due to differences in derivation of the average path and ALH calculation, SCA algorithms do give different values for ALH compared to Hamilton Thorne software. This can cause under-estimation of sperm hyperactivation. Replicate analyses are also possible using later generations of the SCA software.

Flow Cytometer

This is an optional means of reading TUNEL assays (see Chapter 5), e.g. Becton Dickinson FACScan (San Jose, CA, USA) equipped with a 15 mW argon-ion laser for excitation and green FITC fluorescence detection in the FL1 sensor (550 nm dichroic long-pass filter and 525 nm band-pass filter).

Fluorescence Microscope

For visualization of fluorescently labelled lectins (acrosome reaction testing) or TUNEL assays. A dedicated epi-fluorescence microscope system is recommended and must include the appropriate filter sets for the particular fluorescent probes being used:

FITC: excitation at 494 nm (blue); emission at 520 nm (green) and barrier filter (dichroic mirror) at 510–515 nm.

TRITC: excitation at 541 nm (green); emission at 572 nm (red) and barrier filter (dichroic mirror) at 570–580 nm.

H33258: excitation at 343 nm (*u.v.*); emission at 480 nm (blue) and barrier filter (dichroic mirror) at 400 nm.

An attached or integral imaging system is also recommended.

Inverted Microscope

For working with zonae pellucidae (see Chapter 7). For the *hemizona assay*, micromanipulator attachments are required for bisecting the hemizonae and 10× and 40× phase contrast objectives are needed. For the *competitive (intact) zona binding assay*, phase contrast optics giving total magnification of 160× or 250× are needed.

Luminometer

For assaying reactive oxygen species (Chapter 4), e.g. AutoLumat model LB 953 (Berthold Technologies, Oak Ridge, TN, USA).

Macropipetter

For volumes of 1–5 and/or 1–10ml (see Chapter 4).

Magnetic stirrer

For biochemistry assays (see Chapter 4).

Microcentrifuge

For 1.5 ml Eppendorf tubes.

Microtiterplate reader

For biochemistry assays (see Chapter 4).

Multi-step pipetter

For volumes in the range 50–1000 µl (see Chapter 4).

Appendix 3 Home Testing

For over 20 years there has been the possibility that a man could test his semen in the comfort of his own home, and a plethora of commercial products are now available (see Table App 3.1). There are many advantages to at-home testing, including avoiding the sometimes embarrassing and inconvenient attendance at the laboratory to either produce or deliver a semen specimen. In the current environment of the COVID-19 pandemic, home testing would also reduce exposure to risk of infection. Results from home tests are usually available quickly, obviating the need to wait days or sometimes weeks for a laboratory test result.

The primary disadvantage relates to the clinical value of the results from home tests. Semen analysis is a complex diagnostic laboratory procedure and to replicate this in a rapid convenient home test is very challenging [1]. As a consequence, several home tests only estimate sperm number/concentration which, even if accurate, limits the clinical value of the test. Other home tests assess motility as well as providing some estimate of sperm numbers, thus potentially providing results with more clinical relevance.

Some further information on cell-phone-based CASA can be found in Chapter 6 on 'Computer-Aided Sperm Analysis'.

The real issue, however, is that some of the home tests have no significant clinical data accompanying their claims of accuracy and, even when these data have been published, they are usually based on low numbers of patients/specimens. Because the potential of home testing has yet to be rigorously validated, they cannot be used as a replacement for a laboratory semen assessment.

References

1. Björndahl L, Kirkman-Brown J, Hart G, et al. Development of a novel home sperm test. *Hum Reprod* 2006; **21**: 145–9.

2. Cheon WH, Park HJ, Park MJ, et al. Validation of a smartphone-based, computer-assisted sperm analysis system compared with laboratory-based manual microscopic semen analysis and computer-assisted semen analysis. *Invest Clin Urol* 2019; **60**: 380–7.

3. Coppola MA, Klotz KL, Kim KA, et al. SpermCheck® Fertility: an immunodiagnostic home test that detects normozoospermia and severe oligozoospermia. *Hum Reprod* 2010; **25**: 853–61.

4. Castello D, Garcia-Laez V, Buyru F, et al. Comparison of the SwimCount home diagnostic test with conventional sperm analysis. *Adv Androl Gynecol* 2018; **1**: 1–8.

5. Yoon YE, Kim TY, Shin TE, et al. Validation of SwimCount^{TM}, a novel home-based device that detects progressively motile spermatozoa: correlation with World Health Organization 5th Semen Analysis. *World J Men's Health* 2020; **38**: 191.

6. Schaff UY, Fredriksen LL, Epperson JG, et al. Novel centrifugal technology for measuring sperm concentration in the home. *Fertil Steril* 2017; **107**: 358–64.

7. Kobori Y, Pfanner P, Prins GS, Niederberger C. Novel device for male infertility screening with single-ball lens microscope and smartphone. *Fertil Steril* 2016; **106**: 574–8.

8. Agarwal A, Panner Selvam MK, Sharma R, et al. Home sperm testing device versus laboratory sperm quality analyzer: comparison of motile sperm concentration. *Fertil Steril* 2018; **110**: 1277–84.

Table App 3.1 Examples of home-use semen test kits

Test	Method	Readout	Accuracy	Limitations	Primary data with no conflict of interest	Medical device?	Market	Price	Refs
SEEM®	Digital; smartphone camera (CASA-based tracking)	Sperm concentration, total motility	N/A	Lack of published peer-reviewed data (n=1)	Accurate compared with LabCASA, but very small sample size (n=28) and no comparison of accuracy	No	Japan	$45.00	[2]
SpermCheck®	Manual; immunochromatographic assay	Sperm concentration	98%	Only measures one parameter	Strong correlation between results and haemocytometer, correctly identifying 96% of clinical results	FDA	USA	$39.99	[3]
SwimCount™	Manual; colorimetric test	Concentration of progressively motile spermatozoa	95%	Only measures one parameter	95% agreement with Makler chamber analysis reported [4]; sensitivity and specificity of 87.5% and 73.4%, respectively, when compared with laboratory semen analysis [5]	CE, FDA	EU, USA	€49.99	[4,5]
FertilCount®	Manual; colorimetric test by DNA staining	Sperm concentration	97%	Lack of published peer-reviewed data to support product (n=1)	N/A	No	EU	€21.00	N/A
Trak®	Manual; uses centrifuge to analyse sperm concentration	Sperm concentration	97%	Only measures one parameter	Strong correlation with LabCASA analysis reported, but accuracy varies depending on the sperm concentration in the semen sample (ranged from 82.4% to 95.5%)	FDA	USA	$89.99 to $199.99	[6]
Men's Loupe	Manual; ball lens microscope used with smartphone camera	Sperm concentration, total motility	N/A	User must calculate results manually; lens quality is not comparable with LabCASA image quality	High sensitivity and specificity (87.5% and 90.9% respectively) when compared with LabCASA	No	Japan	$15.00	[7]
FertilitySCORE Kit®	Manual; colorimetric test by antibody reaction	Concentration of progressively motile spermatozoa	93%	Only measures one parameter, lack of published peer-reviewed data to support credibility of product	N/A	No	UK	£19.95 to £24.95	N/A

Test	Method	Parameter measured	Reported accuracy	Limitations	Notes	Medical device?	Country	Price	Ref
YO™	Digital; smartphone camera (CASA-based technology)	Concentration of motile spermatozoa	>97%	Only measures one parameter	Reported to be 97.8% accurate when compared with the SQA-Vision device	FDA	USA	$49.95 to $89.95	[8]
ExSeed®	Digital; smartphone camera (CASA-based technology)	Concentration of motile spermatozoa	96%	Lack of published peer reviewed data to support credibility of product	N/A	CE	UK, Denmark	£74.99 to £149.99	N/A
Microscope-based tests, e.g. Micra First Step	Manual; using microscope	Sperm count, total sperm motility, semen volume	N/A	Prone to error as the measurements are made manually by the user via microscope, and calculations must be done manually	N/A	FDA	USA	$85.00	N/A

Reported accuracy is as stated on consumer websites and/or in product information. Medical device? = regulatory approval as a medical device (FDA = US Food and Drug Association, CE = Conformité Européene). Prices obtained from the manufacturer's or re-sellers' websites ($ = USD, € = EUR, £ = GBP). Other abbreviations: n = number of semen samples analysed; N/A = not available; LabCASA = laboratory-computer-aided sperm analysis systems.

The authors gratefully acknowledge the efforts of Róisín Hogan in developing the content of this Table

Appendix 4 Example Andrology Laboratory Forms

Consistent routine is key to achieving reliable results with low variation between different operators, and between different occasions. Elaborated Work Forms help laboratory staff perform the techniques as intended, and such forms can also be used to document which operator was responsible for each of the different parts of the complete semen analysis. This documentation is a basic requirement for quality management in the andrology laboratory.

Comprehensive clinical Report Forms that identify 'abnormal' results and include interpretation guidelines are also important for intelligent use of the results generated by the andrology laboratory.

This Appendix includes examples of such forms.

Table App4.1

Example Laboratory Work Form

Patient name: _____   Date of Birth: _____   Unique ID*: _____

* Social Security Number, Laboratory Patient Number, or other unique identifier   ID controlled by: _____

Sample date: _____   Date of previous ejaculation: _____

Collection time: _____   Complete collection: ☐ Yes   ☐ No

         If not complete, missed: ☐ 1st   ☐ middle   ☐ last part;   approximately ____% of the ejaculate lost

Start of investigations (time): _____   Fresh sample investigator: _____

Liquefaction: ☐ within 30 mins,   ☐ 30–60 min,   ☐ incomplete at 60 min after ejaculation

Volume: _____ ml   Viscosity: ☐ normal;   ☐ increased

Other macroscopic observations: _____

Investigation of the wet preparation:

Estimation of appropriate dilution for concentration: ☐ 1:5,   ☐ 1:10,   ☐ 1:20,   ☐ 1:50

Presence of: ☐ Aggregates   ☐ Agglutinates – dominant region of binding: _____

Motility assessment:	1st drop		2nd drop		Average	Diff |•|* drops	Diff < limit?
	Counts	Percent	Counts	Percent			
rapid (*a*)							
slow (*b*)							
non-progr (*c*)							
immotile (*d*)							
TOTAL		100		100			
Progressive (*a+b*)							
Motile (*a+b+c*)							

*\|•\| = between   Investigator: _____

Determination of sperm concentration: Investigator: _____

Sperm counted in upper left square: _____   1st chamber: Sperm counted _____ in _____ large squares

                                        2nd chamber: Sperm counted _____ in _____ large squares

Total number counted (sum): _____   Difference between counts: _____   OK? ☐ Yes   ☐ No

Divide total number by: _____ = _____ ×10^6/ml   Total sperm number (volume × concentration) = _____ ×10^6/ejac

Table App4.1 (cont.)

Sperm morphology assessment:

	Counts	Percentage	Comments
Ideal			
Abnormal			
TOTAL		**100**	
Head defects			*Percentages are of ALL spermatozoa counted*
Neck/midpiece defects			
Tail defects			
Cytoplasmic residues			
		>100	

Teratozoospermia Index (TZI): _____

Immature germ cells: _____ / _____ spermatozoa = _____ / 100 spermatozoa

Investigator: _____

Sperm vitality assessment:

Number of spermatozoa assessed: _____   Number of live spermatozoa: _____ = _____ % live spermatozoa

Investigator: _____

Assessment of round cells and white blood cells (leukocytes) – *cells in wet preparation*

	Cells counted	No. of microscope fields	Cells/field	Concentration
Round cells				× 10^6/ml
White cells				× 10^6/ml
Spermatozoa				× 10^6/ml

Calculate round cell and leukocyte concentrations as: sperm concentration × (cells/field / spermatozoa/field)

Investigator: _____

Inflammatory cells assessment (peroxidase-positive granulocytes)

Cells counted in counting chamber: _____   Factor to divide cell number by: _____

Calculated concentration = _____ ×10^6/ml   Investigator: _____

Antisperm antibody (ASAB) assessment: Method used: _____

	Reading	Time (min)	Total sperm counted	Sperm with beads (%)	Site
IgG	1			(_____)	
	2			(_____)	
IgA	1			(_____)	
	2			(_____)	

Investigator: _____

General Hospital
Unit for Reproductive Medicine
Andrology Laboratory
Address:
Telephone: E-mail:

patient: **Name**
         ID
partner: (Name)
         (ID)
Ref. Dr:

Print date
Aug 22, 2021

Date:	May 8 '21	Jun 4 '21								Ref.	Unit
Sample No.	2021/1768	2021/1933									
BASIC ANALYSES											
Collection:	m	m								m	-
Complete:	y	y								y	-
Time to invest.:	0.30	0.35								<1.00	h.min
Volume:	3.2	3.7								1.5-6.0	ml
Rapid progr (a):	22	22								>25 or	%
Slow progr (b):	23	39								>50(a+b)	%
Non progr (c):	29	8									%
Immotile (d):	26	31								<60	%
%Live:	74	68								>40	%
Aggregates:	0	0								0-1	a.u.
Round cells:	0.7	0.1								<1	×10⁶/ml
Abst. days:	5	3								2-7	day(s)
Sperm conc.:	115	42									× 10⁶/ml
Sperm count:	368	155								>40	×10⁶/ejac.
Inflam. cells:	0.2	0.0								<1	×10⁶/ml
MORPHOLOGY ASSESSMENT											
% Ideal:	4	12									%
Head	96	81									%
Neck/MP	41	30									%
Tail	27	11									%
Cytpl. Residue:	2	4									%
TZI:	1.73	1.43								<1.60	-
Immature	0	0									
SEMEN BIOCHEMISTRY											
α-glucosidase:	18.0	22.3									mU/ml
α-G-amount:	57.6	82.5								>20.0	mU
Zinc conc.:	1.8	4.4								>1.2	mmol/l
Zinc amount:	5.8	16.4								>2.5	µmol
Fructose conc.:	15.7	18.9								>6.0	mmol/l
Fructose amount:	50.2	69.9								>13.0	µmol
Zinc/Fructose:	0.11	0.24								>0.10	-
ANTISPERM ANTIBODIES											
Test method:	IBT	SpM									
Sperm with beads	8	4								<40	%
localization:	NS	NS									

H = Head; MP = Midpiece; T = Tail; tt = tail tip; any combinations according to actual observations ; NS= none specific

Date	Sample	Comment
May 8 '21	2021/1768	Liquefaction incomplete after 30 min; complete at 60 min
Jun 4 '21	2021/1933	A smaller, isolated gel streak left after 30 min liquefation,

Figure App4.1

Legend: An example of a computer-generated report form where results from up to ten different semen samples from the same patient can be printed, together with basic information of reference ranges, etc. ©2021 LB Andrologikonsult.

Explanatory Notes for the Example Basic Semen Analysis Report Form

Left Text Column

Collection	Coded: M = masturbation; I = interrupted intercourse ('withdrawal'); C = collection condom.
Complete	Coded: Y = yes; N = incomplete. It is advisable to give a text comment (bottom of page) explaining if the first, middle, or last part of the ejaculate was missed, and an approximate estimation of the loss.
Time to invest.	Time to investigation = time between ejaculation and initiation of analysis.
Rapid progr (*a*)	Rapidly progressive spermatozoa (% of all spermatozoa):velocity ≥25 μm/s at 37°C.
Slow progr (*b*)	Slowly progressive spermatozoa (% of all spermatozoa): velocity 5–24 μm/s at 37°C.
Non-progr (*c*)	Non-progressive spermatozoa (% of all spermatozoa): l<5 μm/s at 37°C.
Immotile (d)	Immotile sperm (% of all sperm).
Aggregates	Given in arbitrary units (a.u.): 0, 1, 2, 3 for none, some, many, most.
Abst. days	Days of sexual abstinence before collecting the sample for semen analysis.
Sperm conc.	Sperm concentration.
Sperm count	Total number of spermatozoa in the ejaculate (concentration × volume).
Inflam. cells	Concentration of inflammatory cells (peroxidase-positive cells).
% Ideal	Proportion of spermatozoa with a morphology typical for spermatozoa that are able to reach the site of fertilization, and bind to the zona pellucida.
Head	Proportion of spermatozoa with head morphology that is not consistent with the definition of typical spermatozoa.
Neck/MP	Proportion of spermatozoa with neck/midpiece morphology that is not consistent with the definition of typical spermatozoa.
Tail	Proportion of spermatozoa with tail morphology that is not consistent with the definition of typical spermatozoa.
Cytopl. residue	Proportion of spermatozoa with a cytoplasmic residue that is not consistent with the definition of typical spermatozoa.
TZI	Teratozoospermia Index = average number of abnormal regions in the abnormal (non- typical) spermatozoa; calculated as in the 1992 (third) edition of the WHO Manual.
Immature	Presence of immature germ cells in the ejaculate, expressed as number per 100 spermatozoa.
α-glucosidase	Concentration of marker for epididymal secretion.
α-G-amount	Total amount of epididymal marker in the ejaculate.
Zinc conc.	Concentration of marker for prostatic secretion.
Zinc amount	Total amount of prostatic marker in the ejaculate.
Fructose conc.	Concentration of marker for seminal vesicular secretion.
Fructose amount	Total amount of seminal vesicular marker in the ejaculate.
Zinc/Fructose	Zinc–Fructose molar ratio, indicating the relative contribution of prostatic and seminal vesicular secretions to the ejaculate.
Test method	Method used for anti-sperm antibody assessment, e.g. SpermMar™.
Sperm with beads	Proportion of spermatozoa with antisperm antibodies attached.

Localization   Head, Midpiece, Tail, tt (tail-tip), combinations of these, or NS (non-specific); comment if there is a specific localization of the antibodies.

Columns to the Right of Result Columns

Ref.   Reference limits and ranges. It should be noted that numbers given in this sample form are given as examples only. Each laboratory should determine its own reference ranges and limits. These ranges can be based on frequency distributions of results from fertile and subfertile men, respectively. When no clear cut-off can be determined, a consensus-based decision limit can function as reference.

Unit   Specification of unit used for values presented in each row.

Text Comments

Date, Sample Number, and Comment: text comments regarding additional information obtained from the patient, or during laboratory investigation.

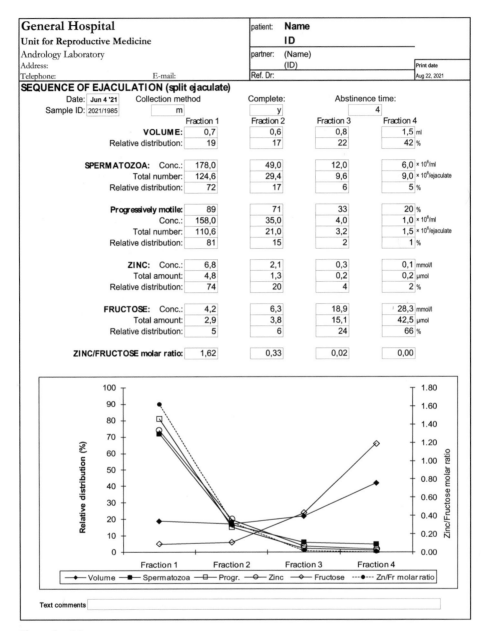

General Hospital		patient:	**Name**		
Unit for Reproductive Medicine			**ID**		
Andrology Laboratory		partner:	(Name)		
Address:			(ID)		Print date
Telephone:	E-mail:	Ref. Dr:			Aug 22, 2021

SEQUENCE OF EJACULATION (split ejaculate)

	Date:	Jun 4 '21	Collection method		Complete:		Abstinence time:		
	Sample ID:	2021/1985	m		y		4		

	Fraction 1	Fraction 2	Fraction 3	Fraction 4	
VOLUME:	0,7	0,6	0,8	1,5	ml
Relative distribution:	19	17	22	42	%
SPERMATOZOA: Conc.:	178,0	49,0	12,0	6,0	$\times 10^6$/ml
Total number:	124,6	29,4	9,6	9,0	$\times 10^6$/ejaculate
Relative distribution:	72	17	6	5	%
Progressively motile:	89	71	33	20	%
Conc.:	158,0	35,0	4,0	1,0	$\times 10^6$/ml
Total number:	110,6	21,0	3,2	1,5	$\times 10^6$/ejaculate
Relative distribution:	81	15	2	1	%
ZINC: Conc.:	6,8	2,1	0,3	0,1	mmol/l
Total amount:	4,8	1,3	0,2	0,2	µmol
Relative distribution:	74	20	4	2	%
FRUCTOSE: Conc.:	4,2	6,3	18,9	28,3	mmol/l
Total amount:	2,9	3,8	15,1	42,5	µmol
Relative distribution:	5	6	24	66	%
ZINC/FRUCTOSE molar ratio:	1,62	0,33	0,02	0,00	

Text comments

Figure App4.2

Legend: An example of a computer-generated report form for a split ejaculate specimen with results in numeric and graphical format. ©2021 LB Andrologikonsult.

Explanatory Notes for the Sample Sequence of Ejaculation Report Form

Collection method, completeness and abstinence time as for the basic semen analysis. This form is based on having the patient collect the three first expelled fractions in the first three containers (Fractions 1–3), and the remainder of the ejaculate in the fourth, last container (Fraction 4).

Relative distribution of volume	The volume in each fraction in relation to the total volume of all fractions.
Progressive motile	Proportion of spermatozoa that were progressively motile in each fraction; used to calculate concentration and total number of progressively motile spermatozoa.
Total number/amount	Calculated from concentration and volume in each fraction.
Relative distribution	Proportion of the measurand in each fraction of the ejaculate; sum of the four fractions = 100%.
Zinc/fructose molar ratio	Contribution of the prostatic marker zinc in relation to the contribution of the seminal vesicular marker fructose.
Graphic representation	Diagram showing relative (%) distribution of volume, spermatozoa, progressively motile spermatozoa, zinc and fructose (left axis), and the zinc/fructose molar ratio (right axis).

Appendix 5 Comparison of Replicate Counts

Acceptable Differences between Replicate Assessments of Proportions

Table App5.1 can be used to facilitate the decision if replicate assessments of proportions (e.g. % motile spermatozoa, % ideal spermatozoa, or % live spermatozoa) can be accepted. Since the recommendation is to count 200 spermatozoa in duplicate (2×200), values are given for this sample size. The table is *not* valid for replicate counts of 100 spermatozoa (i.e. 2×100). The table is calculated from a formula based on the binomial distribution required to determine asymmetrical confidence intervals for proportions (which have absolute minimum and maximum values of 0% and 100%) [1].

Calculate the *average percentage* (rounded with no decimal place) for the replicate assessments, and the *difference* between them. Look up the row corresponding to the average percentage (left column). The difference between the two assessments must be less than or equal to the limit difference given in the right column. If the difference is above the limit, the assessments must be discarded and two new counts made.

Uncertainty of Results due to the Number of Spermatozoa Assessed

Table App5.2 illustrates the uncertainty of results with respect to the number of spermatozoa assessed to obtain the result. The recommended number of assessed cells in each duplicate is 200. In Table App5.2, values are also given for 100 and 200 assessed spermatozoa for comparisons where less than 400 spermatozoa are available for assessment.

Table App5.1

Average %	Limit difference
0	1
1	2
02–03	3
04–06	4
07–09	5
10–13	6
14–19	7
20–27	8
28–44	9
45–55	10
56–72	9
73–80	8
81–86	7
87–90	6
91–93	5
94–96	4
97–98	3
99	2
100	1

Table App5.2

Average percentage found	Total number of spermatozoa assessed		
	400 (2 × 200)	100	200
	95% Confidence Interval		
0	0–1	0–4	0–2
1	0–3	0–5	0–4
2	1–4	0–7	1–5
3	2–5	1–9	1–6
4	2–6	1–10	2–8
5	3–8	2–11	2–9
6	4–9	2–13	3–10
7	5–10	3–14	4–11
8	6–11	4–15	5–13
9	6–12	4–16	5–14
10	7–13	5–18	6–15
11	8–14	6–19	7–16
12	9–16	6–20	8–17
13	10–17	7–21	9–18
14	11–18	8–22	10–20
15	12–19	9–24	10–21
20	16–24	13–29	15–26
25	21–30	17–35	19–32
30	26–35	21–40	24–37
35	30–40	26–45	28–42
40	35–45	30–50	33–47
45	40–50	35–55	38–52
50	45–55	40–60	43–57
55	50–60	45–65	48–62
60	55–65	50–70	53–67
65	60–70	55–74	58–72
70	65–74	60–79	63–76
75	70–79	65–83	68–81
80	76–84	71–87	74–85
85	81–88	76–91	79–90
90	87–93	82–95	85–94
91	88–94	84–96	86–95
92	89–94	85–96	87–95
93	90–95	86–97	89–96
94	91–96	87–98	90–97
95	92–97	89–98	91–98
96	94–98	90–99	92–98
97	95–98	91–99	94–99
98	96–99	93–100	95–99
99	97–100	95–100	96–100
100	99–100	96–100	98–100

When a proportion is determined (as % motile or % ideal spermatozoa), the total number of spermatozoa assessed will influence how certain the result is. The higher the number of spermatozoa that have been examined, the more certain the result will be. This can be expressed as the '95% Confidence Interval' for the obtained proportion. This interval signifies that, with a 95% probability, the true value of the proportion is within the interval.

Example

If the result is 6% ideal spermatozoa after assessing 2 × 200 spermatozoa, then the true proportion is most likely in the range 4–9%. If only 100 spermatozoa had been assessed, the range would be 2–13%. Thus, the uncertainty of the result is much lower when 400 spermatozoa are assessed instead of 100.

Correspondingly, a result of 50% progressively motile spermatozoa has a confidence interval of 45–55% for 400 assessed spermatozoa, but 40–60% when only 100 were assessed.

Acceptable Difference between Replicate Counts

Table App5.3 can be used to facilitate deciding whether replicate assessments of sperm concentration can be accepted.

Calculate the total number of spermatozoa counted and locate the corresponding range in the left column (SUM) of the table. If the difference between the two assessments is less than or equal to the value in the right column (LIMIT) the assessments can be accepted. If the difference between the duplicates is higher than the LIMIT, the assessments must be discarded and two new assessments made. The shadowed part of the table is where, according to recommendations, too few spermatozoa have been counted to achieve a result with less than 10% uncertainty (confidence interval larger than ±10% interval) [1–3].

Table App5.3

SUM	VALUE	SUM	LIMIT
969–1000	61	376–395	38
938–968	60	357–375	37
907–937	59	338–356	36
876–906	58	319–337	35
846–875	57	301–318	34
817–845	56	284–300	33
788–816	55	267–283	32
760–787	54	251–266	31
732–759	53	235–250	30
704–731	52	219–234	29
678–703	51	206–218	28
651–677	50	190–205	27
625–650	49	176–189	26
600–624	48	163–175	25
576–599	47	150–162	24
551–575	46	138–149	23
528–550	45	126–137	22
504–527	44	115–125	21
482–503	43	105–114	20
460–481	42	94–104	19
438–459	41	85–93	18
417–437	40	76–84	17
396–416	39	67–75	16
		59–66	15
		52–58	14
		44–51	13
		38–43	12
		32–37	11
		27–31	10
		22–26	9
		17–21	8
		13–16	7
		10–12	6
		7–9	5
		5–6	4
		3–4	3
		2	2
		1	1
		0	0

Table App5.4

Counted	±%
1	196
5	88
10	62
20	44
30	36
40	31
50	28
60	25
70	23
80	22
90	21
100	20
150	16
200	14
250	12
300	11
400	10
500	9
600	8
700	7
1000	6

Uncertainty of Results in Relation to the Number of Spermatozoa Counted

Table App5.4 illustrates how the certainty, expressed as confidence intervals in relation to counted numbers, of a sperm concentration result depends on the number of spermatozoa actually counted.

If 10 spermatozoa have been counted to get the result 1×10^6/ml in, e.g. a Makler chamber, the confidence of the result is between 0.4 and 1.6×10^6/ml ($1 \times 10^6 \pm 62\%$ according to Table App5.4). Thus, the concentration can vary up to four-fold. If, instead, 100 spermatozoa had been counted (for instance in a haemocytometer with improved Neubauer ruling), the confidence of the result would be between 0.8 and 1.2×10^6/ml ($1 \times 10^6 \pm 20\%$). With the number of spermatozoa in this latter example (i.e. 50 per Neubauer grid area of 5×5 large squares), it would be necessary to assess 100 large squares, or the central grid plus three peripheral areas (each peripheral area is the same size as the central area that consists of 5×5 large squares) in each haemocytometer chamber (see Figure 3.5a), in order to reach a confidence level of $\pm 10\%$ (0.9–1.1×10^6) – or 40 Makler chamber grids.

References

1. Kvist U, Björndahl L, eds. *Manual on Basic Semen Analysis*. ESHRE Monographs 2. Oxford: Oxford University Press, 2002.

2. World Health Organization. *WHO Laboratory Manual for the Examination and Processing of Human Semen*, 6th edn. Geneva: World Health Organization, 2021.

3. International Organization for Standardization. *ISO 23162:2021 Basic Semen Examination – Specification and Test Methods*. Geneva: International Organization for Standardization, 2021.

Index

Note: Page numbers in *Italics* refer to figures and tables

Printed in Great Britain
by Amazon

22484528R00220